Neuroadaptive
SYSTEMS
Theory and Applications

Ergonomics Design and Management: Theory and Applications

Series Editor
Waldemar Karwowski
Industrial Engineering and Management Systems
University of Central Florida (UCF) – Orlando, Florida

Published Titles

Ergonomics: Foundational Principles, Applications, and Technologies
Pamela McCauley Bush

Aircraft Interior Comfort and Design
Peter Vink and Klaus Brauer

Ergonomics and Psychology: Developments in Theory and Practice
Olexiy Ya Chebykin, Gregory Z. Bedny, and Waldemar Karwowski

Ergonomics in Developing Regions: Needs and Applications
Patricia A. Scott

Handbook of Human Factors in Consumer Product Design, 2 vol. set
Waldemar Karwowski, Marcelo M. Soares, and Neville A. Stanton

> Volume I: Methods and Techniques
> Volume II: Uses and Applications

Human–Computer Interaction and Operators' Performance: Optimizing Work
Design with Activity Theory
Gregory Z. Bedny and Waldemar Karwowski

Knowledge Service Engineering Handbook
Jussi Kantola and Waldemar Karwowski

Trust Management in Virtual Organizations: A Human Factors Perspective
Wiesław M. Grudzewski, Irena K. Hejduk, Anna Sankowska, and Monika Wańtuchowicz

Manual Lifting: A Guide to the Study of Simple and Complex Lifting Tasks
Daniela Colombiani, Enrico Ochipinti, Enrique Alvarez-Casado, and Thomas R. Waters

Neuroadaptive Systems: Theory and Applications
Magdalena Fafrowicz, Tadeusz Marek, Waldemar Karwowski, and Dylan Schmorrow

Forthcoming Titles

Organizational Resource Management: Theories, Methodologies, and Applications
Jussi Kantola

Contents

Section I Approaches to Understanding the Neural Network's Functions

Section II Neuroadaptive Systems: Challenges and Applications

Preface

We are pleased to invite all of you to join us in the adventure of studying human neuronal networks and their functions as a basis for neuroadaptive systems. Neuroadaptive systems can be broadly defined as the science and technology of systems responding to neural processes in the brain. Owing to advances in cognitive neuroscience, neuroimaging methods, computational and sensor technologies, and biocompatibility of materials, neuroadaptive systems are a rapidly developing area of study. The neuroadaptive system can be seen as the interaction of two dynamic processes of selecting those neural signal features where the user can supervise and adapt the transformation of these signals into control of a variety of devices. In this context, neuroadaptive systems appear as a spectacular achievement of cognitive neuroscience, modern engineering, and advanced technologies.

This book consists of two sections, "Approaches to Understanding the Neural Network's Functions" and "Neuroadaptive Systems: Challenges and Applications."

The first section comprises six chapters. The first chapter, "Psychological Constructs versus Neural Mechanisms: Different Perspectives for Advanced Research of Cognitive Processes and Development of Neuroadaptive Technologies," written by Joanna Trzopek, Magdalena Fafrowicz, Tadeusz Marek, and Waldemar Karwowski, discusses changes in contemporary sciences and the implications of their findings for both cognitive neuroscience and neuroadaptive technologies.

In the second chapter, "The Neural Cybernetics of Executive Control and Learning," Phan Luu, Don M. Tucker, and Catherine Poulsen present an approach to learning as a secondary phenomenon, subordinate to the first requirement of adaptive behavior, which explains how human actions are regulated (i.e., behaviors) to meet the demands of the environment.

The purpose of the third chapter in this section, "A New Neural Framework for Adaptive and Maladaptive Behavior in Changeable Demands," is to present a model of the development of adaptive or maladaptive behavior in response to constantly changing environmental conditions. The authors, Koryna Lewandowska, Barbara Wachowicz, Ewa Beldzik, Aleksandra Domagalik, Magdalena Fafrowicz, Justyna Mojsa-Kaja, Halszka Oginska, and Tadeusz Marek, in accordance with the assumptions of evolutionism, propose two general goals of human behavior: (1) to maintain effective action fitting with environmental demands through cognitive control of behavior, which includes an estimation of its adequacy and results in updating/modifying behavior if necessary; and (2) to protect systems of the body through fight, flight, or freezing behavior, if the effective action in terms of cognitive control is not possible. Thus, the response to environmental stimuli may proceed on two levels: the more advanced level of cognitive control, which depends on the activity of evolutionarily younger brain structures, such as the neocortex, and the more primitive level associated with the evolutionarily older parts of the brain, such as the amygdala.

The aim of the fourth chapter, "Object Perception versus Target-Directed Manual Actions," by Gregory Króliczak, Cristiana Cavina-Pratesi, and Mary-Ellen Large, is to take a bird's-eye view of the neural underpinning of human object perception and target-directed actions, with an emphasis on grasping, and to discuss when and how the networks that mediate these skills interact during action planning and execution.

In the fifth chapter, "The Neural Control of Visually Guided Eye Movements," Peter H. Schiller discusses the role of different neural circuits and brain areas for control of saccadic eye movements.

The last chapter of this section, "Sleep Deprivation and Error Negativity: A Review and Reappraisal," by Shulan Hsieh, focuses on studies examining the impact of one night of total sleep deprivation on error monitoring by using event-related potentials to complement the usual behavioral measures (e.g., reaction time, accuracy, error rate, and omission rate).

The second section of this book comprises seven chapters devoted to the challenges and applications of neuroadaptive systems. The first chapter of this section, "Augmenting Human Performance," by Kay M. Stanney, examines the general aim of neuroadaptive systems.

The second chapter, "Electroencephalographic Metrics of Workload and Learner Engagement," by Carryl L. Baldwin, Joseph T. Coyne, and James Christensen, discusses how the field of neuroergonomics can be applied in training applications. Several candidate electroencephalographic metrics are discussed and a theoretical framework is presented for using artificial neural networks for real-time learner workload and engagement classification for the purpose of developing neuroadaptive training platforms.

In the third chapter, "Brain–Computer Interfaces: Effects on Brain Activation and Behavior," Sonja C. Kleih, Steve Lukito, and Andrea Kübler provide readers with important results and the most recent findings that have been achieved throughout approximately two decades of research on brain–computer interfaces.

The next chapter, "Neuroadaptive Systems: Challenges and Opportunities in Creating Symbiotic Relationships between Humans and the Machines They Use," by Joseph V. Cohn and Tracey L. Wheeler, explores the underlying rationale for using neuroadaptive systems compared to other kinds of human–machine systems. The impact that recent advances in areas such as neuroimaging, neural decoding, and neural modeling have had and will continue to have on the development and extension of neuroadaptive systems is also discussed.

Heiner Bubb and Martin Wohlfarter's chapter, "Eye-Tracking Data Analysis and Neuroergonomics," deals with the problem of car driving, eye-tracking analysis, and information processing.

The next chapter, "Potential Applications of Systems Modeling Language and Systems Dynamics to Simulate and Model Complex Human Brain Functions," by Waldemar Karwowski, Tareq Z. Ahram, Chris Andrzejczak, Magdalena Fafrowicz, and Tadeusz Marek, focuses on applications of systems modeling language and systems dynamics approaches to modeling and visualizing selected neuroergonomics and cognitive constructs, with the human brain and its capabilities being simulated and analyzed graphically under conditions of a given task or decision-making process.

The final chapter of the book, "Neuroethics: Considerations for a Future Embedded with Neurotechnology," by Joseph R. Keebler, Grant Taylor, Elizabeth Phillips, Scott Ososky, and Lee W. Sciarini, raises questions and concerns in budding neuroscientific areas by exploring possible technological advancements, as well as current-day technologies that can give insight into the way humans may interact with neurotechnological systems in the future.

We hope that we have achieved our aim and that this unique book will give you, the reader, exciting moments of learning and discovery in neuroadaptive systems.

Editors

Magdalena Fafrowicz, PhD, is an assistant professor and the chair of the Eye Movement Laboratory at the Institute of Applied Psychology, Department of Neuroergonomics, Jagiellonian University, Krakow, Poland. She is the author/coauthor of over 60 research publications. Her research interests focus on neural mechanisms of visual attention, error detection, conflict monitoring, diurnal variability of cognitive processes, cognitive and emotional consequences of chronic sleep deficit, and neuroergonomics.

Tadeusz Marek, PhD, is a professor of psychology at Jagiellonian University in Krakow (chairman of the Department of Neuroergonomics and chair of ergonomics and management psychology) and at Warsaw School of Psychology in Warsaw. He is the author/coauthor of over 300 research publications and is the author/editor (coauthor/coeditor) of 22 books. His main research deals with the mental stress and workload, fatigue, professional burn-out, and human functions in relation to the processes of visual attention, cognitive neuroscience, chronopsychology, and neuroergonomics. He is the former president of the Committee on Ergonomics of the Polish Academy of Sciences. He serves as editor-in-chief of *Ergonomia: An International Journal of Ergonomics and Human Factors* and senior editor of *Theoretical Issues in Ergonomics Science*. During 1993–1996, he served on the editorial team for the journal *Ergonomics*. He is a member of many Polish and international learned societies, and collaborates with many scientific centers in Europe, the United States, and Australia.

Waldemar Karwowski, PE, is a professor and chair of the Industrial Engineering and Management Systems Department at the University of Central Florida, Orlando, Florida. He holds an MS (1978) in production engineering and management from the Technical University of Wroclaw, Poland, and a PhD (1982) in industrial engineering from Texas Tech University. He was also awarded the DSc (dr, hab., 2004) in management science by the Institute for Organization and Management in Industry (ORGMASZ), Warsaw, Poland. He is a recipient of honorary doctorate degrees, including those from the South Ukrainian State University of Odessa, Ukraine (2004); Technical University of Koscie, Slovakia (2006); and MIRA Technical University of Moscow, Russia (2007). Dr. Karwowski is a Board Certified Professional Ergonomist. His research, teaching, and consulting activities focus on human systems integration, work systems compatibility, human–computer interaction, prevention of work-related musculoskeletal disorders, management of work systems, agility of manufacturing enterprises, and theoretical aspects of ergonomics science. He currently serves as editor of the *Human Factors and Ergonomics in Manufacturing* and as the editor-in-chief of *Theoretical Issue in Ergonomics Science*.

Dylan Schmorrow, PhD, commander, U.S. naval officer, and an acquisition professional in the Naval Acquisition Corps, is currently serving as associate director of human systems in the Office of the Deputy Undersecretary of Defense (S&T). He is responsible for oversight and coordinate of S&T programs in the human systems technology area, which includes DoD programs in personnel selection, training and leadership, cognitive sciences, interface design, personnel protection, combat feeding, human systems integration, human performance, and cultural and behavioral modeling. He monitors S&T

planning and programming to facilitate applicable insertion into military acquisition programs supporting U.S. warfighters and to support the development of novel S&T to improve capability options. He also serves as the program director for the OSD Human, Social, Culture and Behavioral Modeling Research and Development program that focuses on providing DoD and the U.S. Government with the ability to understand and effectively operate in human/social/culture terrains inherent to nonconventional warfare missions. His interests include advancing neuroscience, human factors, training, autonomy, and decision support technologies to maximize human performance. He frequently collaborates with the National Science Foundation, the National Institutes of Health, the Department of Homeland Security, the Defense Advanced Research Projects Agency, and DoD Services to improve warfighting capabilities and to support academic and industry performers in advancing science and building new technologies.

Contributors

Tareq Z. Ahram
Department of Industrial Engineering
and Management Systems
University of Central Florida
Orlando, Florida

Chris Andrzejczak
Department of Industrial Engineering
and Management Systems
University of Central Florida
Orlando, Florida

Carryl L. Baldwin
Department of Psychology
George Mason University
Fairfax, Virginia

Ewa Beldzik
Department of Neuroergonomics
Jagiellonian University in Krakow
Krakow, Poland

Heiner Bubb
Lehrstuhl für Ergonomie
Technische Universität München
Garching, Germany

Cristiana Cavina-Pratesi
Department of Psychology
Durham University
Durham, United Kingdom

James Christensen
Air Force Research Laboratory
Wright Patterson AFB, Ohio

Joseph V. Cohn
Defense Advanced Sciences
Research Agency
Arlington, Virginia

Joseph T. Coyne
United States Naval Research
Laboratory
Washington, DC

Aleksandra Domagalik
Department of Neuroergonomics
Jagiellonian University in Krakow
Krakow, Poland

Magdalena Fafrowicz
Department of Neuroergonomics
Jagiellonian University in Krakow
Krakow, Poland

Shulan Hsieh
Department of Psychology
and
Institute of Allied Health Sciences
National Cheng Kung University
Tainan, Taiwan

Waldemar Karwowski
Department of Industrial Engineering
and Management Systems
University of Central Florida
Orlando, Florida

Joseph R. Keebler
Team Performance Laboratory
Orlando, Florida

Sonja C. Kleih
Department of Psychology I
University of Würzburg
Würzburg, Germany

and

Graduate School of Neural and
Behavioural Sciences
University of Tübingen
Tübingen, Germany

Gregory Króliczak
Institute of Psychology
Adam Mickiewicz University in Poznan
Poznan, Poland

Andrea Kübler
Department of Psychology I
University of Würzburg
Würzburg, Germany

and

Institute of Medical Psychology and
    Behavioural Neurobiology
University of Tübingen
Tübingen, Germany

Mary-Ellen Large
Department of Psychology
University of Hull
Hull, United Kingdom

Koryna Lewandowska
Department of Neuroergonomics
Jagiellonian University in Krakow
Krakow, Poland

Steve Lukito
Graduate School of Neural and
    Behavioural Sciences
and
Institute of Medical Psychology and
    Behavioural Neurobiology
University of Tübingen
Tübingen, Germany

Phan Luu
Electrical Geodesics, Inc.
and
Department of Psychology
University of Oregon
Eugene, Oregon

Tadeusz Marek
Department of Neuroergonomics
Jagiellonian University in Krakow
Krakow, Poland

Justyna Mojsa-Kaja
Department of Neuroergonomics
Jagiellonian University in Krakow
Krakow, Poland

Halszka Oginska
Department of Neuroergonomics
Jagiellonian University in Krakow
Krakow, Poland

Scott Ososky
Team Performance Laboratory
Orlando, Florida

Elizabeth Phillips
Team Performance Laboratory
Orlando, Florida

Catherine Poulsen
Electrical Geodesics, Inc.
and
Department of Psychology
University of Oregon
Eugene, Oregon

Peter H. Schiller
Department of Brain and
    Cognitive Science
Massachusetts Institute of Technology
Cambridge, Massachusetts

Lee W. Sciarini
Naval Air Warfare Center Training
    Systems Division
Orlando, Florida

Kay M. Stanney
Design Interactive, Inc.
Oviedo, Florida

Grant Taylor
Applied Cognition and Training in
    Immersive Virtual Environments
    Laboratory
Orlando, Florida

Joanna Trzopek
Institute of Applied Psychology
Jagiellonian University in Krakow
Krakow, Poland

Don M. Tucker
Electrical Geodesics, Inc.
and
Department of Psychology
University of Oregon
Eugene, Oregon

Barbara Wachowicz
Department of Neuroergonomics
Jagiellonian University in Krakow
Krakow, Poland

Tracey L. Wheeler
System Planning Corporation
Arlington, Virginia

Martin Wohlfarter
Ergoneers GmbH
Manching, Germany

Section I

Approaches to Understanding the Neural Network's Functions

1

Psychological Constructs versus Neural Mechanisms: Different Perspectives for Advanced Research of Cognitive Processes and Development of Neuroadaptive Technologies

Joanna Trzopek, Magdalena Fafrowicz, Tadeusz Marek, and Waldemar Karwowski

CONTENTS

1.1 Introduction

Over the last century, the predominant research model for science, including naturalistically oriented social sciences and psychology, was physics, which enjoyed undeniable success. At present, however, biology is broadly considered a point of reference for research in cognitive processes. This change is significant as research in physics focusing on general regularities of the physical world inherently excludes the human mind from its investigations. For a long time, this approach has been responsible for perceiving the mind as mysterious and difficult to grasp scientifically (Pinker 1999). On the other hand, all attempts to naturalize mental reality in the physicalist spirit could provoke justified anxiety of antinaturalists opposing this "objectivist" approach (Trzopek 2006). This situation seems [now] to be changing. Edelman (1992) qualify this change as "putting the mind back into nature." As biologically oriented researchers emphasize, the mind is a process whose foundation is a particular biological organization of matter, and as such it can be subjected to both scientific research and explanation with the use of neurobiological tools. Strictly physicalist methods, however fundamental to science, prove insufficient. Although physics constitutes a necessary basis for biology, it does not investigate biological structures, processes, or principles (Edelman 1992, 18–19; Koch 2004, 312). This is particularly evident as biology, in contrast to physics, is characterized by few stringent rules and laws. As a result of natural selection, a whole hierarchy of complex mechanisms has emerged. All this is responsible for the fact that biology-based naturalism differs in its character from the former simplified physicalist naturalism.

Inspired mainly by the progress in research on the human brain, the development of new theoretical constructs and hypotheses is currently proceeding simultaneously in several domains. These include not only biology and neurobiology but also cognitive social psychology and cognitive and neurocognitive sciences. Such development has been possible because of the introduction of new research methods. In neurobiology, these are advanced methods of brain imaging; in cognitive social psychology, controlled research on automatic regulation and cognitive unconsciousness; and, lastly, in cognitivism and neuroscience, the connectionist approach is based on creating artificial neural-like networks.* Not only the growth of knowledge but also the possibility of cooperation and integration of the findings within these domains seems significant. Investigating the issues that so far have been mainly reserved for philosophical reflection has far-reaching consequences.

In his classic textbook on psychology, J. Peter (1986), a Polish psychologist, presented fundamental philosophical debates concerning mainly the essence of the psyche and consciousness (in an ontological sense), the freedom of human behavior, human nature, and the psychophysical problem. For a long time, these issues were not mentioned explicitly in scientific reflection or research. Now they are in the center of scientific (precisely scientific, and not philosophical as was the case before) discussion. Researchers from various fields are actively exploring questions concerning unconsciousness (Damasio 1994, 1999; Edelman 1992; Velmans 2002, 2003), subjectivity (Bargh and Ferguson 2000; Wegner 2002, 2005), will (Libet 2003; Pockett 2004; Wegner 2005), and even the foundations of religiousness and morality (P. M. Churchland 1999; Gazzaniga 2006). It is not only about studying how people *see* these issues (in other words, about frequently conducted studies in psychology on the *feeling* of freedom, subjectivity, agency, etc.), but also about the fundamental question *"what is their salience?"*. The stakes are high as it concerns not only research findings and developments, which, in principle, interest researchers alone, but something much more essential: that is, ourselves (Trzopek 2010).

The scientific approach to the above-discussed problems could impact our culture and institutions in the future. So, we argue that we must change the view of human nature when confronted with new data, which suggests that our commonly accepted view is incorrect or misleading. We would like to quote a few statements as examples illustrating the scientific climate discussed here.

---

* It should be noted that the similarity of connectionist models to the neurobiological "brain architecture" is only partial. Although many advocates of connectionism treat these models as an expression of real implementation of psychological processes (P. M. Churchland 1999; P. S. Churchland 1989; Rumelhart, McClelland, and the PDP Research Group 1986), this analogy should not be taken literally. The models are in many respects different from the way real neural systems work (for more on this topic, see Edelman 1992, 308–309). Irrespective of these differences, however, the connectionist approach and neurobiological research contribute to the criticism of traditional psychological conceptions.

1.2 Contemporary Psychology and Cognitive Neuroscience: New Perspectives

The development of neurobiological research witnessed in recent times, as well as the progress in neuropsychology and neurocognitivism, has confronted scholars with a serious problem, that is, the biological consolidation of collected data. A related task consists of searching for relationships between psychologically defined functions and biological mechanisms and/or brain structures. Increasingly, psychologists are making reference(s) to biological foundations of human functioning. Hence, neurobiological interpretation is offered to behavioral regularities obtained in social research, for example, ideomotor effects (Bargh 2005), or to constructs postulated by cognitive psychology, a case in point being the global workspace (Baars 2003; Dehaene and Naccache 2001) or working memory (Hassin 2005). The view that such cooperation between psychology and neuroscience may enable deeper understanding of widely understood human activity is gaining significant recognition (P. S. Churchland 1989; Edelman 1992). This also brings to light the problem of adequacy of psychological descriptive and explanatory categories that have been applied so far. The categories that draw on folk psychology and dominant cognitive tradition may turn out to be currently discovered qualities of neural processes performed by the brain.

> As P. S. Churchland posits, "the treacherous difficulty here is that we cannot by sure when we are asking the right questions. We do not know whether such categories as 'emotion,' 'declarative memory,' 'procedural memory,' 'learning' and 'consciousness' pick out a unified, single, natural kind, or whether these categories herd together quite motley collections of disparate phenomena." (1989, 152)

The same commentary can refer to other commonly used concepts such as attention or thinking. In this way, using a particular concept may be an expression of a convention assumed by the academic circle and not an indication of unifying processes underlying the notion. Therefore, searching for neural substrates or correlations of defined (traditionally established) psychological processes can be seriously impeded.

The above situation also leads to vital questions about the possible evolution of psychological conceptual frameworks and the future relationship between neuroscience and psychology. At this point, we would like to focus our attention primarily on the former notion that is related to the question about the revision of psychology's basic concepts and theories. The solutions in this field are fundamental for establishing the possibility of developing neuroadaptive technologies based on psychological constructs or on models of neural mechanisms that underlie human behavior. The latter issue that partially raises the problem of autonomy of psychology as science (Bruner 1973; Scriven 1964), though is not less important, goes beyond the scope of the present chapter and will not be discussed here.

While examining the dilemma of "theoretical constructs versus neural mechanism models" presented in studies in the field of neurocognitivism, we can identify two different research approaches: classical and neurocentric. In the classical approach, the starting point is a psychological function defined on the basis of behavioral indicators and described as theoretical constructs. Usually, it is assumed that such a function has a particular structure described by means of simple, commonsense dimensions. A consequence of this approach, which has been deeply rooted in researchers' awareness for years and which stems from the absence of suitable research methods, is a vague, imprecise explanation of investigated phenomena. Many neurocognitivists agree about the weaknesses of their theoretical constructs (e.g., Hancock and Szalma 2003) on which studies of human behavior are grounded. They perceive the results of research conducted in the field of neurocognitivism as a chance to fill the already existing constructs with new content and, thus, to develop, reconstruct, and refine them (Sarter and Sarter 2003; Szalma and Hancock 2002; Scerbo, Freeman, and Mikulka 2003). According to the above-discussed dominant view, it is necessary to assume a reductionist approach in order to make thorough use of the results obtained in the area of neurocognitivism (Hancock and Szalma 2003; Sarter and Sarter 2003). This requires reducing a multidimensional psychological construct to basic cognitive activities closely linked to activity of the brain. It should be noted that the results obtained in the field of neurocognitivism from the perspective of this classical model may be useful only as a sort of a "filler" for existing constructs.

The neurocentric model dispenses with theoretical constructs created on the basis of psychology from the research process (Fafrowicz and Marek 2007, 2009). This new approach offers a different perspective in the research on cognitive processes. In contrast to the classical model, it is not the theoretical construct but the functioning of neural systems that becomes the starting point for the researcher involved in the execution of particular behavioral activities. In this research approach, instead of verifying the rules and laws governing the functioning of the construct, the function and the dynamics of neural structure activity is studied in relation to a specific situation (stimulus situation, task situation, or cognitive situation). The research goal is to identify the neural structure activity patterns that are involved in the performance of a particular task, behavior, or activity. In the neurocentric model, on the one hand, the requirements imposed by the environment are taken into account and, on the other hand, the pattern of neural structure activity related to these requirements is investigated. In this approach, neural mechanisms linked to a specific task or, more generally, activity are the starting point for developing models that embrace both the pattern of neural structure activity and the pattern of behavioral, cognitive, emotional, and perceptual activity.

The process of forming such theoretical constructs today is not homogeneous. A few currents can be distinguished including the branch of traditional cognitivism and the computer metaphor approaches, the branch of cognitive psychology, and the branch of folk psychology.

1.3 Traditional Cognitivism and the Computer Metaphor of Cognitive Processes

From the 1970s, cognitive science started to gain a leading position in the widely understood studies of cognitive processes. Since its advent, this approach aimed to integrate the efforts and achievements of various domains including psychology, linguistics, philosophy, computer science, and cybernetics. Generally, cognitive science constituted a science about systems (units, mechanisms, devices) that can be attributed with the feature of thinking, cognition, or intelligence. Two classes of objects appeared to fulfill this criterion: people and computers. Thus, not surprisingly, the "computer metaphor" came to be used to model cognitive processes of people. Moreover, as Dennett, a cognitive science philosopher of the mind, observes, explaining any computer capabilities is "thoroughly transparent," which constituted one of the most attractive features of the computer metaphor (2005, 43). However, at this point, a question arises about whether the transparency of computing models based on the work of computers actually brings us closer to an adequate explanation of mental/mind phenomena. Before we proceed to the issue, we provide a brief review of the fundamental assumptions of traditional cognitivism (Bobryk 1996; Edelman 1992).

According to the traditional cognitivist approach, cognitive operations can be described entirely in a functional manner just like in the case of a computer program. Both people and computers use symbols that represent external and internal situations. The operations necessary to transform a sequence of input symbols into a sequence of output symbols are called computations. Symbol tokens are formal and arbitrary in character. A symbol is a sign that bears no similarity to the material medium and the represented object. Symbols in the described sense are physical states of matter (such as computer chips or brain cells), which represent objects in the world. The emergence of these objects (so-called access) releases specific activity of the organism/device. Certain symbols are capable of activating other symbols until merger with "retrieval" occurs (the level of effectors). A frequently used analog of computational processes that take place here is the Turing machine (its modern version is a computer). The machine is equipped with a program that enforces certain actions, provided particular conditions are met. In other words, it follows a certain algorithm. Analogically, cognitive processes are treated as sequences of such simple, subjected to rules, operations. The rules determine the order and type of operations that need to be applied in order to achieve a specific cognitive effect. Selfridge labeled these simplest operations "demons" (Lindsay and Norman 1972). Each "demon" is required to react to certain symbols.

Operations on symbols are formal in character, which enables describing human cognition by means of a formalized system. This means that nothing in our brains understands symbols the way we do (i.e., from the perspective of "meaning"). The intelligence of the system emerges from the activity of less complex subsystems (on the lowest level reacting in a zero–one way). In this manner, simple (zero–one, unconscious, and unintentional) computing processes lead to the creation of a complex representation of the world. Particular content (the value of meaning) is revealed via the relationship of a given operation or element with other operations or elements. An element outside the structure of the system cannot have an independent meaning. The algorithms used by the mind, and not the physical structure of the brain, are most important for understanding psychological processes, provided the program works without problems. This constitutes the essence of the functional approach.

Functional models usually assume three levels of description: physical (specific, physical realization of computation), syntactic (rules and operations performed on symbols), and semantic (where the description is given in a mentalistic language of meanings, desires, intentions,* etc.). The second level is suitable for the description and functionalist explanations, as is the case with computers. In this way, the specific construction of a given device is disregarded (whether it is a silicon computer or a biological brain is of no importance) and what is in focus is the set of functions it performs (i.e., what the device *does*).

The discussed assumptions and features of cognitivism have been developed mainly on the ground of the philosophy of cognitive science, developed by its leading representatives such as J. Fodor, H. Putnam, or Z. Pylyshyn (Fodor and Pylyshyn 1988). Nevertheless,

---

* People have the tendency to describe in this language the functioning of even these devices that it is not easy to attribute with mental states or intentionality (Dennett 1991). In this sense, for example, a car "won't" start.

these features and assumptions also exerted considerable influence on empirical cognitive psychology. One of their positive consequences was abandoning simplified behaviorist views. However, these models seem to offer some false assumptions related to the nature of thinking and reasoning or to their relationship with perception.

According to the cognitivist vision, the objects of the external world are grouped in certain fixed, defined categories, and the world is organized in such a way that it can be rearranged by means of models symbolizing specific entities and the relationship between them. The concepts of language are gaining meaning owing to formal, explicit attribution to these categories or relationships. In this way, the system *represents* reality. Mental representations can be identified as true or false depending on whether they faithfully depict reality.* These representations are in the form of inferences and judgments containing concepts and relationships between them. They are often formed in so-called propositional attitudes expressing desires or beliefs. Additionally, it is assumed that "propositional attitudes are functionally discrete, semantically interpretable states that play a causal role in the production of behavior" (Ramsey, Stich, and Garon 2002, 97) and "there is generally some answer to the question of whether a particular belief or memory played a causal role in specific cognitive episode" (Ramsey, Stich, and Garon 2002, 109). The fact that these are discrete states means that "conventional (computational) architecture requires that there be distinct symbolic expressions for each state of affairs that it can represent" (Fodor and Pylyshyn 1988, 51). "Semantically interpretable" suggests that they assume the form of sentences, which enter logical relationships with each other; processing the relationships constitutes thinking.

1.3.1 Why the Computer Metaphor Is Inadequate

Modern neurobiological knowledge, as well as studies on artificial neural networks, indicates that the computer metaphor is most probably inadequate. Arguments supporting the notion are numerous; we will review the most frequently cited. The strongest objections with reference to the discussed model of cognitive functioning were expressed by philosophers and scientists representing the connectionist approach. The approach that resorts to the "brain metaphor" in place of the "computer metaphor" is currently gaining significance in the area of neurocognitive sciences. In connectionist models, the knowledge lies in (excitatory and inhibitory) connections within networks and at a given moment reflects its global activity. The network transforms input information into output information by means of parallel transformations taking place in its hidden layers. It can be said that the force of mutual connections ("weights") of the network functions like a program in the classical computer metaphor. At the same time, this means that neurocognitivist networks are to a certain extent programs that adjust their weights to the nature of incoming information/experiences (Ramsey, Stich, and Garon 2002). This configuration of connections "trained" in the course of life history decides how the network (the brain) will react to the world. It should be noted that in the case of a biological brain this unique adaptation of synaptic connections is governed by both genetic heritage of a given species and the individual experience of the organism (P. M. Churchland 1999; Mischel 2004).

---

* One may notice that this vision concurs with the views of Ludwig Wittgenstein presented in *Tractatus Logico-Philosophicus* (1922). The vision constitutes also a foundation of neopositivist philosophy of science (Trzopek 2006), which, though criticized for years in various respects, still seems to have a stable position in scientific psychology.

Hidden qualities of the artificial neural network are not easily interpreted in a symbolic manner. As P. M. Churchland (2002) emphasizes, there are no neural substrates for sentence-like propositional attitudes such as beliefs or desires, where knowledge depends largely on the overall context rather than on functionally "discrete," stored representations.

> The microstructure of the brain and the recent success of connectionist AI (artificial intelligence) both suggest that our principal form of representation is the high-dimensional activation vector, and that our principal form of computation is the vector-to-vector transformation, effected by a matrix of differently weighted synapses. In place of propositional attitudes and logical inferences from one to another, therefore, we can conceive of persons as the seat of vectorial attitudes and various nonlinear transformations from one vector to another. (P. M. Churchland 2002, 67)

Firstly, as information is encoded in a highly distributed manner, with each connection weight and bias embodying information salient to many propositions, the system lacks functionally distinct, identifiable substructures that are semantically interpretable as a representation of individual propositions (see also Ramsey, Stich, and Garon 2002).

Secondly, it is impossible to maintain a cognitivist division in three description levels. As studies on the nervous system indicate, mental processes are the result of the functioning of highly complex brain structure networks that are found at various levels of the organization. It is not yet known how many levels exist. Neurobiologists suggest a whole spectrum from a molecular and cellular level to the level of the whole organism (P. S. Churchland 1989; Edelman 1992), or even inter-individual level encompassing a set of organisms communicating with one another (Edelman 1992; Gazzaniga 2006). The physical structure and the function are often mutually connected and realized in many ways so that the functionalist division into the physical structure (the subject of biology) and the computing function (the subject of cognitive science) does not reflect the existing relationships.

Thirdly, there is nothing in evolution that would resemble an instruction manual or a program. The brain is not a computer and the world is not a floppy disk (Edelman 1992). The brain is a selectional system in which adaptation takes place *ex post facto*. Categorizations performed by the brain are shaped on the basis of experience of the organism that has at its disposal certain values developed evolutionarily. Edelman (1992) understands "value" as a factor increasing the likelihood of strengthening the synaptic connections that correspond to what proved to be evolutionarily adaptable.* It is also worth mentioning that the structure of the brain is characterized by enormous individual diversity and the human genome is insufficient to clearly determine the future synaptic structure of the brain (Edelman 1992). Although the basic organization is common to all members of the same species, details are the results of epigenetic processes and thousands of accidental events, which create a unique multitude of various dispositions. The behavior of every organism is individual and highly diverse so that no finished set of responses or reactions exhausts the wealth of possible effects. As it is the complex, dynamic, and multifaceted set of neural states that constitutes the foundation of mental processes, it usually cannot be memorized or passed to others in entirety (P. M. Churchland 1999; Damasio 1994; Dehaene and Naccache 2001; Dennett 2005).

---

* It is also possible to develop artificial selectional systems based on the principles governing how the biological brain works. This is the character of Darwin III, a robot constructed in Gerald Edelman's team. Darwin is equipped with a value according to which "light is better than no light"; so in the case of light stimulation, the synapses that are active at the time are reinforced in relation to competing synapses. Consequently, a system is created which, by selection and experience, learns to follow the source of light (Edelman 1992).

Furthermore, it does not seem to be the case that the perception of the world or categorization processes function similarly to the tape in the Turing machine that is obedient to algorithms. First and foremost, the brain and the nervous system cannot be analyzed in isolation from the complex external environment, including the social environment. These interactions are potentially undetermined and their number indefinite. The environment is an open system that cannot be described exhaustively with the use of procedures assumed *a priori*. Individuals interpret events and categories in many (not always consistent) ways, and also human thinking is figurative and metaphorical. Linguistic codes, which are used as descriptors, do not exhaust the sense of expressions. Meanings are not clearly defined and are often variable even for one person.

Fourthly, computer programs are defined by formal syntactic rules. Theories grounded in the computer program metaphor claim that the task of the mind consists of interpreting and processing signals and symbols. Resorting to formalized systems has rendered invaluable service to science, especially physics, although, as Edelman observes, it is an indication of "positioning the mind outside nature," (1992, 316) which is possible as long as the actual functioning of the mind in biological organisms is ignored. The fact that human mind processes *meanings*, which, to a large extent, are the result of social communication, and is characterized by subjective experience, which computers do not possess, creates a serious argument against traditional cognitivism (Searl 1992a,b). It should be noted, however, that the issues of meaning are being raised more and more frequently by neurobiologically oriented researchers (Damasio 1994, 1999; Edelman 1992; Koch 2004).

Fifthly, traditional cognitivism leads to an inevitable, yet uncomfortable question: who performs the discussed operations or who is the programmer assigning meaning to symbols and establishing rules concerning their processing? Various theories of "central executioner" appear to verge dangerously on the unacceptable idea of homunculus. As emphasized by neurobiological scientists, there is no programmer in our head, no self or homunculus, other than the brain as a whole. This whole is interconnected, enabling the integration of information coming from various sources and the development of constantly changing and influencing patterns of assessment and reaction of the organism in response to complex situational and internal factors. An overall pattern of neural activation levels at a given moment generates an image of the present situation including the state of the organism, context, and so on. In other words, according to contemporary knowledge, there is nothing like a "conscious decision center" that could be identified with a particular location or a fixed function of the brain. The situation resembles more that of various coalitions of neurons (Dennett 2005; Koch 2004) competing for influence, where the one, which for different dynamically changing aspects, temporarily gains advantage, becomes conscious, and assumes control in the sense of access to planning, decision making, and so on. The consequence of such an approach is that the subject, as something that would be located between the causes of consciousness and its effects, disappears and is replaced with a collective, dynamic phenomenon that does not require top-down supervision (Dehaene and Naccache 2001). The tasks that the subject would (allegedly) perform are distributed between different centers in the brain. As Dennett vividly puts it: "A good theory of consciousness *should* make a conscious mind look like an abandoned factory . . . full of humming machinery and nobody home to supervise it, or enjoy it, or witness it" (2005, 70; emphasis in original). Notice that according to this approach the "self" or the "subject" does not constitute any supervisory addition to brain functions or mechanisms. It is rather so that the unconscious brain processes in fact create *us* and our feeling of subjectivity. The self conceived of in this way constitutes a certain neural state that is constantly being reconstructed in our brain. The existence of the self guarantees us coherence of perspective and integration of experience; it is also the source of (illusory) belief that we are experts in and owners of the majority of the content of our brain. Biological explanation of consciousness and the self are treated as fundamental tasks facing neurobiology in the twenty-first century (Damasio 1999).

Summarizing the issues presented above, it can be argued that the computer metaphor fails when applied to the real mind. Nevertheless, many theories and psychological constructs have been founded on the assumptions and models of brain functioning which draw on the above metaphor. As an illustration, in the following section, we discuss some of the concepts derived from different areas of psychology: decision making, memory, and attention.

1.4 Decisions, Memory, and Attention: Cognitive Psychology Models from the Perspective of Cognitive Neuroscience

Traditional theories of human decision making, judgments, or pursuing goals are usually based on the so-called principle of maximizing the "subjective expected utility." According to this principle, people while making decisions are able to:

1. Distinguish important attributes of compared objects.
2. Compare the pondered objects in terms of these attributes and their significance.
3. Perform complicated calculation of objects with respect to the mentioned features and their value for the subject.
4. Compare the resulting global assessments of particular objects.
5. Choose the most attractive (useful) option (Tyszka 1992, 284).

The decision situation modeled here is slightly simplified when instead of "maximum expected utility" one introduces the so-called satisfaction principle. The choice then concerns not the best option but the one that satisfies certain minimal expectations. Still, in this case, rather complicated assessments are required. The models discussed here tend to resort to the assumption about the rational course of human cognitive decision-making or motivational activities that follows the logic of accessible information. This refers to the computer metaphor; in this case, the identification of thinking with logical operations. However, as contemporary research (Damasio 1999) indicates, these assumptions are false.

Firstly, it should be pointed out that there is a significant disproportion between the amount of information reaching our senses and that which can be consciously processed. Unconscious processing unburdens us in numerous situations, which we are often unaware of. As Damasio (1994) demonstrated in his research on so-called somatic markers, it is the nonconscious automatic processes, expressed by a more or less conscious feeling that something is or is not appropriate, that lie at the roots of our major decisions. These feelings governing our choices are the result of subconscious perception and previous experiences from similar past situations. The decision that is made within a few seconds on the basis of these perceptions would take consciousness incomparably more time (Dijksterhuis, Aarts, and Smith 2005). Secondly, the research by Damasio (1999), referred to above, also indicates that cognition and emotion are closely intertwined, and that rational processes do not lead to accurate decisions in vital life situations. Thus, the belief about both the rationality of choices made and the decisive role of consciousness seems to reflect the actual situation only to a very limited degree.

Similarly, memory models established on the basis of cognitive psychology may turn out to be equally inadequate. For instance, modern neurobiological knowledge reveals that memory is not a storehouse of coded features or information that can be recalled repeatedly, as in the case of a computer. The brain does not, in principle, memorize relevance-free information that does not relate to previous experiences, values, skills, and so on. Memory belongs to the whole system. Hence, the division of memory into episodic, declarative, procedural, semantic, and so on may prove to be artificial and even misleading (Edelman 1992). It seems that each form of memory requires infinite number of connections between the subject located in a given spatiotemporal reality and the structure of already existing knowledge, which is difficult to describe using insufficient language that resorts to terms such as "storing" or "extracting."

Memory is oriented toward what is essential and is capable of generalization. This, in turn, makes memory imprecise and susceptible to errors, especially in the case of details, not all of which are memorized and stored (Edelman 1992; Gazzaniga 2006). Memory content undergoes changes and reconstruction with time. Recollection consists of re-activation of a part of past mapping, but every time the structure and dynamics of neural population involved in recollection are slightly different, dependent on different factors such as previous memories, present plans, mood, and many others (Casebeer and Churchland 2003).

Similar to decision-making processes and memory processes, attentional processes that are operationalized on the basis of cognitive psychology also appear to be extremely simplified from the perspective of cognitive neuroscience. Let us recall a critical analysis conducted by Fafrowicz and Marek (2007). We quote *in extensio* a fragment of their article presenting the core of the issue.

> The phenomenon of attention in the light of research conducted with the use of neuroimaging technique reveals that it is a system very complex in comparison with how it is depicted with the use of psychological constructs. As a result of the research based on neuroimaging we are aware of many extensive networks of brain regions that subserve different aspects of attentional control. (Fafrowicz and Marek 2007, 1946)

Positron emission tomography and functional magnetic resonance imaging research revealed that (e.g., Posner and Petersen 1990):

1. The attention system is a distinctly isolated anatomic-functional system of the brain.
2. The system is constructed on the basis of the neural network.
3. The separate brain structures constituting the attentional system are responsible for the different functions of attention.

Various anatomic-functional brain structures interact within attentional network. Three different anatomic-functional subsystems of attention have been distinguished (e.g., Berger and Posner 2006; Posner and Petersen 1990; Posner and Raichle 1996):

1. The orienting subsystem responsible for orientation and for shifting of attention.
2. The vigilance subsystem responsible for maintaining the appropriate level of alertness.

3. The executive subsystem responsible for recognition, identification, planning, decision making, error detection, novel responses, dangerous conditions, and overcoming habitual actions (Norman and Shallice 1986).

Each of these subsystems, based on specific structures joined in neural networks, is responsible for executing complex, manifold operations.

The orientating subsystem executes the operations of the attention disengagement, shifting of attention index, and attention engagement. According to the latest research, separate neural networks are responsible for shifting and maintaining attention with reference to locations, features, and objects (Corbetta et al. 2000; Corbetta and Shulman 2002; Hopfinger, Buonocore, and Mangun 2000; Liu et al. 2003; Vandenberghe et al. 2001; Yantis et al. 2002). A similar situation occurs in the case of attention processes with respect to linguistic abilities. Neuroimaging has suggested separate neural systems for syntactic and semantic processing (Myachykow and Posner 2005).

Attention function is closely related to the phenomenon of the inhibition of return (Posner et al. 1985). The phenomenon and the underlying neural mechanisms play a significant role in goal-directed behaviors. The mechanism, inhibition of return, aims at protecting against taking in information from the same area from which information has already been absorbed. In their experiment, Posner and Cohen (1984) proved that inhibition operated with respect to locations. Their findings were later confirmed in other numerous studies (e.g., Klein 2000; Lupianez, Tudela, and Rueda 1999). Recently, Grison et al. (2005) has demonstrated that this phenomenon applies also to objects. According to their research, in the case of locations and locating objects, different mechanisms operated by distinct neural systems underlie the inhibition of return phenomenon.

The executive attention system comprises the mechanisms for monitoring and resolving conflict among responses, thoughts, and feelings (Raz 2004). This network is related also to the subjective impression of mental effort (Fernandez-Duque, Baird, and Posner 2000). The anterior cingulate cortex (ACC) is recognized as a node element of executive attention network. ACC's strong neural connection to limbic, association, and motor cortex explains how this structure's activations influence complex cognitive, motor, and emotional functions such as selective attention, motivation or goal-directed behavior. According to brain activation studies, ACC is also responsible for error processing and responds specifically to occurrences of conflict and error detection.

Several studies have shown activation of the anterior cingulate gyrus and supplementary motor area, the orbitofrontal cortex, the dorsolateral prefrontal cortex, the basal ganglia, and the thalamus during effortful cognitive processing, conflict resolution, error detection, and emotional control (Bush, Luu, and Posner 2000; Fernandez-Duque, Baird, and Posner 2000; Posner and Fan 2004). According to Carter, Botvinick, and Cohen (1999), the anterior cingulate cortex plays the main role in conflict monitoring. However, the anterior cingulate cortex and lateral frontal one are areas where the dopamine receptor systems act (Posner and Fan 2004) suggesting that these structures are involved in learning processes. A growing body of research also shows that several different functional zones of the anterior cingulate cortex are involved in a wide spectrum of mental functions (Fafrowicz and Marek 2007, 2008; Marek et al. 2007; Marek et al. 2008). All this research data draws attention as much more complex phenomenon than it has been assumed in traditional psychological constructs.

Additionally, the attention neural networks go about their business through an orchestration of facilitatory and inhibitory processes. Each attention operation is associated with activation of some structures and inhibition of others. For instance, during activity of the vigilance attention network the executive attention subsystem is inhibited, and the orienting as well as the vigilance attention subsystems show stronger activation. The vigilance and orienting attention subsystems inhibit the activity of the executive attention subsystem (e.g., Marek et al. 2004). As a consequence of the discoveries discussed briefly above, theoretical constructs describing attention that have been in use have several shortcomings.

In view of recent findings in neuroscience, the majority of psychological constructs can be seen as a combination of extremely simplified dimensions, a combination forming a system that is unable to absorb new discoveries owing to its over simplicity. Many of the current models, which resort to such constructs, are too simple to absorb the complexity of new discoveries.

1.5 Concepts of Folk Psychology from the Perspective of Cognitive Neuroscience

For years heated debates have surrounded the status of so-called folk psychology (Greenwood 2002a,b). Generally, according to folk psychology, human behaviors (or more broadly actions) are the result of human beliefs, desires, emotions, or intentions. These categories are often called propositional attitudes.

It should be noted that folk psychology embraces not only our commonsense convictions but also a significant part of psychological personality theories, social psychology (Greenwood 2002a,b), and functionalist cognitivism as long as it uses specifically interpreted categories of "beliefs" and "desires" (P. S. Churchland 1989; Ramsey, Stich, and Garon 2002). The relationship, mentioned earlier, between scientific psychology and folk psychology theories is understandable as every theory has to take as a starting point conceptions and their terminology accessible at a given stage. In the case of scientific psychology, the basis and roots were provided naturally by folk psychology (P. S. Churchland 1989).

The important issue is whether the ideas stemming from commonsense are likely to prevail as the fundamentals of scientific thinking in the future.

> Like other folk theories, folk psychology is not without virtue, and within certain circumscribed domains it has considerable predictive success. . . . On the other hand, it would be astonishing if folk psychology, alone among folk theories, was essentially correct. The mind-brain is exceedingly complex, and it seems unlikely that primitive folk would have lit upon the correct theoretical framework to explain its nature where they failed with . . . life, disease, the stars, and so forth. (P. S. Churchland 1989, 395–396)

However, introducing the categories "beliefs" and "desires" to cognitive psychology may be a source of misunderstanding and could stir confusion concerning the actual reference of the term "folk psychology." A lay or naive understanding of the term may not concur with the way propositional attitudes are treated in cognitive psychology. In our daily experience, we do not treat the knowledge about our own and other people's thinking and behavior in such a formalized manner (Heil 2002). According to P. M. Churchland (1999, 2002) and P. S. Churchland (1989), folk psychology theories held a strong position because for a long time no real alternative was available. Presently, however, the situation is beginning to change. According to P. M. Churchland, "recent advances in connectionist artificial intelligence (AI) and computational neuroscience have provided us with a fertile new framework with which to understand the perception, cognition, and behavior of intelligent creatures" (2002, 52). Because cognition in general gets characterized in a new way, the question of *adequacy* of our commonsense understanding became as important as ever.

The reasoning in this case proceeds along the following lines: beliefs, desires, intentions, and so forth constitute constructs that, in the field of folk psychology, aim to account for behavior. The explanations offered by modern neurocognitivism and neuroscience go beyond these commonsense psychological constructs and explanations. Hence, the accounts that resort to folk psychology categories should be eliminated and replaced with more adequate concepts referring to contemporary scientific theories, in particular those grounded in neurobiology or neurocognitivism. An additional consequence tends to be negation of the legitimacy of treating intentions, desires, or beliefs as fixed realities. Our belief that we possess beliefs and that, in our conduct, we are guided by conscious intentions in such a context would be only an illusion.

Yet it is not so that eliminativism is the only acceptable attitude to folk psychology concepts in the area of current neurocognitivist knowledge. Quoting J. Heil, "it is arguable that connectionism does not, in fact, abandon intentional states and processes, but merely locates these in *patterns* of neural activity rather than in bits of neural hardware or simple state-transitions. Connectionists without philosophical axes to grind certainly seem at home with standard intentional categories" (2002, 133; emphasis in original).

By resorting to the "brain metaphor," connectionism, in this context, would simply be a model underlying the dynamics of human beliefs, desires, or other propositional attitudes different from and better than traditional cognitivism whereas the dispute concerning the adequacy of folk theory would become little more than a dispute about words. This stance seems to be generally in accordance with the views of some neurobiologically oriented researchers for whom taking into account and explaining subjective states (including meanings and intentionality) constitutes an essential issue (Damasio 1994; Edelman 1992). Nevertheless, such approaches do not solve yet another problem which then emerges here, that is, reductionism.

As theoreticians investigating the issue discussed here have pointed out, a former theory does not have to be rejected if a possibility exists of identifying or reducing its terms to the terms of a new theory. In this way, for example, the concept of temperature is identified with or reduced to the concept of kinetic energy. It seems that Heil and neurobiologists propose exactly this. This would require presenting already recognized mental phenomena in the language of neurobiology or neurodynamics (P. M. Churchland 1999). In this way, biological processes that appear to be only corresponding to mental processes when they are fully understood would in reality be treated as identical.

The problem concerns whether such reduction is actually possible and whether it is desired by all interested parties. If they did not yield to such reduction or if there was no hope for it in the foreseeable future, from the standpoint presented here intentional phenomena would be regarded as scientifically barren. If, on the other hand, such reduction was possible it would lead to changes significantly greater than mere translatability of the language of description or explanation. Descending to the neurobiological level means including conscious activities (treated then as material) in the causally closed physical world with its mechanistic and deterministic character. What then becomes problematic is how to reconcile the facts occurring at the brain level with the commonsense psychological belief that we have free will at our disposal and that our actions are an actual result of our conscious intentions, choices, or desires.

Folk psychology-related beliefs about the causes of our behavior are negated also from a different perspective: that of the existence of automatic nonconscious systems regulating behavior, of whose presence and role an individual is rarely aware. In the following section of this chapter, we will take a closer look at these issues that, in the context of rapidly developing social cognition, appear to be leading to a new paradigm in thinking with regard to human behavior.

1.6 A Neurocentric Paradigm in Research on Cognitive Processes

What is then the new way of perceiving the human which stems from the new increasingly popular direction of contemporary research? We could name a few spectacular features that are briefly discussed below. Among them, in particular, are studies on the so-called new unconscious or the unconscious regulation and on automatic as well as controlled processes. The studies provoke serious discussions as they raise the question of conscious agency, the self, and the subject. According to R. Hassin, "each new piece of evidence may carry far-reaching implications for our understanding of consciousness, or to speak more generally our views on what it is like to be human" (2005, 196).

1.6.1 The New Unconscious

The expression used in the subtitle, the "new unconscious," is intended at opposing the associations with the psychodynamic unconscious. By definition, the unconscious represents mental processes that are inaccessible to consciousness, but influence judgment, feelings, and behavior. In the presented point of view, the unconscious constitutes a part of normal functioning, with no need to introduce additional theoretical constructs such as repression, resistance, or management of anxiety. In everyday life, a lot of our actions occur relatively effortlessly, without any special thought or deliberation. As James (1890) pointed out, it is really the case for many cognitive processes. The broader literature concerning this topic show that even complex behavior and other higher mental processes can proceed independently of consciousness and require little attention, effort, and volition. "Indeed, the brain evolution and neuropsychological evidence suggests that the human brain is designed for such independence" (Bargh 2005, 54).

At the beginning, the new unconscious was defined as "cognitive"; later, the term "adaptive" started to be applied. The cognitive unconscious was described for the first time by Kihlstrom in 1987 (Kihlstrom 1987). Since then, a lot of research on implicit perception, implicit cognition, or implicit learning was conducted. With time, research in this area expanded to encompass implicit affect, judgment, or even implicit control, implicit working memory, as well as implicit insights (Hassin 2005).

On the other hand, the term "adaptive" meant that nonconscious thinking is an evolutionary adaptation. "The ability to size up our environments, disambiguate them, interpret them, and initiate behavior quickly and nonconsciously confers a survival advantage and thus was selected for," writes Wilson (2002, 23), the promoter of the concept. The adaptive unconscious is an older system designed to scan the environment and detect patterns. It is in part genetically determined, rooted in early childhood, and it continues to guide human behavior into adulthood.

Relatively recent experimental evidence points to an occasionally deep dissociation between conscious awareness and the mental processes responsible for one's behavior. People are often unaware of the reasons and causes of their own behavior. What they usually become aware of are the *effects* of the functioning of unconscious systems in the form of the *content* of consciousness (*what* they think, *what* they recall, *what* they believe). However, people are unaware of the processes that constitute a real source of these thoughts, feelings, or behaviors (Nisbett and Wilson 1977; Wegner 2002; Wilson 2002; Wilson and Dunn 2004; Wilson, Lindsay, and Schooler 2000). Moreover, people often do not realize the fact of their own unconsciousness.

In his book with a telling title, *Strangers to Ourselves* (2002), Wilson points out the areas where the shortages in knowledge are particularly visible. This is well illustrated by the titles of the chapters "Knowing who we are," "Knowing why," "Knowing how we feel," and "Knowing how we will feel." Wilson also argues that many of people's chronic dispositions, traits, and temperaments are parts of the adaptive unconscious, to which they have no direct access. "Because much of our mental life resides outside of consciousness, we often do not know how we are sizing up the world or even the nature of our own personalities," writes Wilson (2002, 41). Consequently, people are forced to construct theories about their own personalities from other sources: their parents, their culture, or ideas about who they prefer to be. Researchers note a remarkable resemblance between participants in contemporary priming studies in social psychology and patients with some forms of brain damage or deeply hypnotized subjects, who on the spot invent interpretations of their own behavior, to the real causes of which they have no access. In this way, the "self" is also a kind of interpretation made by us (Bargh 2005; Gazzaniga 2006). The lack of knowledge about ourselves is the price we pay for benefits such as effortlessness, speed, economy, and usually also adequacy resulting from possessing the adaptive unconscious (Wilson 2002, 40).

As noted by Wilson, "it makes little sense to talk about a single 'self' when we consider that both the adaptive unconscious and the conscious self has regular patterns of responding to the social world" (2002, 68). The adaptive unconscious tends to be the source of what people *do* while the conscious "self" influences what they usually *say* about themselves, their intentions, the reasons for their actions, and so on. It is notable that other researchers too who are interested in the unconscious regulation spoke of dissociation between "knowing" and "doing" or "intention" and "action" (Bargh 2005). This is responsible for the fact that external observers having access to our actions, but not to our thoughts about ourselves, often predict our future behavior better than we do and have a different opinion about us from the one we hold. If it is really the case it questions methods commonly used in psychology, which is based on self-description: tests, questionnaires, scales, and so on.

1.6.2 Unconscious Regulation

Social psychologists have demonstrated that a wide range of human behavior which is claimed to be under conscious control can be activated unconsciously by contextual cues (for a preview, see Bargh and Ferguson 2000). Recent research on automaticity has provided a new impetus to the study of situational determinants of thought, feeling, perception, and situational control over behavior. This research suggests that situational cues can govern behavior without being consciously processed and without making a deliberate choice of an appropriate course of action.

In this research, the contextual triggers are presented subliminally, but sometimes a mere act of perceiving another person can influence behavior. This "perception–behavior link" refers to unintentional, nonconscious, direct effects of social perception on social behavior (Chartrand, Maddux, and Lakin 2005). According to Bargh, "people are behaving, interacting, and pursuing goals, all apparently without meaning to or knowing they are doing so" (2005, 41). One of the clearest demonstrations of such nonconscious influence is an experiment by Bargh and Pietromonaco (1982), in which people did not know that they had an expectation about a person. The researchers activated a personality trait by flashing words to people at subliminal levels, and found that people used this trait when subsequently interpreting another person's behavior. In another study, activation of the stereotype of professor or the trait intelligence was found to lead to activation of behavioral representations such as "concentrate" or "think," which, in turn, affected actual performance on an intellectual task (Dijksterhuis and Knippenberg 1998). Similarly, unconscious activation of representations such as "old" was found to lead to slow walking (Chartrand and Bargh 1996), and so on. Maybe, one reason why these effects seem magical is our fundamental belief in our conscious will, which is derived in large part from our subjective experience of possessing it (Bargh 2005).

Many empirical findings suggest that mental processes, which are central to our conception of "what it is to be human" (Hassin 2005, 197), occur outside conscious awareness and have no phenomenology. Research has started to yield evidence for nonconscious cognitive processes in the area of automatic evaluation and stereotype. Now, there are systematic data that show that some processes traditionally thought of as conscious and controlled can operate nonconsciously.

Social psychologists have shown that goals and motivations can be activated and pursued without conscious awareness. These effects go far beyond mere priming of behaviors. Nonconscious goals and pursuits possess properties similar to those deemed to be fundamental to conscious motivation, specifically persistence (they can guide behavior over extended periods of time in a changing environment) and resumption after disruption. This means that they can operate in a flexible manner. Flexibility is traditionally perceived as one of the advantages of conscious processes over nonconscious processes (Bargh 2005; Bargh and Ferguson 2000; Hassin 2005). A recent study has demonstrated that self-control (Gollwitzer, Bayer, and McCulloch 2005; Moskowitz et al. 1999), metacognition (Glaser and Kihlstrom 2005) or working memory (Hassin 2005), the mental mechanism that is perhaps most associated with controlled, conscious processing, can operate outside conscious awareness. This suggests that nonconscious mental life is more sophisticated and comprehensive than previously considered. The above discussion allows one to verify many of the concepts and constructs that constitute the foundations of planning and performing training activities as well as design-construction activities in relation to the human–machine system, or, more broadly, the human–technology system. The concept of situational awareness can serve here as a characteristic example.

1.6.3 Automatic and Controlled Processes

Contemporary research in social cognition and cognitive science has raised some very important questions. The main one seems to be expressed in the title of the article by Wegner, "Who is the controller of controlled processes?" (2005). The article opens with Wegner asking a provocative question: "Are we the robots?" The answer is not easy and requires a broader context of discussion.

Current research debates concentrate primarily on "automatic action," "mental mechanisms," or "neural circuits," which are increasingly used to account for human behavior. According to Bargh and Ferguson, prominent researchers in the field, "the social–cognition research on automaticity focuses on processes that correspond to the traditional sense of determinism in much of psychology—processes that do not require conscious choice, intention, or intervention to become active and run to completion" (2000, 928). Furthermore, "automatic processes are seen as more scientifically authentic, reflecting the true nature of humans rather than their conscious and strategic affectations" (Wegner 2005, 22). A key word for the discussed standpoint is "mechanism." It indicates that the accounts of human action and behavior should belong to the same general type of explanations as is used in other natural sciences. According to the position, continued dependence on some version of a conscious self makes psychology suspect as a science.

The distinction between unconscious automatic processes and conscious controlled processes is widely accepted and used in psychology. These notions have been challenged at two fundamental points. First, the old division of actions into controlled (conscious) and automatic (occurring without the participation of consciousness) has been undermined significantly by recent research. Second, the disturbing and, until recently, evaded question, who or what controls controlled processes, has arisen.

Automatic cognitive processes are usually seen as unintentional, nonconscious, ballistic, and effortless. Until recently, these automatic processes were considered to be connected mainly with the unconscious regulation of various activities of a living organism (e.g., we do not consciously control postural movements, such as movements performed while talking, walking, or breathing, not to mention regulating autonomic functions). Controlled processes are thought of as the counterpart of automatic processes; they are intentional, conscious, voluntary, and effortful. In this way, the use of the word "controlled" referred to higher cognitive processes that occurred with the involvement of consciousness (such as planning, switching, inhibition of dominant responses, etc.). These processes were characterized by variety, complexity, and the ability to adapt to changeable requirements of the situation. On the other hand, they were also much slower and less efficient than automatic processes.

But, as Hassin says, control means "manipulation of attention or information that allows the organism to overcome the habitual and to go beyond the immediately available" (2005, 215). Note that if one adopts this functional definition of control, there is no reason to expect that controlled processes would be exclusively conscious. It turns out that the scope of automatic processes is much wider than previously reported. We can automatically evaluate objects, form impressions of other people, make decisions, and control our behavior. Hence, a new concept emerges: "nonconscious controlled processes." The notion of nonconscious processes that occur at higher cognition is somehow disturbing because "it suggests that mental processes, which are central to our conception of what is to be human, occur outside of conscious awareness" (Hassin 2005, 197). However, that is not the only problem connected with the use of the term "controlled processes."

The division of psychological processes into "automatic" and "controlled" proves troublesome also for other reasons. Controlled processes are often regarded as more "personal," that is, representing the action and the will of the subject rather than the case of "mechanically" occurring automatic processes. However, as Wegner claims, "by reintroducing this touch of humanity, the notion of a controlled process also brings us within glimpsing range of a fatal theoretical error—the idea that there is a controller" (2005, 19). In Wegner's view, this supposition undermines the possibility of a scientific theory of psychology by creating an explanatory entity that cannot itself be explained. Hence, the already quoted question in the title of Wegner's article, "Who is the controller of controlled processes?"

According to Wegner (2005), regarding controlled processes as an expression of conscious and free-willed human choices and actions is a kind of ghost in the machine and contains an implicit suggestion of a homunculus.* As Wegner points out, the explanatory value of such constructs resembles appealing to God's will: "Just as we cannot tell what God is going to do, we cannot predict what a free-willing homunculus is likely to do either. There cannot be a science of this" (2005, 20). In the approach presented here, the controlled processes must be understood as mechanistic processes, for example, as in the cybernetic and dynamical processes posited in control theories (Bargh and Ferguson 2000). Thus, concepts of control or intention need to be defined without reference to a controlling agent. "In the attempt to address the way in which the mind worked in conjunction with the environment, cognitive science did not need to invoke concepts such as consciousness, intention, or free will" (Bargh and Ferguson 2000, 928). So, as Wegner points out, "to be accurate, we must speak of apparent mental causation or of virtual agency, rather of intention or of a controller" (2005, 32).

Therefore, although conscious (usually controlled) and unconscious (generally automatic) processes differ in the way they regulate behavior, this by no means suggests that the former are devoid of causes or are in any way "free." A task for cognitive sciences is discovering the determinants and "controllers" of conscious and controlled processes (Bargh and Ferguson 2000, 939 et seq.). In Wegner's words,

> On the fringes of our current understanding lie many phenomena that have not been tractable because the assumption of a real controller makes them seem quite out of the question. These phenomena do seem to exist, and our further thinking about the nature of control, automaticity, and the self can be informed by them. All we need to do is assume, for sake of argument, that we are the robots. (2005, 32)

As the questions about the controlling and hence "real" subject constitute a fatal theoretical error (Wegner 2005, 19), as they refer to an instance, which itself cannot be explained, then in the opinions of some researchers the questions should be replaced with a different, easier-to-solve empirical problem: how is it possible that we have an (false) impression that we (our "self") are the source of action (Wegner 2005, 19)? And also why do such illusions and constructions emerge and what is the actual machinery behind actions ascribed to them?

1.6.4 The Problem of Conscious Will

As Wegner points out in his famous book, *The Illusion of Conscious Will* (2002), experiencing will and conscious agency is an insufficient premise on which to assume their real impact. "The personal experience of agency is not a good foundation for a science of mind" (Wegner 2005, 23). Wegner's theory of apparent mental causation rests on the notion that our experience of conscious will is a construction. We experience ourselves as agents who cause our actions when our minds provide us with the idea of the action that is subsequently observed. Our experience of willing is rooted in a causal attribution process that can be experimentally manipulated. We can thus produce false experience of will (Wegner and Wheatley 1999). Action which is perceived as intentional and free is in fact "produced" by unconscious mental processes; other processes of this type are responsible for consciously appearing thoughts, intentions, and choices. According to Wegner (2002),

---

* Consciousness and sense of agency accompany controlled processes, which are slower and proceed with the involvement of attention, whereas automatic processes lack these characteristic features, allowing for the generation of a "virtual subject," and consequently are perceived as alien, which were not caused by the "self" or escaped attention (Wegner 2002, 2005, 31).

the conscious will is an illusion; the intention is not a cause, but a conscious preview of the action. But this does not mean that the creation of our sense of agency is not important. It provides a marker of our authorship, allowing us to understand, organize, and remember the variety of things we find ourselves doing.

In an important, if indirect, way, research on nonconscious forms of social cognition, behavior, motivation, and control speaks to the question of what consciousness is for. As Bargh claims, "if all of these things can be accomplished without conscious choice or guidance, then the purpose of consciousness (i.e. why it evolved) probably lies elsewhere" (2005, 52). The problem is highly complex and at this point we can only signal its existence.

1.7 A Neurocentric Perspective: A New Opening in Research and Design of the Human–Technology Systems

The neurocentric perspective appears to be opening entirely new possibilities for research on cognitive processes. Resorting to the "brain computer" and creating artificial experimental models of brain functioning and neural-like networks allow AI researchers to test hypotheses and conduct research in areas that so far have been beyond their reach. It concerns issues such as the functioning of consciousness, attention, thinking, and so forth, which can be expressed in neuroinformative and reductive categories (P. M. Churchland 1999, 2002).

On the other hand, the categories, usually artificial, rigid, and simplifying, which have been developed by psychologists so far, seem to succumb in the confrontation with the complexity, plasticity, and wealth of neural mechanisms described by neurobiologically oriented researchers. This may lead to certain unexpected consequences, that is, the appreciation of the role of a subjective phenomenal experience.* Subjective facts may become a point of reference for neurobiological research (Varela 1999; Lutz and Thompson 2003). In this way, new knowledge concerning the functioning of the mind/ brain emerges somehow at a meeting point of three disparate research traditions, experience phenomenology, organism behavior, and phenomena occurring at neural level (Damasio 1994, 1999; Koch 2004; Lutz and Thompson 2003; Varela 1999). It may suggest that an *adequate* (in the sense of being better adapted to the possibility of actual cognition) theory of cognitive processes, which would seek to describe and explain significant properties of the human and employ the knowledge to create neuroadaptive technologies, is still to a large extent *in statu nascendi*, and its development will be contingent on the results of currently undertaken research in which new areas and directions embracing human behavior in the context of neural activity rather than the context of constructs created on the basis of external indicators and measures of human behavior have been delineated.

The neurocognitive perspective, which refers to the neurocentric model in research and design of human–technology systems, offers an opportunity to determine the patterns of neural systems activity that are characteristic of various types of loading and task requirements under a variety of working conditions. Thus, new activity areas for cognitive ergonomics, engineering, and sciences devoted to organization and management

---

* At the same time, the phenomenal level of description should not be confused with what tends to be called "folk psychology"; the latter is generally understood as a certain theory equipped with particular features.

can be outlined. These new research possibilities contribute to the emergence of new disciplines, namely, neuroergonomics, augmented cognition, and neuroengineering. Within these areas, the primary research and design engineering focus on the patterns of neural systems activity related to human performance at work. As a result, research and design activities can be focused on state-of-the-art technologies that allow the development of neuroadaptive systems. The specificity of the neurocentric approach determines the future directions and progress in the fields of neuroergonomics and neuroengineering.

1.7.1 Neuroergonomics: A Neurocentric Approach to the Management of Complex Work Environments

Research on neuroergonomics was initiated almost two decades ago (e.g., Fafrowicz, Marek, and Noworol 1993), but a clear identification of the new way of treating the human–technology relationships took place relatively recently. In 2003, the journal *Theoretical Issues in Ergonomics Science*, published by Taylor & Francis, presented a dozen articles in a special issue devoted to neuroergonomics (Parasuraman 2003). This issue of the journal can be regarded as a sort of a creed for the new subdiscipline within ergonomics. The official proclamation of the new branch, according to Parasuraman (2003), was preceded by a lengthy discussion conducted on the Internet.

One of the first conferences that focused on neuroergonomics in a significant way was the XVth Triennial Congress of the International Ergonomics Association held in Seoul in 2003. A special plenary paper was dedicated to issues on neuroergonomics (Marek 2003). Also several articles in a three-volume publication, *International Encyclopedia of Ergonomics and Human Factors* (Karwowski 2006), were devoted to neuroergonomics. Research reports on neuroergonomics have appeared in journals such as *Ergonomics* (Marek and Fafrowicz 2007). A major monograph entitled *Neuroergonomics: The Brain at Work*, edited by Parasuraman and Rizzo, consisting of 24 chapters, discussed the methods used within the field of neuroergonomics and application of neuroergonomics to the neurorehabilitation processes (Parasuraman and Rizzo 2007).

Neuroergonomics focuses on exploring the functioning of neural systems involved in the performance of work tasks (activities). Its main objective is to study relationships of work performed by the human, the structure and content of tasks, and corresponding neural systems. Neural structures, their function and activity dynamics, which set the limits of human unfailing functioning, are studied. Neuroergonomics seeks to identify the limits of neural systems efficiency involved in performing work. This research approach takes into account, on the one hand, the requirements imposed by work tasks and, on the other hand, the parameters defining neural efficiency. The neural mechanisms underlying work activities become (inform the perspective of neuroergonomics) a starting point for designing work, its content, work tasks, workstations, or the entire systems. The classical methods used for work design take into consideration the requirements imposed by particular technologies and behavioral effectiveness indicators of the humans involved in the work processes. In the neuroergonomics approach, the criterion of behavioral effectiveness is replaced with the criterion of neural process efficiency linked with the functioning of particular neural structures. The traditional approach, out of necessity, contained many simplifications and oblique assumptions. At present, the introduction of noninvasive methods of registering the functioning of brain structures enables more precise identification and description of the neural network involved in task performance. The research subject of neuroergonomics is the analysis of neural process parameters implemented by specific neural structures of the brain during task performance. The configuration of the parameters and the constellation of neural structures engaged in task performance impose constraints on neural efficiency for a given task type.

Among some of the most important neuroergonomics studies are those on neural indicators of cognitive load present in work process (e.g., Baldwin 2003; Just, Carpenter, Miyake 2003, Gevins and Smith 2003), neural indicators enabling the monitoring of the operator's state in the conditions of vigilance and surveillance (e.g., Fafrowicz, Marek, and Noworol 1993; Hitchcock et al. 2003; Warm and Parasuraman 2007), neural indicators of systems design that display various types of information in human–work systems (e.g., Sanderson et al. 2003), neural indicators of spatial navigation and orientation (e.g., Sapiers and Maguire 2007), neural mechanisms enabling the control of physical effort levels (Karwowski et al. 2007), and diurnal variability in activity patterns of neural mechanisms of attention (Fafrowicz 2006; Marek et al. 2010). Of particular significance, in the context of studies on limiting potential sources of errors related to human factors, is research on neural systems responsible for execution and control of actions and error detection (e.g., Fu and Parasuraman 2007; Grafman 2007).

1.7.2 Neuroengineering and Neuroadaptive Systems

Many engineering design activities geared toward utilizing various physiological parameters in the construction of human–work systems have been undertaken successfully in the 1980s. Such activities were labeled biocybernetics (e.g., Donchin 1980; Gomer 1981). At the turn of the twenty-first century, together with the development of noninvasive imaging methods of neural brain functions, the main focus of engineering activity moved decisively toward neural processes (neuroengineering). The works exploiting electroencephalogram signals in the human–computer interaction were groundbreaking efforts in the new field of neuroengineering (e.g., Donchin, Spencer, and Wijesinghe 2000; Pfurtscheller and Neuper 2001). These undertakings initiated the development of neuroadaptive technologies including neuroadaptive interfaces.

Studies on neuroadaptive technologies, or, more generally, neuroadaptive systems, are currently conducted in many laboratories worldwide (e.g., Hettinger et al. 2003; Scerbo, Freeman, and Mikulka 2003). The focus of such research efforts is on designing systems sensitive to changes in the states of neural modules responsible for the execution of particular functions. For instance, the "B-alert" company is working on systems supporting situational awareness (Berka et al. 2005). Advanced designs offer systems that are steered and controlled directly by the states of specific neural modules. At present, this is undoubtedly one of the most fascinating challenges facing neuroengineering, that is, creating new quality conditions for shaping the structure of work systems and their content.

Neuroadaptive technologies are opening up completely new perspectives in research linked to rehabilitation of people with disabilities and to widely understood disability adjustment and compensation for disability. A review of spectacular achievements in this field is presented in the monograph *Neuroengineering*, edited by DiLorenzo and Gross (2008), which illustrates important directions of research that results in the construction of various neuroadaptive prostheses or neuroadaptive technological systems that enable people with disabilities to function effectively beyond their ability areas.

Significant achievements in the area were reported already at the turn of the twenty-first century and concerned a wide spectrum of activities. One can summon the construction of neuroadaptive limb prostheses (e.g., Riener 2007), the development of various corrective or compensatory systems for defects and deficits of the visual or auditory organs (e.g., Poggel, Merabet, and Rizzo 2007), and, finally, the introduction of technological systems improving the interaction of people with disabilities with a computer (Hettinger et al. 2003; Pfurtscheller, Scherer, and Neuper 2007).

The research activities presented in this chapter are characterized by the neurocentric approach to system design. It appears that this very approach is responsible for the success of such research efforts.

References

Baars, B. J. 2003. How brain reveals mind. Neural studies support the fundamental role of conscious experience. *Journal of Consciousness Studies* 10 (9–10):100–14.

Baldwin, C. L. 2003. Neuroergonomics of mental workload: New insights from the convergence of brain and behaviour in ergonomics research. *Theoretical Issues in Ergonomics Science* 4 (1–2):132–41.

Bargh, J. 2005. Bypassing the will: Toward demystifying the nonconscious control of social behavior. In *The New Unconscious*, edited by R. Hassin, J. Uleman, and J. Bargh, 37–58. New York: Oxford University Press.

Bargh, J. and M. J. Ferguson. 2000. Beyond behaviorism: On the automaticity of higher mental processes. *Psychological Bulletin* 126 (6):925–45.

Bargh, J. and P. Pietromonaco. 1982. Automatic information processing and social perception: The influence of trait information presented outside of conscious awareness on impression formation. *Journal of Personality and Social Psychology* 43:437–49.

Berger, A. and M. I. Posner. 2006. Attention and human performance: A cognitive neuroscience approach. In *International Encyclopedia of Ergonomics and Human Factors*, edited by W. Karwowski, 594–9. London and New York: Taylor & Francis.

Berka, C., D. Levendowski, P. Westbrook, G. Davis, M. N. Lumicao, C. Ramsey, M. M. Petrovic, V. T. Zivkovic, and R. E. Olmstead. 2005. Implementation of a closed-loop real-time EEG-based drowsiness detection system: Effects of feedback alarms on performance in a driving simulator. Paper presented at the *Proceedings of the 1st International Conference on Augmented Cognition held in conjunction with the 11th International Conference on Human–Computer Interaction*, Las Vegas, NV, July 22–27, 2005.

Bobryk, J. 1996. *Acts of Consciousness and Cognitive Processes*. Wroclaw: Leopoldinum.

Bruner, J. 1973. *Going Beyond the Information Given*. New York: Nortons.

Bush, G., P. Luu, and M. I. Posner. 2000. Cognitive and emotional influences in the anterior cingulate cortex. *Trends in Cognitive Sciences* 4:215–22.

Carter, C. S., M. M. Botvinick, and J. D. Cohen. 1999. The contribution of the anterior cingulate cortex to executive processes in cognition. *Reviews in Neuroscience* 10:49–57.

Casebeer, W. D. and P. S. Churchland. 2003. The neural mechanisms of moral cognition: A multiple-aspect approach to moral judgment and decision-making. *Biology and Philosophy* 8 (1):169–94.

Chartrand, T. L. and J. A. Bargh. 1996. Automatic activation of impression formation and memorization goals: Nonconscious goal priming reproduces effects of explicit task instructions. *Journal of Personality and Social Psychology* 71:464–78.

Chartrand, T. L., W. W. Maddux, and J. L. Lakin. 2005. Beyond the perception–behavior link: The ubiquitous utility and motivational moderators of nonconscious mimicry. In *The New Unconscious*, edited by R. Hassin, J. Uleman, and J. A. Bargh, 334–61. New York: Oxford University Press.

Churchland, P. M. 1999. *The Engine of Reason, the Seat of the Soul. A Philosophical Journey into the Brain*. Cambridge: The MIT Press.

Churchland, P. M. 2002. Folk psychology and the explanation of human. In *The Future of Folk Psychology. Intentionality and Cognitive Science*, edited by J. Greenwood, 51–69. Cambridge: Cambridge University Press.

Churchland, P. S. 1989. *Neurophilosophy. Toward a Unified Science of the Mind/Brain*. Cambridge: The MIT Press.

Corbetta, M., J. Kincade, J. M. Ollinger, M. P. McAvoy, and G. L. Shulman. 2000. Voluntary orienting is dissociated from target detection in human posterior parietal cortex. *Nature Neuroscience* 3:292–7.

Corbetta, M. and G. L. Shulman. 2002. Control of goal-directed and stimulus-driven attention in the brain. *Nature Reviews Neuroscience* 3:201–15.

Damasio, A. 1994. *Descartes Error. Emotion, Reason, and the Human Brain*. New York: Grosset/Putman.

Damasio, A. 1999. *The Feeling of What Happens: Body and Emotion in the Making of Consciousness*. Orlando: Harcourt Brace.

Dehaene, S. and L. Naccache. 2001. Towards a cognitive neuroscience of consciousness: Basic evidence and workspace framework. *Cognition* 79:1–37.

Dennett, D. 1991. *Consciousness Explained*, Boston, MA: Little, Brown.

Dennett, D. 2005. *Sweet Dreams. Philosophical Obstacles to a Science of Consciousness*. Cambridge: The MIT Press.

Dijksterhuis, A., H. Aarts, and P. Smith. 2005. The power of the subliminal persuasion and other potential application. In *The New Unconscious*, edited by R. Hassin, J. Uleman, and J. A. Bargh, 77–106. New York: Oxford University Press.

Dijksterhuis, A. D. and A. van Knippenberg. 1998. The relation between perception and behavior, or how to win a game of Trivial Pursuit. *Journal of Personality and Social Psychology* 74:865–77.

Donchin, E. 1980. Event-related potentials: Inferring cognitive activity in operation settings. In *Biocybernetics Applications for Military Systems*, edited by E. Gomer, 35–42. Long Beach, CA: McDonnell Douglas.

Donchin, E., K. M. Spencer, and R. Wijesinghe. 2000. The mental prosthesis: Assessing the speed of a P300-based brain-computer interface. *IEEE Transactions on Rehabilitation Engineering* 8:174–9.

Dupuy, J. P. 1999. Philosophy and cognition: Historical roots. In *Naturalizing Phenomenology. Issues in Contemporary Phenomenology and Cognitive Sciences*, edited by J. Petitot, F. Varela, B. Pachoud, and J. M. Roy, 539–51. California: Stanford University Press.

Edelman, G. 1992. *Bright Air, Brilliant Fire: On the Matter of Mind*. New York: Basic Books.

Fafrowicz, M. 2006. Operation of attention disengagement and its diurnal variability. *Ergonomia: An International Journal of Human Factors and Ergonomics* 28 (1):13–31.

Fafrowicz, M. and T. Marek. 2007. Quo vadis, neuroergonomics. *Ergonomics* 50 (11):1941–9.

Fafrowicz, M. and T. Marek. 2008. Attention, selection for action, error processing, and safety. In *Ergonomics and Psychology: Developments in Theory and Practice*, edited by O. Y. Chebykin, G. Bedny, and W. Karwowski, 203–18. New York: CRC Press.

Fafrowicz, M. and T. Marek. 2009. Cognitive neuroscience and psychology—New quality in research. *Annals of Psychology* 12 (1):27–35.

Fafrowicz, M., T. Marek, and C. Noworol. 1993. Changes in attention disengagement process under repetitive visual discrete tracking task measured by oculographical index. In *The Ergonomics of Manual Work*, edited by W. S. Maras, W. Karwowski, J. S. Smith, and L. Pacholski, 433–6. London: Taylor & Francis.

Fernandez-Duque, D., J. A. Baird, and M. I. Posner. 2000. Executive attention and metacognitive regulation. *Conscious Cognition* 9:288–307.

Fodor, J. and Z. Pylyshyn. 1988. Connectionism and cognitive architecture: A critical analysis. *Cognition* 28:3–71.

Fu, S. and R. Parasuraman. 2007. Event-related potentials (ERPs) in neuroergonomics. In *Neuroergonomics. The Brain at Work*, edited by R. Parasuraman and M. Rizzo, 32–50. New York: Oxford University Press.

Gazzaniga, M. 2006. *The Ethical Brain. The Science of Our Moral Dilemmas*. New York, London, Toronto, and Sydney: Harper Perennial.

Gevins, A. and M. E. Smith. 2003. Neurophysiological measures of cognitive workload during human-computer interaction. *Theoretical Issues in Ergonomics Science* 4 (1–2):113–31.

Glaser, J. and J. Kihlstrom. 2005. Compensatory automaticity: Unconscious volition is not an oxymoron. In *The New Unconscious*, edited by R. Hassin, J. Uleman, and J. Bargh, 171–95. New York: Oxford University Press.

Gollwitzer, P., U. Bayer, and K. McCulloch. 2005. The control of the unwanted. In *The New Unconscious*, edited by R. Hassin, J. Uleman, and J. Bargh, 485–515. New York: Oxford University Press.

Gomer, F. 1981. Physiological systems and the concept of adaptive systems. In *Manned Systems Design*, edited by J. Moral and K. F. Krais, 257–63. New York: Plenum Press.

Grafman, J. 2007. Executive functions. In *Neuroergonomics. The Brain at Work*, edited by R. Parasuraman and M. Rizzo, 159–77. New York: Oxford University Press.

Greenwood, J. 2002a. Introduction: Folk psychology and scientific psychology. In *The Future of Folk Psychology. Intentionality and Cognitive Science*, edited by J. Greenwood, 1–21. Cambridge: Cambridge University Press.

Greenwood, J. 2002b. Reason to believe. In *The Future of Folk Psychology. Intentionality and Cognitive Science*, edited by J. Greenwood, 70–92. Cambridge: Cambridge University Press.

Grison, S., K. Kessler, M. A. Paul, H. Jordan, and S. P. Tipper. 2005. Object- and location-based inhibition in goal-directed action. In *Attention in Action*, edited by G. W. Humphreys and M. J. Riddoch, 171–208. Hove and New York: Psychology Press.

Hancock, P. A. and J. L. Szalma. 2003. The future of neuroergonomics. *Theoretical Issues in Ergonomics Science* 4 (1–2):238–49.

Hassin, R. 2005. Nonconscious control and implicit working memory. In *The New Unconscious*, edited by R. Hassin, J. Uleman, and J. Bargh, 196–222. New York: Oxford University Press.

Heil, J. 2002. Being indiscrete. In *The Future of Folk Psychology. Intentionality and Cognitive Science*, edited by J. Greenwood, 120–34. Cambridge: Cambridge University Press.

Hettinger, L. J., P. Branco, L. M. Encarnacao, and P. Bonato, P. 2003. Neuroadaptive technologies: Applying neuroergonomics to the design of advanced interface. *Theoretical Issues in Ergonomics Science* 4 (1–2):220–37.

Hitchcock, E. M., J. S. Warm, G. Matthews, W. N. Dember, P. K. Shear, L. D. Tripp, D. W. Mayleben, and R. Parasuraman 2003. Automation cueing modulates cerebral blood flow and vigilance in a simulated air traffic control task. *Theoretical Issues in Ergonomics Science* 4 (1–2):89–112.

Hopfinger, J. B., M. H. Buonocore, and G. R. Mangun. 2000. The neural mechanisms of top-down attentional control. *Nature Neuroscience* 3:284–91.

James, W. 1890. *The Principles of Psychology*. New York: Holt.

Just, M. A., P. A. Carpenter, and A. Miyake. 2003. Neuroindices of cognitive workload: Neuroimaging, pupillometric and event-related potential studies of brain work. *Theoretical Issues in Ergonomics Science* 4 (1–2):56–88.

Karwowski, W., ed. 2006. *International Encyclopedia of Ergonomics and Human Factors*. London and New York: Taylor & Francis.

Karwowski, W., B. Sherehiy, W. Siemionow, and K. Gielo-Perczak. 2007. Physical neuroergonomics. In *Neuroergonomics. The Brain at Work*, edited by R. Parasuraman and M. Rizzo, 221–38. New York: Oxford University Press.

Kihlstrom, J. F. 1987. The cognitive unconscious. *Science* 237:1445–52.

Klein, R. M. 2000. Inhibition of return. *Trends in Cognitive Sciences* 4:138–47.

Koch, Ch. 2004. *The Quest for Consciousness: A Neurobiological Approach*. Englewood: Roberts & Company Publishers.

Libet, B. 2003. Can conscious experience affect brain activity? *Journal of Consciousness Studies* 10 (12):24–41.

Lindsay, P. H. and D. A. Norman. 1972. *Human Information Processing*. New York: Harcourt Brace Jovanovich, Inc.

Liu, T., S. D. Slotnick, J. T. Serences, and S. Yantis. 2003. Cortical mechanisms of feature-based attentional control. *Cerebral Cortex* 13:1334–43.

Lupianez, J., P. Tudela, and C. Rueda. 1999. Inhibitory control in attentional orientation: A review about inhibition of return. *Cognitiva* 11:23–44.

Lutz, A. and E. Thompson. 2003. Neurophenomenology. Integrating subjective experience and brain dynamics in the neuroscience of consciousness. *Journal of Consciousness Studies* 10 (9–10):31–52.

Marek, T. 2003. Attention—Neuroergonomics point of view. In *Ergonomics in the Digital Age*, edited by M. K. Chung, 1–4. Seoul: The Ergonomics Society of Korea.

Marek, T. and M. Fafrowicz. 2007. Quo vadis, neuroergonomics? *Ergonomics* 50 (11):1941–9.

Marek, T., M. Fafrowicz, K. Golonka, J. Mojsa-Kaja, H. Oginska, and K. Tucholska. 2007. Neuroergonomics, neuroadaptive technologies, human error, and executive neuronal network. In *Ergonomics in Contemporary Enterprise*, edited by L. M. Pacholski and S. Trzcieliński, 13–27. Madison: IEA Press.

Marek, T., M. Fafrowicz, K. Golonka, J. Mojsa-Kaja, H. Oginska, K. Tucholska, A. Urbanik, E. Beldzik, and A. Domagalik. 2010. Diurnal patterns of activity of the orienting and executive attention neuronal networks in subjects performing a Stroop-like task: An fMRI study. *Chronobiology International, The Journal of Biological and Medical Rhythm Research* 27 (5):945–58.

Marek, T., M. Fafrowicz, K. Golonka, J. Mojsa-Kaja, K. Tucholska, H. Oginska, T. Orzechowski, and A. Urbanik. 2008. Changes of the anterior cingulated cortex activity due to prolonged simulated driving—An fMRI case study. In *Conference Proceedings—Applied Human Factors and Ergonomics Conference (AHFE)*, edited by W. Karwowski and G. Salvendy. Miami, FL: USA Publishing.

Marek, T., M. Fafrowicz, and J. Pokorski. 2004. Mechanisms of visual attention and driver error. *Ergonomia: An International Journal of Human Factors and Ergonomics* 26:201–8.

Mischel, W. 2004. Toward an integrative science of the person. *Annual Review of Psychology* 55:1–22.

Moskowitz, G., P. Gollwitzer, W. Wasel, and B. Schaal. 1999. Preconscious control of stereotype activation through chronic egalitarian goals. *Journal of Personality and Social Psychology* 77 (1):167–84.

Myachykow, A. and M. I. Posner. 2005. Attention in language. In *Neurobiology of Attention*, edited by L. Itti, G. Rees, and J. K. Tsotsos, 324–9. Amsterdam: Elsevier.

Nisbett, R. and T. Wilson. 1977. Telling more than we can know: Verbal reports on mental processes. *Psychological Review* 84:231–59.

Norman, D. A. and T. Shallice. 1986. Attention to action: Willed and automatic control of behavior. In *Consciousness and Self-Regulation*, edited by R. J. Davidson, G. E. Schwartz, and D. Shapiro, 1–18. New York: Plenum.

Parasuraman, R., ed. 2003. Special issue: Neuroergonomics. *Theoretical Issues in Ergonomics Science* 4:1–249.

Parasuraman, R. and M. Rizzo, eds. 2007. *Neuroergonomics: The Brain at Work*. Oxford and New York: Oxford University Press.

Pfurtscheller, G. and C. Neuper. 2001. Motor imagery and direct brain-computer communication. *Proceedings of the IEEE* 89: 1132–4.

Pfurtscheller, G., R. Scherer, and C. Neuper. 2007. EEG based brain-computer interface. In *Neuroergonomics. the Brain at Work*, edited by R. Parasuraman and M. Rizzo, 315–28. New York: Oxford University Press.

Pieter, J. 1986. *Introduction to Psychology*, Warszawa: PIW.

Pinker, S. 1999. *How the Mind Works*. London: Penguin Books.

Pockett, S. 2004. Does consciousness cause behaviour? *Journal of Consciousness Studies* 11 (2):23–40.

Poggel, D. A., L. B. Merabet, and J. F. Rizzo. 2007. Artificial vision. In *Neuroergonomics. The Brain at Work*, edited by R. Parasuraman and M. Rizzo, 329–59. New York: Oxford University Press.

Posner, M. I. and Y. Cohen. 1984. Components of visual orienting. In *Attention and Performance X*, edited by H. Bouma and D. G. Bouwhuis, 531–56. Hillsdale, NJ: Lawrence Erlbaum Associates.

Posner, M. I. and J. Fan. 2004. Attention as an organ system. In *Topics in Integrative Neuroscience: From Cells to Cognition*, edited by J. R. Pomerantz and M. C. Crair, 31–61. Cambridge, UK: Cambridge University Press.

Posner, M. I. and S. E. Petersen. 1990. The attention system of the human brain. *Annual Reviews of Neurosciences* 13:25–42.

Posner, M. I., R. D. Rafal, L. S. Choate, and J. Vaughan. 1985. Inhibition of return: Neural bias and function. *Cognitive Neuropsychology* 2:211–28.

Posner, M. I. and M. E. Raichle. 1996. *Images of Mind*. New York: Scientific American Library.

Ramsey, W., S. Stich, and J. Garon. 2002. Connectionism, eliminativism, and the future of folk psychology. In *The Future of Folk Psychology. Intentionality and Cognitive Science*, edited by J. Greenwood, 93–119. Cambridge: Cambridge University Press.

Raz, A. 2004. Anatomy of attentional networks. *The Anatomical Record* 281B:21–36.

Riener, R. 2007. Neurorehabilitation robotics and neuroprosthetics In *Neuroergonomics. The Brain at Work*, edited by R. Parasuraman and M. Rizzo, 346–57. New York: Oxford University Press.

Rumelhart, D., J. McClelland, and the PDP Research Group. 1986. *Parallel Distributed Processing*, vols 1 and 2. Cambridge: The MIT Press.

Sanderson, P., A. Pipingas, F. Danieli, and R. Silberstein. 2003. Process monitoring and configural display design: A neuroimaging study. *Theoretical Issues in Ergonomics Science* 4 (1–2):151–74.

Sarter, N. and Sarter, M. 2003. Neuroergonomics: Opportunities and challenges of merging cognitive neuroscience with cognitive ergonomics. *Theoretical Issues in Ergonomics Science*, 4 (1–2):142–50.

Sapiers, H. J. and E. A. Maguire. 2007. A navigational guidance system in the human brain. *Hippocampus* 17 (8):618–26.

Scerbo, M. W., F. G. Freeman, and P. J. Mikulka. 2003. A brain-based system for adaptive automation. *Theoretical Issues in Ergonomics Science* 4 (1–2):200–19.

Scriven, M. 1964. Views of human nature. In *Behaviorism and Phenomenology. Contrasting Bases for Modern Psychology*, edited by T. W. Wann, 163–83. Chicago: University of Chicago Press for William Marsh Rice University.

Searle, J. S. 1992a. *The Rediscovery of the Mind*. Cambridge: MIT Press.

Searle, J. S. 1992b. *Minds, Brains and Science*. London: Penguin Books.

Szalma, J. L. and P. A. Hancock. 2002. On mental resources and performance under stress. Unpublished white paper, University of Central Florida.

Trzopek, J. 2006. *Philosophy of Psychology. Naturalistic and Antinaturalistic Foundation of Contemporary Psychology*. Krakow: UJ Press.

Trzopek, J. 2010. The new conception of human nature in scientific psychology. In *The Great Theory of Personality. End or Beginning?*, edited by A. Tokarz, 49–70. Lublin-Nowy Sacz: KUL Press.

Tyszka, T. 1992. Choices: Valuation and strategy. In *Psychology and Cognition*, edited by M. Materska and T. Tyszka, 283–308. Warszawa: PWN.

Uleman, J. 2005. Becoming aware of the new unconscious. In *The New Unconscious*, edited by R. Hassin, J. Uleman, and J. Bargh, 3–15. New York: Oxford University Press.

Vandenberghe, R., D. R. Gitelman, T. B. Parrish, and M. M. Mesulam. 2001. Location- or feature-based targeting of peripheral attention. *Neuroimage* 14:37–47.

Varela, F. 1999. The specious present: A Neurophenomenology of time consciousness. In *Naturalizing Phenomenology. Issues in Contemporary Phenomenology and Cognitive Sciences*, edited by J. Petitot, F. Varela, B. Pachoud, and J. M. Roy, 266–316. California: Stanford University Press.

Velmans, M. 2002. How could conscious experiences affect brains? *Journal of Consciousness Studies* 9 (11):3–29.

Velmans, M. 2003. Preconscious free will. *Journal of Consciousness Studies* 10 (12):42–61.

Warm, J. S. and R. Parasuraman. 2007. Cerebral hemodynamics and vigilance. In *Neuroergonomics. The Brain at Work*, edited by R. Parasuraman and M. Rizzo, 146–58. New York: Oxford University Press.

Webel, C. and T. Stigliano. 2004. Are we beyond good and evil? Radical psychological materialism and the "cure" for evil. *Theory and Psychology* 14:81–103.

Wegner, D. 2002. *The Illusion of Conscious Will*. Cambridge, MA and London, England: The MIT Press.

Wegner, D. 2005. Who is the controller of controlled processes? In *The New Unconscious*, edited by R. Hassin, J. Uleman, and J. Bargh, 19–30. New York: Oxford University Press.

Wegner, D. M. and T. P. Wheatley. 1999. Why it feels as if we're doing things: Sources of the experience of will. *American Psychologist* 54:480–92.

Wilson, T. 2002. *Strangers to Ourselves. Discovering the Adaptive Unconscious*. Cambridge, MA and London, England: Harvard University Press.

Wilson, T. and E. Dunn. 2004. Self-knowledge: Its limits, value, and potential for improvement. *Annual Review of Psychology* 55:493–518.

Wilson, T., S. Lindsay, and T. Schooler. 2000. A model of dual attitudes. *Psychological Review* 107 (1):101–26.

Wittgenstein, L. 1922. *Tractatus Logico-Filosophicus*. New York: Harcourt, Brace & Company, Inc.

Yantis, S., J. Schwartzbach, J. T. Serences, R. L. Carlson, M. A. Steinmetz, J. J. Pekar, and S. M. Courtney. 2002. Transient activity in human parietal cortex during attentional shifts. *Nature Neuroscience* 5:995–1002.

2

Neural Cybernetics of Executive Control and Learning

Phan Luu, Don M. Tucker, and Catherine Poulsen

CONTENTS

2.1 Introduction

In this chapter, we approach learning as a secondary phenomenon, subordinate to the first requirement of adaptive behavior, which is how to regulate actions (i.e., behaviors) to meet the demands of the environment. Although the distinction may be considered purely semantic and needless, we argue that this distinction is critically important. The purpose of this distinction is to address the basic mechanisms of adaptive behavior and frame learning within an organismic framework, wherein all "cognitive" processes are understood to arise from motivational control of action. Moreover, the framework permits us to draw upon constructs that are applicable to animals as well as humans, demonstrating the basic organization of brain function.

We start with an introduction to the cognitive concept of executive control in learning. We then review evidence for the existence of two neural systems with distinct cybernetic control mechanisms for the regulation of actions. We demonstrate how these two systems, when functioning properly, account for learning and performance. Throughout the chapter, we review the neuroscience evidence for how activity within these two systems is investigated and measured.

2.2 Executive Control and Learning

2.2.1 Cognitive Neuroscience Models

In 1986, Norman and Shallice proposed an influential cognitive model of executive control to describe how actions are regulated. This model posits that there are multiple subsystems that regulate behavior. The first is a contention scheduling system that regulates behaviors via selections of "schemas." A schema is a vaguely defined cognitive construct that is conceptually equivalent to the idea of an internal model, based on past experiences, of the external world. A schema is selected by the contention scheduling system via local inhibition of competing schemas. Once selected, actions are executed in an automated fashion, as part of the activated schema.

When there is conflict between a selected schema and environmental demands, a supervisory system was proposed to intervene so that a contextually appropriate schema can be selected. The supervisory system, Norman and Shallice (1986) argued, has access to the overall representation of the environment and goals of the person. Moreover, they define situations in which this system should be engaged, including planning and decision making, error correction, response novelty, danger, and overcoming of habitual responses. Essentially, these situations require learning what to do because actions (practiced or automated) that were adaptive are no longer relevant.

The Norman and Shallice model was an influential cognitive model, but it did not address the neural substrates of the subsystems and processes. With widespread availability of noninvasive neuroimaging technologies (such as functional magnetic resonance imaging), this model was used by scientists to study control mechanisms of the human brain. It became immediately apparent that certain aspects of the frontal lobe, such as the medial prefrontal cortex and the anterior cingulate cortex (ACC; see Figure 2.1), were involved in executive control (see Posner and DiGirolamo 1998), consistent with classic neurological evidence (Mesulam, 1985).

Because of the ACC's demonstrated involvement in experimental tasks such as the Stroop task, wherein subjects are required to name the color of a conflicting word (such as the word "red" written in blue ink), it was believed that the ACC was involved in the executive control of attention (Posner and Dehaene 1994; Posner and DiGirolamo 1998), a construct that is consistent with Norman and Shallice's supervisory system construct. These early findings of ACC involvement in executive attention dominated cognitive neuroscience in the 1990s partly because, to cognitive scientists, attention was a process considered central to understanding cognition and behavior.

More recently, the view of the ACC has changed along with the notion of executive control. There is now good evidence that the ACC is not involved in executive attention per se, but rather in the detection of conflict, such as the conflict generated by naming the color of the word "red" printed in blue ink (Botvinick, Cohen, and Carter 2004). Conflict in these types of paradigm is reflected in delayed reaction times when naming the conflicting ink color compared to naming the ink color that is not conflicting with reading the word. Once detected, conflict is resolved by the lateral prefrontal cortex (Miller and Cohen 2001). As an example, when subjects were provided with instructions at the beginning of each trial in a Stroop task, the lateral prefrontal cortex showed increased activation in response to color-naming instruction trials whereas it did not for word-reading instruction trials (MacDonald et al. 2000). This pattern was not found in the ACC. Rather, the ACC was more active *during* the performance of conflicting trials. This finding was presented as evidence

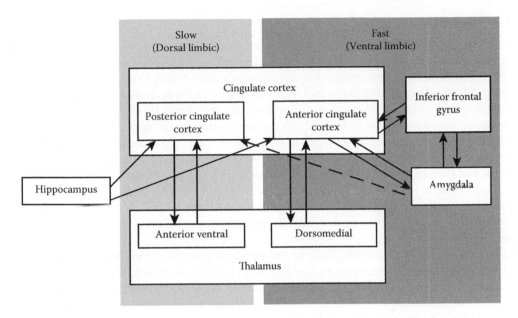

FIGURE 2.1
Schematic of brain structures involved in learning. The fast learning system is engaged early in learning and certain structures of this system has been identified to be involved in executive control, including the anterior cingulate cortex and inferior frontal gyrus.

for the role of the lateral prefrontal cortex in cognitive control. Thus, the construct of executive control has been separated into two components: conflict detection and cognitive control. Parcellating executive control in this manner avoids the inherent homunculus problem by distributing control across brain regions.

Skilled performance as automatized actions, which in the Norman and Shallice model ensues from schema activation, was originally studied extensively using motor learning paradigms. Skilled performance, however, must cut across many situations that involve mapping sensory input to motor output. It is only recently that this has been addressed (Chein and Schneider 2005). Building on the famous Schneider and Shiffrin (1977) model of controlled and automatic information processing, Chein and Schneider (2005) presented evidence that there are domain-general brain regions that are involved in early stages of learning and these regions drop out with practice. Although not invoking the concept of executive control per se, they did identify, from a meta-analytic study, brain regions involved in the early stages of learning; these include the medial prefrontal cortex (including the ACC and pre-supplementary motor area), the lateral prefrontal cortex, posterior parietal cortex, and the occipito-temporal regions. After practice, a subset of those areas engaged in early learning is further activated in addition to the posterior cingulate cortex (PCC) and precuneus. Using dense-array electroencephalography measures we have observed similar activity in the medial prefrontal cortex associated with early learning and in the PCC associated with extended practice (Luu, Tucker, and Stripling 2007; Luu et al. 2009).

To summarize, cognitive neuroscience research has identified two networks implicated in performance: a frontal network (medial and lateral prefrontal cortex, including the ACC) that is engaged in control processing required in early learning and situations where habitual responses must be overridden, and a more posterior network (PCC and precuneus) that is recruited in skilled performance following extensive practice.

2.2.2 Neural Systems Model

We now turn to evidence from animal learning studies that do not invoke cognitive constructs of attention or cognitive control to understand adaptive behavior and yet they can account for the same phenomena that cognitive science aspires to elucidate. Further, they reveal additional insights into the motivational nature of these dual systems. The evidence we review here is based on discrimination learning in rabbits by the work of Gabriel and colleagues (e.g., see Gabriel et al. 2002). In discrimination learning paradigms, an animal is presented with either a stimulus (such as an auditory tone) that predicts (CS+) the delivery of a reward or punishment or one that does not (CS–). The animal must make a response (CR) to the CS+ in order to obtain a reward or avoid the punishment. Through training, the animal learns to discriminate between the CS+ and CS–. Gabriel and colleagues have used this paradigm along with microelectrode recordings of neuronal activity implanted into various brain regions to understand the brain systems involved in discriminating CS+ from CS–.

Gabriel and colleagues (1986, 2002) found neurons that are differentially active for CS+ and CS– as a result of learning in cortical and subcortical structures; these include the ACC and PCC, hippocampus, amygdala, and mediodorsal (MD) and anterior ventral (AV) nuclei of the thalamus. This differentiation is characterized predominantly by increases in neuronal activity in response to CS+ after learning, rather than by a significant decrease in neuronal activity to CS–.

Particularly striking is the finding that these structures form spatiotemporal networks responsible for regulating learning at different stages. The ACC, amgydala, and MD are involved in the early stages of learning, wherein learning requires effort to override habitual or automated responses that are usually primed in an obligatory manner by incoming stimuli. The PCC, hippocampus, and MD form a network involved in the late stages of learning; this system codes the regularity of the learning situation, which requires repeated exposure and performance, to provide a context for action.

Lesions to the early and late learning networks affect acquisition and asymptotic/automated performance, respectively, clearly showing that these systems control unique aspects of learning. They are not, however, completely independent with regard to their contributions to learning (Gabriel, Sparenborg, and Stolar 1986). For example, even though the hippocampus is clearly part of the late learning system because of its critical role in contextual coding, it uniquely contributes to new learning (even though it does not show the training-induced activity that differentiates CS+ from CS– until the later stage of learning) by inhibiting actions that are no longer appropriate in new learning conditions.

This model of learning put forth by Gabriel and colleagues was built with evidence from animal studies, independent of cognitive constructs or data derived from human studies, and yet it contains characteristics of executive control processes described by cognitive neuroscientists. In particular, it has features very similar to what Chein and Schneider (2005) proposed: that learning can be separated into two stages with overlapping neural structures. Moreover, this animal-derived model can account for executive control processes without having to address the homunculus problem because executive control is simply the process of associative learning in the early stages, regulated by interruption of ongoing plans (i.e., automated actions) when expected outcomes are violated. After repeated exposure to the same learning situation, new regularities are extracted and come to form the context for action. Context, as represented within the late learning system, is akin to the concept of a schema.

Thus far, we have described these systems as if they are devoid of motivational influence. To the student of the brain, it is readily apparent that the brain structures of the two systems are essentially limbic structures. Limbic structures are relatively old, phylogenetically speaking, and they receive not only convergent sensory information but also visceral/internal information from midbrain and brainstem structures about the state of the organism (MacLean 1993). Therefore, the question naturally is, "How are these systems regulated by motivationally significant information?" Here, again, the work of Gabriel and colleagues (see Poremba and Gabriel 1997; Smith et al. 2002) is particularly illuminating.

In animal research, motivation is commonly assessed by measuring the animal's approach or avoidance behavior in response to a stimulus, and it is believed that these approach and avoidance tendencies are regulated by neural systems that are common across the vertebrate kingdom. Examining the role of the dual systems in avoidance discrimination learning (e.g., performing an action in response to a CS+ to avoid a shock), Poremba and Gabriel (1997) found that the amygdala was critically important in the early stage of learning. If the amygdala was destroyed or inactivated, animals showed profound deficits for learning within the first day of training compared to control animals, and they did not show the increased neuronal responses to CS+ in either the ACC or the MD. However, they could still be trained to performance criterion (i.e., they were able to learn). Once the animal had learned and was highly trained, amygdalar lesions did not affect performance. Of note is that the amygdala not only contributed to early learning, it also seemed to facilitate learning in the late-stage circuit in avoidance learning (Smith et al. 2002). However, it is important to note that while it facilitates late-stage learning, this effect is still gradual compared with the rapid learning that occurs in the early system.

In contrast to avoidance discrimination learning, approach discrimination learning (e.g., performing an action in response to a CS+ to receive a reward) does not depend on the amygdala and only indirectly on the early system. Smith et al. (2002) showed that in control animals, approach discrimination learning during the early stages was not associated with differential neuronal encoding of CS+ and CS− (i.e., increased activity to CS+) in structures such as the ACC, as it is with avoidance discrimination learning. Nevertheless, these animals demonstrated the normal learning curve. That is, they were quickly able to learn to approach the reward stimulus (e.g., drinking spout) when presented with the CS+. When structures of the early learning network were lesioned (such as the MD), these lesioned animals showed profound deficits in early learning, although they were able to learn to criterion levels after extended training. Smith et al. (2002) interpreted these findings to indicate the importance of the fast learning network in associating the CS− with no reward in approach learning such that approach behavior can be inhibited, even though changes in neuronal activity in response to CS− is not encoded by structures of this network per se.

Therefore, it appears as if new learning, as regulated by the early learning system, is driven by discrepancies, and these discrepancies are evaluated along a dimension of negative affect (such as fear and anxiety). That is, under situations in which ongoing, well-practiced, or automated behaviors are no longer appropriate (i.e., those situations that cognitive scientists have argued require executive control), expectations of correct actions and their associated rewards are violated. In both avoidance and approach learning, it is the negatively valenced (CS+ for avoidance and CS− for approach) stimuli that are important to learning.

2.3 Learning as Action Regulation

Whether we examine human or animal evidence, there appear to exist, at some fundamental level of cerebral organization, dual systems responsible for adapting behavior to environmental demands. This argues for a deeper understanding of how adaptive behavior is regulated and organized. Specifically, it requires that we look for the reasons why adaptive behavior is regulated in exactly this way: fast versus slow learning. Here, we want to point out the subtle distinction between learning and action regulation. While both terms refer to the process of adapting behavior to changing environmental demands, we believe learning often carries with it too many cognitive constructs that may not generalize across animals. Action regulation, on the other hand, places emphasis on the goal that an animal strives to achieve, which is to adjust behavior to environmental demands, and is a more neutral term with regard to cognitive constructs. Moreover, as its emphasis is on action control, cybernetic concepts are readily applicable.

Cybernetics is a scientific discipline that aims to understand the role of variable feedback in guiding systems toward a goal. As we will show, the cybernetic approach to understanding action regulation will reveal some fundamental insights into brain function because it gives us a way to understand a curious, yet, fundamental principle of vertebrate cortical organization. If we understand this organization, we understand the brain's cybernetics and, thus, adaptive behavior.

Here, we state the main ideas of our proposal to guide the reader through complicated lines of evidence that can only be presented briefly. First, cortical organization is organized along two lines: a dorsal line that emphasizes output and a ventral line that emphasizes input. From a cybernetic perspective, these lines translate to feedforward and feedback modes, respectively, of action regulation. From a cognitive perspective, these modes of control provide models, based on the history of an organism, of how the world is expected to be in the future (feedforward) and a check against this model in order to adapt behavior to changes (feedback).

2.3.1 Cortical Evolution and Cybernetic Control

The origin of the mammalian neocortex is a controversial topic in comparative neuro-anatomy. Evidence from modern evolutionary developmental biology has now clearly demonstrated that neocortical neurons are derived from primitive proliferation zones near the cerebral ventricles (see Rakic 2009). Yet, it remains to be elucidated as to how the neocortical fields come to be organized along two lines that have their roots in ancient cortical fields: the olfactory and hippocampal cortices. It has long been recognized that the entire cortical mantle can be described as organized into two distinct cortical trends: a *mediodorsal* trend with roots in the hippocampus and a *ventrolateral* trend with roots in the olfactory cortex (Sanides 1970). The initial evidence for such organization was based on the study of the cellular distribution and myelination characteristics of the cortical fields. With the development of modern methods for tracing cortical connectivity, it became clear that cortical communication is also organized along these two trends (Pandya, Seltzer, and Barbas 1988).

Relative to the present topic of action regulation and learning, the ACC, PCC, and hippocampus are the core limbic structures of the mediodorsal trend and the orbitofrontal cortex and insula are core limbic structures of the ventrolateral trend. Subcortically, on the basis of connection evidence, the AV belongs with the mediodorsal trend and the MD and amygdala are grouped with the ventrolateral trend. Each trend emphasized, during cortical evolution, the development of different cell types. The mediodorsal trend emphasized development of large pyramidal cells distributed in output layers of the cortex, whereas the ventrolateral trend emphasized granular cells distributed in input layers (Sanides 1970; Pandya, Seltzer, and Barbas 1988). The differential emphasis on output and input functions may lay the foundation for different modes of cybernetic control.

One of the most influential findings in cognitive neuroscience was that visual processing can be separated into two pathways: one for spatial and the other for object processing (Ungerleider and Mishkin 1982). Independent of the model proposed by Sanides (1970), researchers noted that the spatial processing pathway involved cortical fields located in the mediodorsal trend and that object processing engaged cortical fields of the ventrolateral trend. An alternative proposal to the function of the dual pathways for perception argued that the mediodorsal trend is better described as specialized for perception in the service of action because motor-related functions are inherently tied to spatial information processed within this trend (Goodale and Milner 1992). Yet, we know that motor functions are not the purview of just the mediodorsal trend. Certainly, action must also be influenced and guided by object-related information, and there are premotor and motor fields that lie within the ventrolateral trend.

Using the cortical organizational framework of Sanides (1970) to understand the body of evidence on motor control, Goldberg (1985) proposed that each trend has different modes of motor control. The mediodorsal trend is involved in feedforward control of actions, wherein internal models of the world guide actions. These internal models are essentially contextually based models derived from configural–spatial processing capabilities of the hippocampus and PCC. In contrast, the ventrolateral trend is involved in feedback control, guided by object-related information.

2.4 Learning Reinterpreted within the Framework of Cybernetic Control

As argued above, the functional organization of the cortical mantle, including perception, learning, memory, and action control, is dictated by the differential emphasis of output versus input functions during cortical evolution. The most coherent way to understand the consequence of this emphasis is through cybernetic control, as proposed by Goldberg (1985). We now revisit the dual-systems learning model within this cybernetic framework.

Neuroanatomical evidence clearly shows that cortical organization is separated along a dorsal–ventral axis whereas the dual-systems model cleaves the brain into anterior/posterior sectors. This difference, we argue, is because the dual-systems model accounts for a higher-level phenomenon, namely learning. On the basis of the cybernetic control model, however, we see that the fast-learning anterior system is regulated by both feedback and feedforward control. In fact, it is exactly the interaction of these two systems that permits fast learning. Fast learning requires a model of the world that constitutes the basis of action. This model is a feedforward model. It is only against this background that discrepancies can be detected, which is a function of feedback control. Feedback control is based on discrepancies between the model and actual outcomes. A corollary, supported by the evidence from avoidance and approach learning, is that the feedforward model inherently possesses a positive hedonic tone and that feedback control is intrinsically negative.

The slow-learning system, we argue, mainly reflects the function of feedforward control. This mediodorsal system extracts regularities over repeated exposure to the learning situation, thereby providing the context for actions. This context not only provides a model for automated performance but also provides the basis for the generation of new models, by the ACC, to guide new learning. In this sense, feedforward control extends history into the future to guide action. It is a unique form of expectancy, one that probabilistically estimates the future (i.e., a hypothesis).

Using this same cybernetic framework, we can also understand skilled (i.e., automatic) performance and executive control in a new light. Again, skilled performance appears to be primarily regulated by the mediodorsal system. It is worth emphasizing here that we refer to skilled performance produced through learning rather than the kinds of automatic behavioral responses that may be innately elicited by a particular class of stimuli for a given species, such as the inherent responses to threat or food objects. Thus, skilled performance can be understood to result from a stable model of the action context, and this is mainly directed by feedforward control. While it could be argued that an animal can demonstrate skilled performance to a CS+ as a result of simple learning of stimulus–response pairing, this skilled performance must occur within the relevant context, otherwise automated performance to the CS+ would occur in all situations, which would be maladaptive.

Executive control, while critically dependent on detection of discrepancies (and therefore feedback control), is again dominated by feedforward control. Executive control is required in numerous situations and yet there are no inherent discrepancies. An example is when subjects are required to generate movements internally (as opposed to responses determined by a stimulus) or to make decisions under uncertainty. It has been shown that these situations engage the ACC and related structures of the medial prefrontal cortex (Haggard 2008). These situations are considered underdetermined in that actions are not specified by stimuli per se. Underdetermined situations require an internal target of action, such as the unique form of expectancies generated by feedforward control.

2.5 Summary and Conclusion

We have proposed a unified model of learning and performance that draws upon human cognitive neuroscience, animal learning, and evolutionary neuroanatomy research and theory. This model identifies early and late learning systems that differentially draw upon the engagement of two neuroanatomical networks: a ventrolateral network (orbital frontal and insular cortex, amygdala, and MD) that is inherently negative in hedonic tone and provides feedback control through detection of discrepancy and threat; and a mediodorsal network (ACC, PCC, hippocampus, and AV) that is inherently positive in hedonic tone and operates through feedforward control based on a contextual model accrued through experience. This broad perspective offers a more coherent, integrated view of human learning and performance, one that reconciles purely cognitive constructs with neuroanatomical and neurofunctional organization, animal learning evidence, and motivational controls. In doing so, it eliminates the homunculus problem, which has plagued cognitive science explanations of performance, by identifying the triggering of executive control functions to the interaction of these basic ventral–dorsal neuroanatomical networks and their inherent motivational control biases.

Acknowledgment

This project was supported by the Office of Naval Research HPT&E Program.

References

Botvinick, M. W., J. D. Cohen, and C. S. Carter. 2004. Conflict monitoring and anterior cingulate cortex: An update. *Trends in Cognitive Sciences* 8:539–46.

Chein, J. M. and W. Schneider. 2005. Neuroimaging studies of practice-related change: fMRI and meta-analytic evidence of a domain general control network for learning. *Cognitive Brain Research* 25:607–23.

Gabriel, M., L. Burhans, A. Talk, and P. Scalf. 2002. Cingulate cortex. In *Encyclopedia of the Human Brain*, edited by V. S. Ramachandran, 775–91. Amsterdam: Elsevier Science.

Gabriel, M., S. P. Sparenborg, and N. Stolar. 1986. An executive function of the hippocampus: Pathway selection for thalamic neuronal significance code. In *The Hippocampus*, edited by R. L. Isaacson and K. H. Pribram, 1–39. New York: Plenum.

Goldberg, G. 1985. Supplementary motor area structure and function: Review and hypotheses. *Behavioral and Brain Sciences* 8:567–615.

Goodale, M. A. and D. A. Milner. 1992. Separate visual pathways for perception and action. *Trends in Neurosciences* 15:20–5.

Haggard, P. 2008. Human volition: Towards a neuroscience of will. *Nature Reviews Neuroscience* 9:934–46.

Luu, P., M. Shane, N. L. Pratt, and D. M. Tucker. 2009. Corticolimbic mechanisms in the control of trial and error learning. *Brain Research* 1247:100–13.

Luu, P., D. M. Tucker, and R. Stripling. 2007. Neural mechanisms for learning actions in context. *Brain Research* 1179:89–105.

MacDonald, A. W., J. D. Cohen, V. A. Stenger, and C. S. Carter. 2000. Dissociating the role of the dorsolateral prefrontal and anterior cingulate cortex in cognitive control. *Science* 288:1835–8.

MacLean, P. D. 1993. Introduction: Perspectives on cingulate cortex in the limbic system. In *Neurobiology of the Cingulate Cortex and Limbic Thalamus*, edited by B. A. Vogt and M. Gabriel, 1–15. Boston: Birkhauser.

Mesulam, M. M. 1985. Patterns in behavioral neuroanatomy: Association areas, the limbic system, and hemispheric specialization. In *Principles of Behavioral Neurology*, edited by M. M. Mesulam, 1–70. Philadelphia: Davis Co.

Miller, E. K. and J. D. Cohen. 2001. An integrative theory of prefrontal cortex function. *Annual Review of Neuroscience* 24:167–202.

Norman, D. A. and T. Shallice. 1986. Attention to action: Willed and automatic control of behavior. In *Consciousness and Self-Regulation*, edited by R. J. Davidson, G. E. Schwartz, and D. Shapiro, 1–18. New York: Plenum.

Pandya, D. N., B. Seltzer, and H. Barbas. 1988. Input-output organization of the primate cerebral cortex. *Comparative Primate Biology* 4:39–80.

Poremba, A. and M. Gabriel. 1997. Amygdalar lesions block discriminative avoidance learning and cingulothalamic training-induced neuronal plasticity in rabbits. *Journal of Neuroscience* 17:5237–44.

Posner, M. I. and S. Dehaene. 1994. Attentional networks. *Trends in Neurosciences* 17:75–9.

Posner, M. I. and G. DiGirolamo. 1998. Executive attention: Conflict, target detection and cognitive control. In *The Attentive Brain*, edited by R. Parasuraman, 401–23. Cambridge: MIT Press.

Rakic, P. 2009. Evolution of the neocortex: A perspective from developmental biology. *Nature Reviews Neuroscience* 10:724–35.

Sanides, F. 1970. Functional architecture of motor and sensory cortices in primates in the light of a new concept of neocortex evolution. In *The Primate Brain: Advances in Primatology*, edited by C. R. Noback and W. Montagna, 137–208. New York: Appleton-Century-Crofts.

Schneider, W. and R. M. Shiffrin. 1977. Controlled and automatic human information processing: I. Detection, search, and attention. *Psychological Review* 84:1–66.

Smith, D. M., J. H. Freeman, Jr., D. Nicholson, and M. Gabriel. 2002. Limbic thalamic lesions, appetitively motivated discrimination learning, and training-induced neuronal activity in rabbits. *Journal of Neuroscience* 22:8212–21.

Ungerleider, L. G. and M. Mishkin. 1982. Two cortical visual systems. In *Analysis of Visual Behavior*, edited by D. J. Ingle, M. A. Goodale, and R. J. W. Mansfield, 549–86. Cambridge: MIT Press.

3

A New Neural Framework for Adaptive and Maladaptive Behaviors in Changeable and Demanding Environments

Koryna Lewandowska, Barbara Wachowicz, Ewa Beldzik, Aleksandra Domagalik, Magdalena Fafrowicz, Justyna Mojsa-Kaja, Halszka Oginska, and Tadeusz Marek

CONTENTS

3.1 Introduction

In a constantly changing world, the ability to learn, develop skills, and adapt to new conditions is probably the most important capability that allows for effective functioning in the social and professional environment.

The purpose of this chapter is to present a simplified model of developing adaptive or maladaptive behavior in response to constantly changing environmental conditions. We propose, in accordance with the assumptions of evolutionism, two general goals of human behavior: (1) to maintain effective action fitting with environmental demands through cognitive control of behavior, which includes estimation of its adequacy and adjustment of behavior if necessary; (2) to protect systems of the organism through fight, flight, or freezing behavior, if an effective action in terms of cognitive control is not possible. Thus, the response to environmental stimuli may be proceeded at two levels: a more advanced level of cognitive control, which depends on the activity of evolutionarily younger brain structures, such as the neocortex, and a more primitive level associated with evolutionarily older parts of the brain, such as the amygdala (e.g., MacLean 1985).

Taking into consideration the evolution theory, neuroscience findings, and the knowledge and assumptions presented in two models briefly described below, we propose a new neural framework for responding to changeable demands of the environment. It involves three separate neural systems responsible for evaluating the conformity/discrepancy between individual resources and environmental demands, generating or maintaining the adequate behavioral pattern, and preventing such states/conditions in which no adequate behavior is possible. The proposed framework can explain human functioning under unstable conditions and, additionally, may be helpful in understanding pathological changes in the brain caused by maladaptive adjustments and behaviors.

3.1.1 Models of Cognition and Behavior

It seems that, in terms of everyday activities, generally it is better to control impulsive reactivity and to provide cogitative self-management that allows for the achievement of far-reaching goals (Carver, Johnson, Jurmann 2009). The division into cognitive control of behavior and often unconscious, impulsive reactivity, the younger and older evolutionarily brain structures, is reflected by many theories and models that describe our cognition and behavior. The core idea is that people simultaneously process information in two ways: one more primitive and basic, and the second more sophisticated and advanced. For instance, in terms of visual attention, the processing is controlled both by cognitive (top-down) factors, such as knowledge, expectation, and current goals, and by bottom-up factors that reflect sensory stimulation.

Corbetta and Shulman (2002) suggest that top-down and bottom-up processing can be associated with two separate neural pathways. Top-down regulation of attention is goal-directed and allows for volitional selection of stimuli. They reported that the process of voluntarily directed visual attention (which is modulated by stimuli detection) is controlled by the bilaterally organized dorsal frontoparietal network. The main structures of this network are the intraparietal sulcus and the frontal eye field (FEF), where the main neurotransmitter is acetylocholine. The bottom-up process is related to the reflexive stimulus-driven attention. The involuntary response to stimuli, which have potentially major significance for the organism, corresponds to the right-lateralized ventral frontoparietal network. The main structures of this network are the temporoparietal junction and the ventral frontal cortex, where the main neurotransmitter is norepinephrine. The Ventral frontoparietal network seems to act as a breaker of ongoing cognitive activity when a relevant stimulus occurs.

A slightly different and more elaborated model of self-regulation and selection of behavioral programs was recently presented by Tops et al. (2010). They proposed two pathways of information processing: ventrolateral and mediodorsal. The ventrolateral pathway proceeds from the olfactory cortex through the orbital frontal lobe and the lateral frontal cortex to the ventral premotor and motor cortices. This network is thought to facilitate a tight momentary control or an inhibition of behavior in order to process the aspects of stimuli. The ventrolateral pathway in this model is also responsible for focusing attention on potential discrepancies, threats, and rewards. Its activation may support perseverative cognition. However, it might guide further learning owing to frustration as well. The main neuromodulator of this system is dopamine. Tops et al. (2010) proposed to link this pathway to the reactive behavioral programs. The mediodorsal pathway starts from the cingulate gyrus and runs through the medial frontal cortex and the dorsolateral prefrontal cortex (DLPFC) to the premotor and motor areas. This system is associated with global attention, working memory, and gradual learning. It provides proactive context-dependent behavioral programs, in which predictions of possible results of behavior guide the action toward a goal. The main neuromodulator of this system is norepinephrine.

In summary, both models assume an existence of two separate neural networks, which operate simultaneously in order to mediate human behavior. According to models described above and to recent research findings, we present a new neural framework for adaptive behavior, assuming that the dorsal and evolutionarily younger parts of the brain are associated with cognitive control, whereas the ventral and older parts of the brain are linked to more reactive, impulsive, and emotional processing. Therefore, we propose that the ventral and older brain parts may be involved in prevention, whereas the dorsal and younger parts in evaluation and maintenance of an effective action.

3.2 A New Neural Framework for Responding to Changeable Demands of the Environment

In the proposed neural framework, the generation of adaptive and effective responses that meet environmental demands is achieved by three neural systems: the evaluative, the adaptive-compensative, and the preventive systems (Figure 3.1). The evaluative system (ES) provides an estimation of the ability to perform effective response to a stimulus or a set of stimuli. The second, that is, the adaptive-compensative system (ACS), is responsible for learning, updating, and generating efficient patterns of behavior that allows goal achievement. The role of the third system, that is, the preventive system (PS), is to protect an organism by triggering off fight, flight, or freezing behavior. Generally, the interactions within the systems can be described as follows. If an effect of the ES evaluation is positive, the existing pattern of behavior will be activated as a reaction to a stimulus or a set of stimuli. If the system reports an expectancy violation, then the ACS will be activated in order to improve or to generate efficient behavioral pattern or to activate a compensation mechanism. Finally, if the pattern of behavior fitting the environmental demand does not exist (i.e., the ES estimation is negative), or the amount of one's resources stymies its generation (the ACS failure), then the PS will be activated in order to prevent potential harm. Each of the systems will be described in detail in the following sections.

3.2.1 The Evaluative System

The first proposed system, which determines effective control over behavior and efficient functioning in the environment, is the ES. Its role is to estimate whether the pattern of behavior exists and whether it is adequate to meet the demands of the environment. The ES also evaluates whether the level of performance is appropriate and whether there is a discrepancy between the expectations and the actual outcomes of an action. Besides, in case the adequate behavioral pattern does not exist, the ES evaluates whether there is enough resources to generate it. In other words, the ES is particularly engaged in conflict detection, action monitoring, and expectancy violation through an

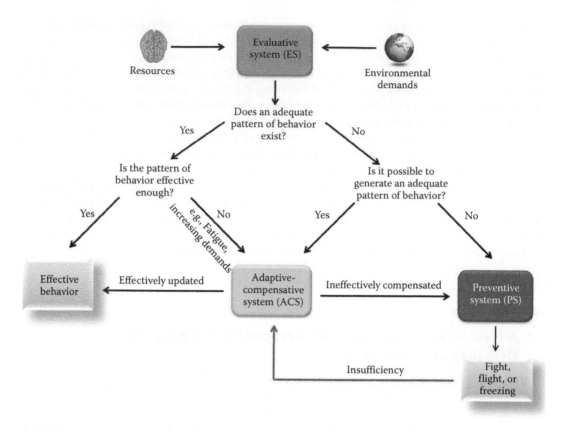

FIGURE 3.1
The evaluative, adaptive-compensative, and preventive systems (ES, ACS, and PS, respectively).

evaluation of signals from the inner and outer surroundings, including an individual's resources and environmental demands. We propose the following neural structures to be involved in the evaluation process: the anterior cingulate cortex (ACC), as its main component, with cooperation of the parietal lobe (PL) and presupplementary motor area (preSMA).

3.2.1.1 Neural Substrates of the ES

The ACC is a part of the medial frontal cortex. The consistent findings show that this brain structure is involved in error detection and conflict monitoring (Botvinick et al. 2004). This assumption has come from an observation of error-related negativity (ERN or Ne), a component of error-related potential (ERP), in electroencephalography studies, which is generated when an incorrect response occurs (Falkenstein et al. 1991; Gehring et al. 1993). The ERN is related to error processing during response execution and reflects a difference in neural processing between erroneous responses and correct responses in speeded response time tasks. Recently, another error-related negativity component has been found (Holroyd et al. 2009). A very similar negative response is observed when feedback information is given to an unaware error. This ERP's component was called "feedback ERN" (fERN) in contrast to the previously discovered "response ERN" (rERN). Electrophysiological source analyses indicated the ACC to be the neural source of both rERN and fERN (Luu et al. 2003). Moreover, Miltner et al. (2003) confirmed the source being ACC as they demonstrated the existence of the "magnetic equivalent of the ERN" (mERN) generated within the region. In an event-related functional magnetic resonance imaging (fMRI) experiment, Holroyd et al. (2004) also showed that the error responses and error feedback activated the ACC. More direct evidence that the ERN is generated by the ACC has been provided through trial-by-trial couplings of electroencephalography (EEG) and fMRI signals (Debener et al. 2005).

In terms of cognitive psychology, the role of the ACC would be to detect conflict in information processing in order to trigger off a mechanism of compensation and cognitive control or to improve a level of concentration of attention (Botvinick et al. 2004). Therefore, the activity of the ACC most likely manifests itself in sensitivity to a stimuli and response incompatibility with previously set expectations and in sensitivity to the outcomes inconsistent with anticipated results of an action. As Botvinick et al. (2004) indicated, in experimental conditions the increase of neural activity in the ACC can be observed in subjects who carry out tasks: (1) requiring a choice between several equally valid responses, (2) requiring the inhibition of dominant reaction, or (3) in which an error of commission is made.

As mentioned before, conflict detection by the ACC triggers off mechanisms of cognitive control and concentration of attention. One of the manifestations of this process, the Gratton effect, can be observed during performance of the Flanker task (Eriksen and Erisken 1974), which examines the resistance to a distraction. In situations where stimuli are incongruent, the response time is extended. Response time, however, is relatively shorter, if the previous set of stimuli was also incongruent. Another effect, which is thought to be the behavioral manifestation of intensified cognitive control, is the Stroop interference (Stroop 1935). Apparently, the lower a frequency of incongruent stimuli, the longer the response times. These phenomena may be a sign of the strengthening of mechanisms of top-down control and attention in response to the detection of conflict reported by the ACC (Botvinick, Cohen, and Carter 2004).

In studies in which a task-related interference appears, increase in activity is usually observed not only in the ACC but also in the preSMA (Haupt et al. 2009), which is often enlisted as part of a well-known frontoparietal circuit responsible for cognitive control (e.g., Hon et al. 2006). Recent findings of van Maanen et al. (2011) indicate that preSMA is especially involved in maintaining a lower level of response caution and shows greater activation when speed is at a premium than during accuracy-stressed trials of the task, which require more response caution (more information is required before a decision is made). Thus, together with the ACC, preSMA is involved in conflict management.

The ACC might be divided into two parts: dorsal and ventral. The dorsal ACC (dACC) is thought to be involved in cognitive processing, whereas the ventral ACC, consisting of rostral (rACC) and subgenual components, has been shown to be linked to emotional processing (Etkin et al. 2006). The dACC is connected with brain areas that are thought to be involved in top-down control implementation, such as DLPFC (Kim, Kroger, and Kim 2011), whereas the ventral ACC is connected with the amygdala (Stefanacci and Amaral 2002). "Cognitive" and "affective" subdivisions, as some researchers call these subregions (Bush, Luu, and Posner 2000), are also interconnected. These findings are consistent to some extent with the findings of Polli et al. (2005) which suggest that the dACC contributes to performance optimization whereas both rACC and dACC activation mediates performance evaluation. As researchers have shown, errors in performance of antisaccade tasks were preceded by failure in bilateral deactivation of the rACC. Therefore, the decrease in rACC activity during demanding cognitive tasks (Bush, Luu, and Posner 2000) seems to be necessary for proper cognitive performance. On the contrary, clinical studies have shown that the rACC may be involved in active adjustment in cognitive tasks following the occurrence of the response conflict in previous trials (di Pellegrino, Ciaramelli, and Làdavas 2007). In the study by di Pellegrino, Ciaramelli, and Làdavas (2007), patients with lesions in the rACC region showed neither difference, depending on the conflict level in the performance of the Simon task, nor significant post-error slowing. However, this contradiction may arise from the difference in construction of these two experiments: di Pellegrino, Ciaramelli, and Làdavas (2007) noted the role of the rACC in the adjustment of the task performance in which stimulus conflict was repeated (e.g., incongruent task that followed incongruent ones), whereas Polli et al. (2005) focused more on optimizing the task performance at its beginning.

However, it is important to note that dACC activation can be observed during the performance of various cognitive tasks such as the Stroop or Flanker task (Botvinick, Cohen, and Carter 2004; Mohanty et al. 2007; Ochsner et al. 2009). Recent findings of Schulz et al. (2011) have shown that dACC activity contributes also to the top-down control of the preparatory process. In this study, 16 healthy right-handed adults were asked to perform a cued Go/No-Go task. Results showed increased activity to the cue stimulus informing about direction of the target in the dACC and other brain areas such as the DLPFC, frontal operculum, cerebellum, and sensory and motor cortices. Moreover, left cues activated the right dACC whereas right cues activated the left dACC. Such activation may be understood in terms of preparatory selection of a motor program of context-appropriate responses, which is consistent with our model.

In terms of conflict processing, another interesting finding has been made recently. Kim, Kroger, and Kim (2011) have shown that conflict detection activates the dACC on two levels: perceptual and responsive. In this study, participants were asked to perform a Stroop task. Results indicate that the caudal part of the dACC (cdACC) is involved in perceptual conflict, whereas the rostral part of the dACC (rdACC) is engaged in response conflict. Thus, as Kim, Kroger, and Kim (2011) proposed, the dACC can be divided into two functionally different subregions: the cdACC, monitoring conflict in stimuli perception, and the rdACC, monitoring conflict in response selection. Taken together, it seems to be appropriate to say that the dACC is strongly involved in the process of cognitive evaluation whether or not the response to a stimulus or a set of stimuli is contextually adequate.

As mentioned, Bush, Luu, and Posner (2000) suggested the existence of "affective" subdivision of the ACC (perigenual ACC, including the rostral and subgenual areas), which is connected to the basolateral amygdala (BLA; Stefanacci and Amaral 2002) and the periaqueductal gray and nucleus accumbens (Bush, Luu, and Posner 2000). The rACC plays a role in the widely understood emotional information processing (Bush 2004). Activity changes in this part of the ACC can be observed in affective disorders, including depression (e.g., Yoshimura et al. 2010) and posttraumatic stress disorder (e.g., Shin et al. 2001), which also confirms that the rACC is involved in emotional processing. Increase of activation in the rACC during the performance of affective tasks (including conflict-related activity) is nowadays commonly known, though still not fully explained. Besides, the rACC is known to be involved in error commission, that is, detection of another expectancy violation in cognitive tasks (Holroyd et al. 2004).

Etkin et al. (2006) have studied the engagement of the rACC in high conflict resolution tasks. In an fMRI study, they used an emotional conflict task (modification of Stroop task—pictures of happy or fearful faces with the word "happy" or "fear" on it). Results showed that when the incongruent trials were repeated (high conflict resolution), the amygdala activity decreased and the rACC activity increased (it was especially high when earlier conflicts were successfully resolved); when incongruent trials followed congruent ones (low conflict resolution), the amygdala and DLPFC activities increased and the rACC activity was rather low. Etkin et al. (2006) indicated that the rACC is involved in coping with emotional conflict and may be engaged in the top-down inhibition of the amygdala during the high conflict resolution trials (which may be implemented to reduce emotions).

The role of the ACC in conflict monitoring and its evaluative function has been widely studied (for a review, see Botvinick et al. 2004). Many fMRI findings indicate greater rACC activity in response to errors than to correct responses (Holroyd et al. 2004). Some of the EEG studies indicate that the response error-related negativity (Ne100, rERN) may come from both the rACC and the dACC (Luu et al. 2003). Yet, other studies indicate that both the rERN and the fERN come only from the caudal or the dorsal ACC (Holroyd et al. 2004; van Veen and Carter 2002a). Nevertheless, links are visible between emotionality and ERN amplitude—negative affect increases the amplitude of ERN (Gehring, Himle, and Nisenson 2000; Hajcak, McDonald, and Simons 2004). Moreover, ERN amplitude is changed in patients with affective disorders such as obsessive-compulsive disorders or anxiety (Hajcak, McDonald, and Simons 2004; Holroyd et al. 2004). These studies may indirectly indicate that rACC may have an influence on amplitude of ERN. Therefore, Luu and Pederson (2004) suggested that the ERN reflects the affective consequences of expectancy violation.

Because the affective component in conflict monitoring is clearly seen, Botvinick et al. (2004) and Luu and Pederson (2004) have indicated that the ACC plays a role in evaluating the motivational or affective consequences of expectancy violation. Not all of the aforementioned studies directly refer to the rACC, but its seems to be justified to propose it for this role, when taking into account its engagement in the reward circuit (Wacker, Dillon, and Pizzagalli 2009) and many links to affect. This assumption is consistent with an fMRI finding that has shown increased activity in the rACC as a loss-related response to errors commission, although, interestingly, activity in the rACC did not increase when participants failed to gain owing to error commission (Taylor et al. 2006). In the study by Taylor et al. (2006), a cognitive task similar to the Flanker task with three different types of cues at the beginning of each trial (monetary gain, monetary loss, and "null"—failure to gain) was used. Their results indicate involvement of the rACC in emotional responses to errors.

Thus, the rACC seems to be involved in a widely understood evaluation of an error including the affective consequence of expectancy violations in cognitive tasks. In addition, the rACC is also involved in managing emotional conflict (Etkin et al. 2006). In summary, it seems that the rACC is responsible for the emotional aspects of performance and its integration with the cognitive aspect.

The PL, the last structure of the ES, was shown to be involved in saccades (Simon et al. 2002), attention (Corbetta and Shulman 2002), and visuospatial and numerical processing (Dehaene et al. 2003; Hubbard et al. 2005). It also receives and integrates sensory information from various parts of the body and creates representations of their position in order to plan the motor reactions (Gross and Graziano 1995). Recent findings of Lee et al. (2006) suggest that both the posterior PL and the ACC activity increases during performance of complex cognitive reasoning tasks. It was found that stronger activity in the posterior PL correlates with a higher level of intelligence (measured by Raven's Advanced Progressive Matrices and WAIS-R) during performance of such reasoning tasks. Moreover, not only the ACC but also the posterior PL seems to be engaged in conflict monitoring, respectively, first at the level of response and second at the level of stimulus representation (Liston et al. 2006). The study by Liston et al. (2006) indicates that increased posterior parietal cortex activity on a given trial was associated with enhanced performance on a subsequent trial. It was also found that both the PL and the rACC elicit late (250–400 ms) subcomponent of the Pe (error positivity following the ERN), which manifests aspects of error processing (van Veen and Carter 2002b). Considering all mentioned reports, we suggest that the PL, owing to its co-engagement in error processing, conflict monitoring, and its role in sensory and spatial information processing, is also involved in evaluation of adequacy/discrepancy between one's resources and environmental demands.

3.2.1.2 *The ES in Action*

The ACC, preSMA, and PL are involved in both stimulus/response conflict monitoring and error evaluation (Botvinick et al. 2004; Haupt et al. 2009; Kim, Kroger, and Kim 2011; Liston et al. 2006). It is worth emphasizing the relationship between the ACC and both the cognitive sphere (Ochsner et al. 2009) and the emotional sphere (mainly the emotional evaluation of expectancy violation; Luu and Pederson 2004). With respect to our model, the influence of the dACC on strengthening top-down regulation (Botvinick et al. 2004, Kim, Kroger, and Kim 2011), especially the top-down control of the preparatory process of motor programs of context-appropriate responses (Schulz et al. 2011), seems to be particularly important. Besides, the mediating role of the ACC in the top-down mechanism of monitoring the action is consistent with our suggestion that its main function is evaluation. What is more, the ACC is involved in early stages of compensatory behaviors by triggering off a change of behavior when outcomes are not as expected (Bush et al. 2002; Shima and Tanji 1998), which is also in line with our suggestions.

3.2.2 The Adaptive-Compensative System

The second neural system we propose is an adaptive-compensative system (ACS). It is involved in preparing successful responses that fit environmental and situational demands through adaptation of an individual's available resources and generation of new behavioral pattern. The ES estimates the extent to which a developed pattern of behavior meets the demands of the environment.

If a pattern of behavior is efficient, it remains unchanged as long as it is effective enough to support the achievement of one's goals. Environmental conditions and demands constantly change. Hence, the pattern of behavior should be flexible enough and easily modifiable if such a need occurs. Similarly, individual internal conditions may vary and change the quantity or quality of available resources. The cause of that variation may be multiple factors, such as time of the day and phase of the circadian rhythm (Marek et al. 2010a; Schmidt et al. 2007), sleep deficit (Durmer and Dinges 2005; Fafrowicz et al. 2010), fatigue (Marek et al. 2010b), health, or mood.

When the change in an environment or in an organism occurs and execution of behavior must be continued, the role of the ACS is to recruit additional resources to support satisfactory level of performance. Therefore, the compensation, which should lead to the maintenance of a successful response in changing outer and inner conditions, is an extension of already existing behavioral pattern. A new component of behavioral pattern must be synchronized with the old ones. It should be noted that the more components, the more difficult it is for the organism to synchronize them in a proper way. Finally, the system may be unable to prepare and maintain adequate response, what results in maladaptive strategies.

We propose that at least three neural structures are involved in generating effective behavioral patterns: (1) DLPFC, (2) the basal ganglia (BG), and (3) the hippocampus. In the next section, we will briefly focus on their functions.

3.2.2.1 Neural Substrates of the ACS

The prefrontal cortex (PFC) is a part of the frontal lobe, which is thought to be responsible for executive functions understood in terms of "goal formation, planning, carrying out goal directed plans and effective performance" (Jurado and Rosselli 2007, 213). Additionally, models of the PFC system usually attribute to it three functions: active maintenance, top-down control, and rapid updating. Especially, rapidly updating of what is being maintained seems to be crucial for behavioral flexibility (O'Reilly 2006). According to the literature, we assume that this ability is mediated by interaction between the DLPFC and the BG (McNab and Klinberg 2008; O'Reilly and Frank 2006).

The DLPFC was shown to be involved in behavioral goal selection, set-shifting, and planning, including monitoring, manipulation, and integration of information (Jurado and Rosselli 2007; Tanji and Hoshi 2008). It is widely known to be responsible for organizing items in working memory, specifically for maintaining representations of intentions and rules in working memory (Miller and Cohen 2001) and strengthening an inter-items association in long-term memory by processing them in working memory (Blumenfeld and Ranganath 2006). The DLPFC is also thought to implement and support cognitive control by inhibition of processing of distractive stimuli (Barbas and Zikopoulos 2007) and stereotyped responses (Kadota et al. 2010) in order to perform voluntary, planned activities (MacDonald et al. 2000).

Another function that seems to be linked with the DLPFC is the ability to use feedback about previous actions to guide future behavior (Barcelo and Knight 2002). This ability can be seen as an effect of comparison made between action and its eventual outcome in working memory (Genovesio, Brasted, and Wise 2006). As Weissman, Perkins, and Woldorff (2007) suggested, recruitment of the DLPFC is also important for cognitive control in the social context because of its involvement in evaluating the social outcomes of other people's behavior and estimating whether one person's intentions are consistent with another person's actions. According to them, the DLPFC may be responsible for incorporating social outcomes of observed behavior into planning of our own future behavior.

While enumerating functions of the DLPFC, it should be noted that the results of studies suggest that this structure's functions are strongly lateralized. The right DLPFC was shown to be one of the several brain structures involved in anticipation of aversive stimuli (Nitschke et al. 2006) and in mediating negative attitudes (Wood et al. 2005), whereas the left DLPFC was found to be involved in verbal processing (Jurado and Rosselli 2007). Furthermore, results of the study by Grimm et al. (2008) showed that left DLPFC hypoactivity is associated with negative emotional judgment, whereas right DLPFC hyperactivity is related to attentional modulation in patients with major depressive disorder.

Kerns et al. (2004), in the fMRI study, observed a relationship between control-related activation of the right DLPFC and the amount of post-error slowing, which is considered to reflect an increase in cognitive control in the form of a tendency to compensate an error by being slower and more careful. Thus, after recognizing an error, people are able to adjust their behavior to reduce or prevent future errors. The degree of post-error slowing is related to the ERN (Debener et al. 2005), that is the greater ERN's amplitude, the slower people tend to be on trials following the error (van Veen and Carter 2006). Marco-Pallarés et al. (2008), in an EEG study, investigated the neuropsychological mechanisms involved in post-error slowing using ERP analysis. The results suggest that the adaptive actions after commission of an error may be evoked by a neural circuit involving the right DLPFC and the inferior parietal cortex. Considering the above findings, it seems appropriate to say that DLPFC plays a key role in assessing possible outcome, planning, performing, and maintaining behavior consistent with learnt rules, in order to achieve far-reaching goals.

The second neural substrate of the ACS, the BG, is associated with a variety of functions, including action selection, action gating, motor preparation, timing, exploratory behavior, goal-oriented behavior, working memory, procedural learning related to routine behaviors, mediating acquisition of stimulus–response associations, reward processing, and reward-based learning (Chakravarthy, Joseph, and Bapi 2010; Stocco, Lebiere, and Anderson 2010). In the context of ACS, some special functions of the BG should be noted. For example, it is widely known, that striatal activity is modulated by reward signals (Tobler, Fiorillo, and Schultz 2005). Specifically, the BG are supposed to provide additional reward-related information that mediates goal-oriented activity in the PFC (Chakravarthy, Joseph, and Bapi 2010). Moreover, many aspects of BG functioning could be understood in terms of selection of action/information and inhibition of competing programs (Redgrave, Prescott, and Gurney 1999). Activity of the BG is thought to be, especially, important for filtering out stimuli that should not be included in the set maintained in the working memory (Hazy, Frank, and O'Reilly 2006; McNab and Klinberg 2008; O'Reilly and Frank 2006). As Montague, Hyman, and Cohen (2004) have shown, a phasic dopamine burst is involved in this process by opening the gate for information and, thus, permitting updating of goal-oriented activity in the PFC. Information from the BG, namely from the ventral tegmental area, is transmitted to the cortex via the dopaminergic pathway (Cohen, Braver, and Brown 2002). Taken together, the process of transferring reward-related information by dopamine signal to the cortex may be crucial for decision making by selecting which information should be held and updated in the working memory in order to maintain goal-oriented behavior.

In the wide context of gaining experience and the development of behavioral patterns compatible with environmental demands, it should be also remembered that the BG are involved in stimulus–response acquisition (Packard and Knowlton 2002) and skill acquisition, which is based on practice and results in the development of automatic procedures (Doyon, Penhune, and Ungerleider 2003). As Atallah et al. (2007) have shown, two different parts of the BG are critical for skill acquisition in rats. The ventral striatum is critical for learning, whereas the dorsal part is crucial for performance. What is important, practice can improve already existing patterns of performance by eliminating intermediate processing steps that require cognitive control (Stocco, Lebiere, and Anderson 2010). Therefore, a greater amount of cognitive resources may be used to develop an extension of behavioral patterns in situation of increasing environmental demands.

The third neural element of ACS is the hippocampus. Since the operation performed on patient H.M., functions of this structure were widely investigated and linked to declarative memory and consolidation of memory traces (Squire 1992), spatial memory and navigation, episodic memory (Burgess, Maguire, and O'Keefe 2002), and novelty detection as a result of building context representation (Vinogradova 1995). The role of the hippocampus in the theory of declarative memory is thought to be time-limited (Squire and Alvarez 1995). This theory assumes that memory traces are gradually reorganized and consolidated after learning. The process of consolidation in such terms relies on time-dependent interaction between the hippocampus and long-term memory storage located within the neocortex. Eventually, this process leads to stabilization of originally labile memory traces in the neocortex. When the process of consolidation is completed, activity in the hippocampus is no longer required or involved in recall. Thus, the hippocampus is understood here as a basal brain structure for the ability to learn and for memory storage. An important extension of the declarative memory theory called the "relational processing" theory was proposed by Cohen and Eichenbaum (1993). Their main assumption was that declarative memory involves processing the relations between different items. At the level of encoding, this mechanism enables access to stored information in situations quite different from those of original learning. According to Cohen and Eichenbaum (1993), storage of individual items is located in the perihinal and parahippocampal cortex; the hippocampus is thought to be responsible for relational processing.

O'Reilly and Rudy (2001) proposed a slightly different view on hippocampal function. They suggested that the role of the hippocampus is to rapidly acquire information about a specific experience by building and storing "configural associations" between elemental stimuli that occur at one time, which leads to the development of conjunctive representation of a new experience. What is more, the hippocampal formation also minimizes the interference between aspects of a new experience and similar old experiences in the process of "pattern separation" in order to facilitate an effective processing in the cortex, or in other words, slow cortical learning. The hippocampus separates patterns of experiences by using a relatively small number of highly selective units to represent an input pattern (so-called sparse representation). This assumption is consistent with the findings showing that experience-dependent hippocampal growth is possible (Clayton and Soha 1999; Maguire et al. 2000). Furthermore, hippocampal formation is also involved in the process of "pattern completion," which enables activation of a stored pattern that represents previous experience by a subset of cues from that experience, in order to support memory retrieval. Thus, the hippocampus must balance two countervailing functions: "pattern separation" and "pattern completion." What researchers additionally pointed out is that even if the hippocampus is damaged, learning is still possible as the cerebral cortex detects combinations of stimuli that appear repeatedly, although much slower.

At least three mechanisms of learning are thought to be linked with the hippocampus. One of them is based on the process of neurogenesis in the dentate gyrus (Shors et al. 2001); the second one depends on expression of the brain-derived neurotrophic factor (Hall, Thomas, and Everitt 2000); and the third one is an activity-dependent AMPA/NMDA-receptor-dependent, associative synaptic plasticity based on the mechanism of long-term-potentiation (for a review, see Whitlock et al. 2006).

All the aforementioned theories and information indicate that the function of hippocampal formation is understood in terms of memory, contextual learning, and the acquisition of experience. Consequently, the correct functioning of this structure seems to be important or even crucial for the process of adaptation and effective functioning in an environmental context.

3.2.2.2 *Interactions within the System*

As proposed earlier, the combined activity of described structures, namely DLPFC, BG, and hippocampal formation, serves as a neural substrate of the ability to adapt to changeable outer and inner environmental conditions by using efficient cognitive control and motor performance. Previous findings have shown that these structures are involved in instrumental conditioning, reversal learning, planning, and feedback learning (Moustafa and Gluck 2011). Furthermore, many computational models have focused on simulating the function of corticostriatal (e.g., O'Reilly and Frank 2006) and corticohippocampal (e.g., O'Reilly and Norman 2002) connections. Although there is less information about the function of a hippocampal–striatal pathway, at least two anatomical pathways connect hippocampal formation with the BG (e.g., Shen and Tsai 1995). The first one runs from the hippocampus to the ventral striatum via the subiculum; the second one runs from the hippocampus to the PFC, which sends further information to the BG. In addition, a relatively recent study has shown simultaneous hippocampus and BG activity during a sequence learning task performance (Albouy et al. 2008). Various neurotransmitters are involved in the transmission of information within this system. Amongst them, two seem to be the most important: dopamine and acetylocholine. It is important to note that the role of dopamine depends on brain area. Research findings have shown that in the BG phasic dopamine is important for stimulus–response and feedback learning (Tsai et al. 2009), whereas in the PFC dopamine signal is essential for working memory and attention (Iba and Sawaguchi 2003).

We are not the first to point out that the PFC, hippocampal formation, and the BG work as a neural network to perform efficient motor and cognitive processing. The model proposed by Moustafa and Gluck (2011) presents the same brain structures organized in a functional network and playing different computational roles. In their model, the hippocampus is responsible for stimulus–stimulus representational learning. Information about stimuli is sent from hippocampal formation to the BG—the key structure for stimulus–response and reinforcement learning—and the PFC, which in their model is linked to stimulus selection. In our model, these three brain structures serve as a neural circuit responsible for functions of adaptation and compensation, where the hippocampus is seen as a basal structure for memory and contextual learning, the DLPFC is seen to be responsible for maintaining goal-oriented processing, and the BG is seen to mediate information gating and skill acquisition. We assume that interactions between these three structures may lead to generation of a new behavioral pattern, which fits environmental demands, or to extension of an already existing pattern in order to maintain a satisfactory level of performance.

3.2.2.3 The ACS in Action

If the ES estimates a behavioral program as effective enough, the ACS will decrease its activity. In an opposite situation, when the ES detects a discrepancy between the expected and actual results of behavior, the ACS will remain activated in order to generate new or extend existing behavioral patterns. Such a situation could happen if one does not dispose adequate resources to generate an efficient behavioral program owing to the biological and genetic constitution or social context. If we are not able to create such a pattern of reaction to a stimulus or to a set of stimuli that will allows us to control the situation, then stress and anxiety arise. Consequently, maladaptive behaviors may develop as a result of an attempt to cope with overwhelming demands.

The described concept is consistent with the results of research indicating that the PFC area is involved in regulation of the hypothalamic–pituitary–adrenal axis (HPA axis) (Diorio, Viau, and Meaney 1993), whose role is to control an organism's response to stress and regulate various body processes. As de Kloet (2003) has suggested, physical impact of specific stressors on animals may depend either on whether they can perform any adaptable response to escape or on whether they must endure it. In humans, planning and decision making in higher brain structures and an individual's perception of an experience with regard to past experience of similar events strongly influence whether a specific stimulus or a set of stimuli has a positive or negative effect on performance. In addition, Lupien and Lepage (2001) also suggested that the PFC and the hippocampus are parts of the regulatory HPA feedback circuitry. In other words, components of the ES and the ACS may implement a top-down control that can result in decreased HPA axis activity. What is more, there is an inverted U-shaped function between the level of acute stress and the working memory linked to the DLPFC (Elzinga and Roelofs 2005; Lupien, Gillin, and Hauger 1999), which suggests that this function too is stress-dependent.

In our model, we also propose that the behavioral pattern may become ineffective in a situation where one must continue its execution, and a chronic fatigue occurs as an effect. In such a situation, the resources at disposal are reduced, and the maintenance of behavior is becoming increasingly difficult for the organism. Therefore, prolonged compensation in this case leads to chronic stress due to the environmental demands that eventually exceed an individual's resources and to the lack of ability to control the situation. As a result, stress-related maladaptive strategies may develop.

At this point it is vital to note that in scientific literature the link between stress and the hippocampus has been emphasized: McEwen, Weiss, and Schwartz (1968) showed that the area with the highest density of receptors for corticosteroids (hormones involved in stress response) in the rodent brain was the hippocampus. Lupien and Lepage (2001) in their review enlisted four major arguments that confirm significant impact of stress hormones on memory, learning, and hippocampal structure. The first one relates to the finding of McEwen, Weiss, and Schwartz (1968)—the presence of glucocorticoid receptors in the hippocampus. The second one is based on findings that showed significant negative impact of high levels of stress on declarative memory. The third one concerns the fact that the chronic exposure to high levels of stress may cause an atrophy of this structure. For example, Vyas, Shankaranarayana Rao, and Chattarji (2002) have shown that, in rats, chronic immobilization stress induces dendritic atrophy and debranching in pyramidal neurons of the hippocampal CA3 component. The fourth argument relates to findings showing that stress can decrease the level of neurogenesis in the dentate gyrus.

Another hypothesis suggests that hippocampal dysfunction might be the effect of increased synaptic glutamate levels, the main excitatory neurotransmitter in the brain, which can lead to excitotoxicity—the pathological process in which neurons are damaged by excessive stimulation (Ortuño-Sahagún et al. 2012). Studies have shown that chronic lithium treatment, which was shown to protect neurons in conditions of increased glutamate levels (Coyle and Duman 2003), increases cell proliferation in the dentate gyrus of the rodent brain (Chen et al. 2000) and prevent cells of the hippocampal CA3 component from dendritic shrinkage (Wood et al. 2004). What is more, the effects of glutamate activity parallel the effects of stress on learning and can be presented as an inverted U-shaped function.

As we emphasized before, efficient cognitive and motor processing is a key factor for effective adaptation to the demands of the environment and runs through the generation of patterns of behavior fitting these demands by the ACS. However, under conditions of prolonged activity, which may cause fatigue and stress, the pattern of behavior may become less effective. In such a situation, the ES reports a discrepancy between expectations and the actual outcomes of behavior. This information causes the activation of the ACS in order to improve behavioral pattern. Note that such an assumption is consistent with a recent finding showing co-activation of the cdACC and the DLPFC, structures that are involved in response conflict and triggering top-down control in order to override prepotent responses, during performance of the Stroop task (Kim, Kroger, and Kim 2011).

Lupien and Lepage (2001) proposed that combined implication of stress and the HPA axis related to hippocampal atrophy in various disorders (e.g., posttraumatic stress disorder or depression) may be an effect of "decreasing capacity of the individual to respond to environmental demands," which is stress-induced. Indeed, prolonged glutamate overstimulation of the hippocampus can cause damage to this structure through the process of excitotoxicity (Ortuño-Sahagún et al. 2012). As the hippocampus seems to be a crucial structure for learning, memory formation, and usage of stored information, damage of this brain area is a serious loss for an individual. Therefore, we assume that in conditions where continuing the performance would not be sufficient to meet environmental demands, the third proposed neural system—the PS—activates in order to prevent this damage. We also assume that the PS will take control over the behavior, if the ES estimates that the pattern of behavior fitting with the environmental demand does not exist or the situation/amount of resources stymies its generation.

3.2.3 The Preventive System

When an adequate pattern of behavior cannot be found/generated or adjusted, the stress related to the maladaptive strategies appears. We suggest that in such situations the ES "signalize" to the PS that the situation is life-threatening or can induce pathological changes in the brain, for instance, excitotoxic neuronal damage of the hippocampus.

Switching on the PS is intrinsically linked to strong emotional tension. Hence, the activity of the PS is mostly related to rapid, often violent behaviors that should immediately end the situation. Sometimes, it is better to inhibit the response if running away from the situation or dissolving it rapidly is impossible. Therefore, the preventive activity may lead to three different types of behavior: fight, flight, or freezing. Choosing one of these possibilities depends on many factors (e.g., anticipated outcomes, such as rewards and losses) and is determined by the environmental conditions, individual features, and subjective attitude (based on earlier personal experience). Such an evaluation is most likely provided by the ACC and partially by the orbitofrontal cortex (e.g., Gottfried, O'Doherty, and Dolan 2003).

3.2.3.1 Neural Substrates of the PS

The main neural structure of the PS is the amygdala. This structure was found to be involved in emotional learning, reprocessing, and responses as well as in the emotional modulation of the memory (Phelps and LeDoux 2005). According to research findings, the amygdala is in particular responsible for detection of threat (Satterthwaite et al. 2011), anger reaction, and fear conditioning (Holahn and White 2004) and it mediates maternal attitudes and sexual behaviors. Moreover, it seems to play an important role in expressing sex differences in emotional and sexual functioning (Hamann 2005; Hamann et al. 2004).

The amygdala consists of several structurally and functionally separated nuclei, of which the most important are the lateral nucleus, the basal nucleus, and the central nucleus (LeDoux 2007). The functional differentiation of amygdala nuclei is still not clear, but it seems that the lateral nucleus of the amygdala is the main input from sensory pathways (visual, auditory, somatosensory, olfactory, and taste) and receives information about threat. Some findings have shown that during fear conditioning the long-term potentiation appears in the lateral nucleus of the amygdala (Clugnet and LeDoux 1990); thus, it is also considered as an important region for fear conditioning. The basal nucleus of the amygdala gets inputs both from the lateral amygdala and from the orbitofrontal cortex (Satterthwaite et al. 2011). It seems to elicit (or not) the reaction to the signalized threat (Gottfried, O'Doherty, and Dolan 2003; Holland and Gallagher 2004), which depends on the context, probably provided by the orbitofrontal cortex (information about risk assessment and reward value; see Roitman and Roitman 2010). If the situation is classified as a real threat, the basal nucleus seems to "activate" the central nucleus (LeDoux 2007). Moreover, the basal nucleus has a projection to the striatum and, therefore, is likely to be engaged in controlling actions. The central nucleus may be an effecter for emotional and associated physiological responses. It is supposed to be involved in the reaction of conditioned fear, such as startling and freezing (Jhou 2005; Vermetten and Bremner 2002).

The amygdala has projections to numerous parts of the brain, for instance, to the basal forebrain, thalamus, brainstem, hippocampus (Phelps 2004), cingulate gyrus, and neocortex (areas in the frontal and temporal lobes) (Krolak-Salmon et al. 2004; Vermetten and Bremner 2002). It also receives projections from many structures, including frontal, insular, cingulate, and temporal lobes (Stefanacci and Amaral 2002). Some of these projections seem to be particularly important for the PS. Amygdala inputs to the hypothalamus and brainstem are thought to mobilize components of autonomic response (Ulrich-Lai and Herman 2009) and the cholinergic projections to the basal forebrain are thought to enhance generalized arousal (Pessoa 2010). The amygdala also has projections to all areas of the hippocampus (CA1, CA2, CA3) (Amaral 1986), which are suggested to enhance memories of particularly dangerous life episodes in order to avoid unpleasant situations in the future (Phelps 2004). Reciprocally, it receives projections from CA1 of the hippocampus (Saunders, Rosene, and Van Hoesen 1988) and has feedforward and feedback connections with areas of the lateral PFC, including the DLPFC (Ghashghaei and Barbas 2002). Moreover, there are numerous reciprocal connections between the BLA and the rACC (Stefanacci and Amaral 2002). This fact stands in line with our suggestion that the rACC evaluates the affective consequences of expectancy violation and is generally involved in emotional information processing. Projections to the neocortex may indirectly mediate focusing of attention on danger stimuli (so-called stimulus-driven attention; Corbetta and Shulman 2002).

3.2.3.2 *The Generalized Idea of Preventive Behaviors*

Stress-related signals are transmitted to the amygdala via the catecholaminergic (e.g., adrenaline, noradrenaline, dopamine) pathway from the vagus nerve to the nucleus of the tractus solitaris and then, via the main noradrenergic pathway, to the amygdala (Sapolsky 2003). Thus, as mentioned before, in a situation of escalated distress, activity of the amygdala is mostly limited to the reactive, often violent attempts to dissolve the problem. Hence, we suggest that the first factor of the PS is emotions associated with perceived stress. We believe that emotional tension enables a rapid response to the life-threatening situation or to the prolonged inefficiency of the ACS, which might lead to excitotoxicity of the hippocampus. The second, crucial factor of the activity of the PS is a behavior strengthened by emotions.

The emotional factor of the PS is involved in both the recognition and emotional evaluation of the stressor and in enhancing autonomic components of the stress response due to the amygdala's connection with the HPA axis via the locus coeruleus (Ulrich-Lai and Herman 2009). As mentioned, projections from the amygdala to the hypothalamus and thalamus and mainly reciprocal connections with the brainstem (pons and medulla) facilitate the amygdala's role in autonomic response (LeDoux et al. 1988; Ulrich-Lai and Herman 2009). Because the sympathetic part of the autonomic system is essential for the fight or flight action, interactions between the central nucleus and the brainstem seems to be involved in controlling emotional reactions (including freezing in the presence of threat) (Amorapanth, LeDoux, and Nader 2000). Animal studies confirm the involvement of the central or basal nucleus of the amygdala in a startle reaction, which resembles such a freezing (Campeau and Davis 1995). Moreover, almost all of the nuclei of the amygdala projects to the bed nucleus of the stria terminalis (BNST). This so-called extended amygdala is involved in generalized anxiety, stress responses, and control of instrumental behaviors (Walker, Toufexis, and Davis 2003). Nevertheless, the role of the striatum is much more complicated. Recent findings have shown that the ventral pallidum (a part of the striatum) and the posterior hippocampus are involved in the identification of an unrelated threat emotion, whereas the amygdala and the orbitofrontal cortex respond to threat-related information (Satterthwaite et al. 2011). The study by Satterthwaite et al. (2011) also indicates a specific role of the amygdala in threat identification. The important set of connections, which arises from the basal nucleus and leads to the striatum (i.e., BNST), is involved in controlling anxiety-like actions and behaviors, such as running to safety ("flight") (LeDoux 2007). Furthermore, facilitating the autonomic response is essential for a rapid action in which the amygdala is involved.

Therefore, the emotional factor of the amygdala's activity is directly connected with the factor crucial for prevention—an action. As claimed before, we suggest that the PS may dissolve the problem in three different ways by flight, fight, or freezing. Flight-type action means withdrawing from the problem situation. When the threat is real or when the ACS cannot find a pattern of behavior that would fit to the demands at work or in private life, one of the possible actions is to escape. Another possibility is to omit the problem, for instance, by ignoring the task and engaging in another one. The second type of action that the PS can evoke is fight. It is an impulsive and usually aggressive behavior, which is aimed to dissolve the problem by disrupting it or forcing its change. This behavior is associated with high risk, such as exposure to unpleasant social feedback, but it can be beneficial. Both flight and fight are typical actions to stress.

The PS may evoke an inhibition of reaction called freezing. In this type of reaction, extremely high emotional tension and vigilance can occur, despite the lack of movement. As mentioned before, freezing may have one of three backgrounds: (1) a type of reaction that aims to focus attention and to find the best behavior; (2) a type of reaction that dissolves the problem; or (3) a real inability to react, which is sometimes related to numbing. The first type of freezing is a short-term response inhibition due to appearance of the stressful, unexpected situation. It is sometimes defined as a period of watchful immobility and in animal studies is treated as an augmentation of the startle reflex by a fearful stimulus. Owing to its hypervigilance component, it seems to resemble an extended orientation reflex, followed by one of the previously discussed behavior: fight, flight or, if there are enough resources, any behavior that fits the demands. Hence, it is a state that gives the opportunity to focus attention, evaluate the threat, and choose the optimal action. Studies on the startle reaction induced by the corticotrohpin-releasing factor indicate a possible role of the ventral hippocampus in this type of reaction (Lee and Davis 1997), which is consistent with our assumption that startle is a "behavior" that allows one to search for information and to select the most adequate behavior. Secondly, we suggest that freezing may be a type of reaction that dissolves the problem. Refraining from the response, in fact, may be a behavior that is beneficial itself, as in the case of pretending to be dead or simply refraining from movement because of life-threatening situations. For instance, staying motionless when one is attacked by a dog is this type of reaction. This is a temporary behavior that, under more favorable circumstances, can be converted into any other. Last of all, freezing may be the manifestation of a real inability to react where neither an adequate pattern of behavior exists nor flight or fight can be applied. This may be related to maladaptive behaviors such as learned helplessness. However, changing freezing behavior to an action may become possible if the environment or resources change (e.g., the restoration of resources due to sleep) and the ACS would come with a solution. Nevertheless, there is a serious risk of an atrophy of the hippocampus due to prolonged extensive activity. We postulate that the prolonged inability to solve the problem leads to the system pathology as well as insufficient fight or flight actions. Some findings indicated that an inability to react leads to neuroendocrine responses other than fight or flight (Pacák and Palkovitz 2001), which may suggest its different influence on degenerative changes in the brain. Moreover, it seems that there are different neurological correlates of startle reaction to an unexpected stimulus and of conditioned freezing behavior caused by predictable stimuli. Whereas the startle reaction enhanced by light or the corticotropin-releasing hormone seems to be dependent on the BNST (Davis et al. 1997) but not on the amygdala (Choi and Brown 2003), the fear-potentiated one remains largely dependent on the amygdala (Choi and Brown 2003; Davis et al. 1997; Fendt 2001; Holahn and White 2004). It is consistent with our suggestion that a freezing reaction is heterogeneous.

3.2.3.3 The PS in Action

We suggest that the PS is activated in two situations: when the ES "signalizes" a discrepancy between environmental demands and one's resources needed to generate an adequate response fitting those demands and when, despite prolonged attempts to improve or update existing patterns of behavior, the ACS remains ineffective. In the first situation, an inability to generate an effective behavioral pattern may be because of the lack of resources or because of a life-threatening situation. Respectively, the role of the PS is to prevent the changes that might occur in the brain (there are no changes in the hippocampus when the immobilization is short-term; Mitra et al. 2005) or to protect an organism by rapidly ending such a situation. When the situation must be endured and the ACS prolonged, attempts to find or adjust the pattern of behavior remain ineffective; the hippocampus may be overstimulated and finally damaged because of excitotoxicity. Therefore, we postulate that in such a case the third system is activated in order to prevent the damage of that crucial area for functioning.

It is stated that some factors such as sleep deficit influence not only the ability of the ACS to manage adaptive behavior (Durmer and Dinges 2005; Fafrowicz et al. 2010) but also the level of PS reactivity. According to a study by Yoo et al. (2007), the activity of the amygdala in response to negative stimuli was higher in the sleep-deprived condition than the rested state. They found significantly greater amygdala connectivity with autonomic-activating centers of the brainstem (e.g., locus coeruleus) and a loss of functional connectivity with the medial PFC. The findings are in agreement with our assumptions that the PS is more easily activated under sleep deprivation than in rested wakefulness, as a result of the reduction of both to top-down control by the ACS and/or the feedback on whether the amygdala should react provided by the ES.

In conclusion, we postulate that the third system is activated to prevent potential harm. It might be related to a life-threatening situation as well as to damage the structure that is extremely needed from the evolutionary point of view—the hippocampus. However, it is worth noting that both situations may be dissolved by fight or flight (and sometimes by freezing) and both, if unsolved, can lead to pathology caused by the prolonged inability to react or response inefficiency.

3.3 Degenerative Changes in the Brain Caused by Stress-Related Maladaptive Behaviors

Maladaptive behaviors related to prolonged stress may lead to degenerative changes in the brain. Stress arises when the ES reports a discrepancy between an individual's resources and environmental demands. When neither the ACS is able to generate an adequate pattern of behavior nor the PS can dissolve the situation through fight, flight, or freezing behavior, stress leads to degenerative changes in the brain.

Stress enhances secretion of glucocorticoids, resulting in changes in the size and density of dendritic trees in the BLA, which has many glucocorticoid receptors (Mitra et al. 2005; Mitra and Sapolsky 2008; Vyas, Shankaranarayana Rao, and Chattarji 2002). The same level of stress facilitates long-term potentiation in the amygdala and simultaneously leads to dendritic atrophy in the hippocampus (Sapolsky 2003). The study by Mitra et al. (2005) has shown different changes in the amygdala during acute and chronic stress. A single episode of stress related to the inability to react leads to an increase in spine density of the BLA but not to the generation of new dendrites. These changes are gradual and simultaneous to the observed progressive development of anxiety-like behavior. On the other hand, chronic immobilization stress was shown to cause dendritic hypertrophy in the BLA (Vyas, Shankaranarayana Rao, and Chattarji 2002), including both a rise of new dendrites and an increase in spine density noticeable on the very next day after chronic stress (Mitra et al. 2005). The animal studies that involved injecting corticosterone into the amygdala instead of exposing animals to immobilization stress showed similar hypertrophy of dendritic trees in acute and chronic stress (Mitra and Sapolsky 2008). On the contrary, chronic but not immobilization stress leads to different changes from long-term "stucking" in the same stressful situation. Studies in rats indicate that chronic "unpredictable" stress (due to numerous different stressors) leads to an atrophy of the BLA (Vyas, Shankaranarayana Rao, and Chattarji 2002), whereas all types of immobilization stress seem to cause its hypertrophy (Mitra et al. 2005; Vyas, Shankaranarayana Rao, and Chattarji 2002). Furthermore, only long-lasting immobilization leads to atrophy of dendrites and debranching in the CA3 region of the hippocampus (Vyas, Shankaranarayana Rao, and Chattarji 2002). Consistent with these findings, in humans the chronic exposure to stressful stimuli that cannot be avoided may cause maladaptive behaviors such as learned helplessness as well as depressive symptoms, occupational burnout, and other emotional and motivational disorders. In conclusion, it seems that only the long-term inability to react to a difficult situation (helplessness) is neurotoxic for the hippocampus and causes hypertrophy of the BLA. As aforementioned, the BLA is involved in controlling reaction to the stressful situation and is important for the stress-induced facilitation of learning. Hence, perhaps its hypertrophy decreases the possibility of controlling reactions and reinforces freezing reaction based on helplessness. In case of chronic stress, where there is a possibility to react, the structure of the amygdala is also changed, yet ambiguous.

In case of ACS and PS inefficiency, many degenerative changes in the brain may develop. To a certain extent, fear-induced fainting may be the last possibility to avoid these changes. Bracha et al. (2005) state that a propensity to fainting may be linked to evolutionary conditioned, fear-induced allelic polymorphism. As they suggested, fainting could facilitate human survival during periods of inescapable threat in the past. Perhaps, fainting may be protective in life-threatening situations, but it also might serve as an organism's defense reaction when neither the adequate pattern of behavior nor the fight, flight, or freezing behavior can be applied.

3.4 Summary

The ability to adapt quickly to the changing demands of the environment is crucial for effective functioning in a variety of contexts. The model we proposed comprises three

TABLE 3.1

Characteristics of the Systems Involved in Responding to Changeable Demands of the Environment

Systems	Neural Structures	Functions
Evaluative system (ES)	Caudal part of the dorsal ACC (cdACC) Rostral part of the dorsal ACC (rdACC) Rostral ACC (rACC) Parietal lobe (PL) Persupplementary motor area (preSMA)	Evaluating the conformity/discrepancy between human resources and environmental demands and evaluating the efficiency of behavior
Adaptive-compensative system (ACS)	Dorsolateral prefrontal cortex (DLPFC) Basal ganglia (BG) Hippocampus	Generating or maintaining the effective pattern of behavior which meets the environmental demands
Preventive system (PS)	Amygdala	Preventing threats and pathological changes in the brain by triggering fight, flight, or freezing behavior in situations where there is no possibility of finding an adequate behavior

strongly interconnected neural systems whose common goal is to respond adequately to changeable demands of inner and outer conditions (Table 3.1).

The ES is involved in conflict monitoring and in the widely understood evaluation of expectancy violation, including its cognitive, motivational, and emotional aspects. The main role of that system is to signalize the discrepancy between the existing pattern of behavior (if any) and the environmental demands and to evaluate whether the problem may be managed. We suggested that, from an evolutionary point of view, there are two important functions: to protect systems of the organism and to maintain effective actions that fit the environmental demands. The ACS should generate the adequate pattern of behavior through cognitive control. It may also adjust previously existing behavioral programs to compensate changes in demands or resources. Because of its engagement in cognitive control, which is needed to gain rewards in life, it is especially important to human beings. Additionally, one part of this system—the hippocampus—is involved in memory processes and, therefore, has a crucial role in "survival" (effectively maintaining further environmental demands) owing to its major role in storage and usage of past experiences.

The PS should protect the organism. It is linked to the autonomic system that enables rapid, even violent reactions. That system is involved in fight, flight, or freezing behaviors in case of life-threatening and/or prolonged stressful situations that can induce pathological changes in the brain. To conclude, we propose an evolutionary-based model that describes adaptive or maladaptive functioning of humans in changeable and demanding environments.

Acknowledgment

This paper was prepared as a part of research supported by grant from the Polish Ministry of Science and Higher Education 2011/01/B/HS6/00446 (2011–2014).

References

Albouy, G., V. Sterpenich, E. Balteau, G. Vandewalle, M. Desseilles, T. Dang-Vu, A. Darsaud et al. 2008. Both the hippocampus and striatum are involved in consolidation of motor sequence memory. *Neuron* 58 (2): 261–72.

Amaral, D. G. 1986. Amygdalohippocampal and amygdalocortical projections in the primate brain. *Advances in Experimental Medicine and Biology* 203: 3–17.

Amorapanth, P., J. E. LeDoux, and K. Nader. 2000. Different lateral amygdala outputs mediate reactions and actions elicited by a fear-arousing stimulus. *Nature Neuroscience* 3 (1): 74–9.

Atallah, H. E., D. Lopez-Paniagua, J. W. Rudy, and R. C. O'Reilly. 2007. Separate neural substrates for skill learning and performance in the ventral and dorsal striatum. *Nature Neuroscience* 10 (1): 126–31.

Barbas, H. and B. Zikopoulos. 2007. The prefrontal cortex and flexible behavior. *The Neuroscientist* 13 (5): 532–45.

Barcelo, F. and R. T. Knight. 2002. Both random and perseverative errors underlie WCST deficits in prefrontal patients. *Neuropsychologia* 40: 349–56.

Blumenfeld, R. S. and Ch. Ranganath. 2006. Dorsolateral prefrontal cortex promotes long-term memory formation through its role in working memory organization. *The Journal of Neuroscience* 26 (3): 916–25.

Botvinick, M., T. Braver, N. Yeung, M. Ullsprger, C. Carter, and J. Cohen. 2004. Conflict monitoring: Computational and empirical studies. In *The Cognitive Neuroscience of Attention*, edited by M. Posner, 91–104. New York: Guilford Press.

Botvinick, M., J. D. Cohen, and C. Carter. 2004. Conflict monitoring and anterior cingulate cortex. *Trends in Cognitive Sciences* 8 (12): 539–46.

Bracha, H. S., A. S. Bracha, A. E. Williams, T. C. Ralston, and J. M. Matsukawa. 2005. The human fear-circuitry and fear-induced fainting in healthy individuals. The paleolithic-threat hypothesis. *Clinical Autonomic Research* 15: 238–41.

Burgess, N., E. A. Maguire, and J. O'Keefe. 2002. The human hippocampus and spatial and episodic memory. *Neuron* 35: 625–41.

Bush, G. 2004. Multimodal studies of cingulate cortex. In *The Cognitive Neuroscience of Attention*, edited by M. Posner, 207–17. New York: Guilford Press.

Bush, G., P. Luu, and M. I. Posner. 2000. Cognitive and emotional influences in anterior cingulated cortex. *Trends in Cognitive Sciences* 4: 215–22.

Bush, G., B. Vogt, J. Holmes, A. M. Dale, D. Greve, M. A. Jenike, and B. R. Rosen. 2002. Dorsal anterior cingulate cortex: A role in reward-based decision making. *Proceedings of the National Academy of Sciences of the United States of America* 99: 523–8.

Campeau, S. and M. Davis. 1995. Involvement of the central nucleus and basolateral complex of the amygdala in fear conditioning measured with fear-potentiated startle in rats trained concurrently with auditory and visual conditioned stimuli. *The Journal of Neuroscience* 15 (3): 2301–11.

Carver, C. S., S. L. Johnson, and J. Jurmann. 2009. Two-mode models of self-regulation as a tool for conceptualizing effects of the serotonin system in normal behavior and diverse disorders. *Current Directions in Psychological Science* 18 (4): 195–9.

Chakravarthy, V. S., D. Joseph, and R. S. Bapi. 2010. What do the basal ganglia do? A modeling perspective. *Biological Cybernetics* 103 (3): 237–53.

Chen, G., G. Rajkowska, F. Du, N. Seraji-Bozorgzad, and H. K. Manji. 2000. Enhancement of hippocampal neurogenesis by lithium. *Journal of Neurochemistry* 75: 1729–34.

Choi, J.-S. and T. H. Brown. 2003. Central amygdala lesions block ultrasonic vocalization and freezing as conditional but not unconditional responses. *The Journal of Neuroscience* 23 (25): 8713–21.

Clayton, N. S. and J. Soha. 1999. Memory in avian food-storing and song learning: A general mechanisms or different processes. *Advances in the Study of Behavior* 28: 115–74.

Clugnet, M-Ch. and J. E. LeDoux. 1990. Synaptic plasticity in fear conditioning circuits: Induction of LTP in the lateral nucleus of the amygdala by stimulation of the medial geniculate body. *The Journal of Neuroscience* 10 (8): 2818–24.

Cohen, J. D. T. S. Braver, and J. W. Brown. 2002. Computational perspectives on dopamine function in prefrontal cortex. *Current Opinion in Neurobiology* 12: 223–9.

Cohen, N. J. and H. Eichenbaum. 1993. *Memory, Amnesia and the Hippocampal System.* Cambridge, MA: MIT Press.

Corbetta, M. and G. Shulman. 2002. Control of goal-directed and stimulus driven attention in the brain. *Nature Reviews Neuroscience* 3: 201–15.

Coyle, J. T. and R. S. Duman. 2003. Finding the intracellular signaling pathways affected by mood disorder treatments. *Neuron* 38: 157–60.

Davis, M., L. M. Walker, and Y. Lee. 1997. Amygdala and bed nucleus of stria terminalis: Differential roles in fear and anxiety measured with the acoustic startle reflex. *Philosophical Transactions of the Royal Society of London B: Biological Sciences* 352: 1675–87.

Debener, S., M. Ullsperger, M. Siegel, K. Fiehler, D. Y. von Cramon, and A. K. Engel. 2005. Trial-by-trial coupling of concurrent electroencephalogram and functional magnetic resonance imaging identifies the dynamics of performance monitoring. *The Journal of Neuroscience* 25: 11730–7.

Dehaene, S., M. Piazza, P. Pinel, and L. Cohen. 2003. Three parietal circuits for number processing. *Cognitive Neuropsychology* 20: 487–506.

de Kloet, E. R. 2003. Hormones, brain and stress. *Endocrine Regulations* 37: 51–68.

Diorio, D., V. Viau, and M. J. Meaney. 1993. The role of the medial prefrontal cortex (cingulate gyrus) in the regulation of hypothalamic-pituitary-adrenal responses to stress. *The Journal of Neuroscience* 13: 3839–47.

di Pellegrino, G., E. Ciaramelli, and E. Làdavas. 2007. The Regulation of cognitive control following rostral anterior cingulate cortex lesion in humans. *Journal of Cognitive Neuroscience* 19 (2): 275–86.

Doyon, J., V. Penhune, and L. G. Ungerleider. 2003. Distinct contribution of the corticostriatal and cortico-cerebellar systems to motor skill learning. *Neuropsychologia* 41 (3): 252–62.

Durmer, J. and D. Dinges. 2005. Neurocognitive consequences of sleep deprivation. *Seminars in Neurology* 25 (1): 117–129.

Elzinga, B. M. and K. Roelofs. 2005. Cortisol-induced impairments of working memory require acute sympathetic activation. *Behavioral Neuroscience* 119 (1): 98–103.

Eriksen, B. and C. Erisken. 1974. Effects of noise letters upon the identification of target letters in a nonsearch task. *Perception and Psychophysics* 16 (1): 143–9.

Etkin, A., T. Egner, D. M. Peraza, E. R. Kandel, and J. Hirsch. 2006. Resolving emotional conflict: A role for the rostral anterior cingulated cortex in modulating activity in the amygdala. *Neuron* 51: 1–12.

Fafrowicz, M., H. Oginska, T. Marek, K. Golonka, J. Mojsa-Kaja, and K. Tucholska. 2010. Chronic sleep deficit and performance of a sustained attention task—An EOG study. *Chronobiology International* 27 (5): 934–44.

Falkenstein, M., J. Hohnsbein, J. Hoorman, and L. Blanke. 1991. Effects of crossmodal divided attention on late ERP components: nError processing in choice reaction task. *Electroencephalography and Clinical Neurophysiology* 78: 447–55.

Fendt, M. 2001. Injections of the NMDA receptor antagonist AP5 into the lateral nucleus of the amygdala block the expression of fear-potentiated startle and freezing. *Journal of Neuroscience* 21: 4111–5.

Gehring, W. J., B. Goss, M. G. H. Coles, D. E. Meyer, and E. Donchin, E. 1993. A neural system for error detection and compensation. *Psychological Science* 4: 385–90.

Gehring, W. J., J. Himle, and L. G. Nisenson. 2000. Action monitoring dysfunction in obsessive-compulsive disorder. *Psychological Science* 11: 1–6.

Genovesio, A., P. J. Brasted, and S. P. Wise. 2006. Representation of future and previous spatial goals by separate neural populations in prefrontal cortex. *The Journal of Neuroscience* 26: 7305–16.

Ghashghaei, H. T. and H. Barbas. 2002. Pathways for emotion: Interactions of prefrontal and anterior temporal pathways in the amygdala of the rhesus monkey. *Neuroscience* 115 (4): 1261–79.

Gottfried, J. A., J. O'Doherty, and R. J. Dolan. 2003. Encoding predictive reward value in human amygdala and orbitofrontal cortex. *Science* 301: 1104–7.

Grimm, S., J. Beck, D. Schuepbach, D. Hell, P. Boesiger, F. Bermpohl, L. Niehaus, H. Boeker, and G. Northoff. 2008. Imbalance between left and right dorsolateral prefrontal cortex in major depression is linked to negative emotional judgment: An fMRI study in severe major depressive disorder. *Biological Psychiatry* 63 (4): 369–76.

Gross, C. G. and M. S. A. Graziano. 1995. Multiple representations of space in the brain. *The Neuroscientist* 1 (1): 43–50.

Hajcak, G., N. McDonald, and R. F. Simons. 2004. Error-related psychophysiology and negative affect. *Brain and Cognition* 56: 189–97.

Hall, J., K. L. Thomas, and B. J. Everitt. 2000. Rapid and selective induction of BDNF expression in the hippocampus during contextual learning. *Nature Neuroscience* 3 (6): 533–5.

Hamann, S. 2005. Sex differences in the responses of the human Amygdala, *Neuroscientist* 11 (4): 288.

Hamann, S., R. A. Herman, C. L. Nolan, and K. Wallen. 2004. Men and women differ in amygdala response to visual sexual stimuli. *Nature Neuroscience* 7 (4): 411–6.

Haupt, S., N. Axmacher, M. X. Cohen, C. E. Elger, and J. Fell. 2009. Activation of the caudal anterior cingulate cortex due to task-related interference in an auditory Stroop paradigm. *Human Brain Mapping* 30: 3043–56.

Hazy, T. E., M. J. Frank, and R. C. O'Reilly. 2006. Banishing the homunculus: Making working memory work. *Neuroscience* 139: 105–18.

Holahn, M. R. and N. M. White. 2004. Intra-amygdala muscimol injections impair freezing and place avoidance in aversive contextual conditioning. *Learning & Memory* 11: 436–46.

Holland, P. C. and M. Gallagher. 2004. Amygdala-frontal interactions and reward expectancy. *Current Opinion in Neurobiology* 14: 148–55.

Holroyd, C. B., O. E. Krigolson, R. Baker, S. Lee, and J. Gibson. 2009. When is an error not a prediction error? An electrophysiological investigation. *Cognitive, Affective and Behavioral Neuroscience* 9: 9–70.

Holroyd, C. B., S. Nieuwenhuis, R. B. Mars, and M. G. H. Coles. 2004. Anterior cingulate cortex, selection for action, and error processing. In *The Cognitive Neuroscience of Attention*, edited by M. Posner, 219–31. New York: Guilford Press.

Hon, N., R. A. Epstein, A. M. Owen, and J. Duncan. 2006. Frontoparietal activity with minimal decision and control. *The Journal of Neuroscience* 26 (38): 9805–9.

Hubbard, E. M., M. Piazza, P. Pinel, and S. Dehaene. 2005. Interactions between number and space in parietal cortex. *Nature Reviews Neuroscience* 6: 435–47.

Iba, M. and T. Sawaguchi. 2003. Involvement of the dorsolateral prefrontal cortex of monkeys in visuospatial target selection. *Journal of Neurophysiology* 89 (1): 587–99.

Jhou, T. 2005. Neural mechanism of freezing and passive avoidance behaviors. *The Journal of Comparative Neurology* 493: 111–4.

Jurado, M. B. and M. Rosselli. 2007. The elusive nature of executive functions: A review of our current understanding. *Neuropsychological Review* 17: 213–33.

Kadota, H., H. Sekiguchi, S. Takeuchi, M. Miyazaki, Y. Kohno, and Y. Nakjima. 2010. Dorsolateral prefrontal cortex in the inhibition of stereotyped responses. *Experimental Brain Research* 203: 593–600.

Kerns, J., J. Cohen, A. MacDonald, R. Cho, A. Stenger, and C. Carter. 2004. Anterior cingulate conflict monitoring and adjustments in control. *Science* 303: 1023–6.

Kim, C., J. K. Kroger, and J. Kim. 2011. A functional dissociation of conflict processing within anterior cingulate cortex. *Human Brain Mapping* 32 (2): 304–12.

Krolak-Salmon, P., M.-A. Hénaff, A. Vighetto, O. Bertrand, and F. Mauguière. 2004. Early amygdala reaction to fear spreading in occipital, temporal, and frontal cortex: A depth electrode ERP study in human. *Neuron* 42: 665–76.

LeDoux, J. 2007. The amygdala. *Current Biology* 17 (20): 868–74.

LeDoux, J., J. Iwata, P. Cicchetti, and D. J. Reis. 1988. Different projections of the central amygdaloid nucleus mediate autonomic and behavioral correlates of conditioned fear. *The Journal of Neuroscience* 8 (7): 2517–29.

Lee, K. H., Y. Y. Choi, J. R. Gray, S. H. Cho, J. H. Chae, S. Lee, and K. Kim. 2006. Neural correlates of superior intelligence: Stronger recruitment of posterior parietal cortex. *NeuroImage* 29 (2): 578–86.

Lee, Y. and M. Davis. 1997. Role of the septum in the excitatory effect of corticotropin-releasing hormone on the acoustic startle reflex. *The Journal of Neuroscience* 17 (16): 6424–33.

Liston, C., S. Matalon, T. A. Hare, M. C. Davidson, and B. J. Casey. 2006. Anterior cingulate and posterior parietal cortices are sensitive to dissociable forms of conflict in a task-switching paradigm. *Neuron* 50 (4): 643–53.

Lupien, S. J., C. Gillin, and R. L. Hauger. 1999. Working memory is more sensitive than declarative memory to the acute effects of corticosteroids: A dose–response study. *Behavioral Neuroscience* 113 (3): 420–30.

Lupien, S. J. and M. Lepage. 2001. Stress, memory and the hippocampus: can't live with it, can't live without it. *Behavioral Brain Research* 127: 137–58.

Luu, P. and S. M. Pederson. 2004. The anterior cingulate cortex. Regulating actions in context. In *The Cognitive Neuroscience of Attention*, edited by M. Posner, 232–42. New York: Guilford Press.

Luu, P., D. M. Tucker, D. Derryberry, M. Reed, and C. Poulsen. 2003. Electrophysiological responses to error and feedback in the process of action regulation. *Psychological Science* 14: 47–54.

MacDonald, A. W., J. D. Cohen, V. A. Stenger, and C. S. Carter. 2000. Dissociating the role of the dorsolateral prefrontal and anterior cingulated cortex in cognitive control. *Science* 288: 1835–8.

MacLean, P. D. 1985. Brain evolution relating to family, play and the separation call. *Archives of General Psychiatry* 42: 405–17.

Maguire, E. A., D. G. Gadian, I. S. Johnsrude, C. D. Good, J. Ashburner, R. S. Frackowiad, and C. D. Frith. 2000. Navigation-related structural changes in the hippocampus of taxi-drivers. *Proceedings of the National Academy of Sciences of the United States of America* 98: 4398–403.

Marco-Pallarés, J., E. Camara, T. Münte, and A. Rodríguez-Fornells. 2008. Neural mechanisms underlying adaptive actions after slips. *Journal of Cognitive Neuroscience* 20: 1595–610.

Marek, T., M. Fafrowicz, K. Golonka, J. Mojsa-Kaja, H. Oginska, K. Tucholska, A. Urbanik, E. Beldzik, and A. Domagalik. 2010a. Diurnal patterns of activity of orienting and executive attention neuronal networks in subjects performing a Stroop-like task—An fMRI study. *Chronobiology International* 27 (5): 945–58.

Marek, T., M. Fafrowicz, K. Golonka, J. Mojsa-Kaja, H. Oginska, K. Tucholska, E. Beldzik, A. Domagalik, and A. Urbanik. 2010b. Effort, fatigue, sleepiness, and attention networks activity—An fMRI study. In *Human-Computer Interaction and Operators' Performance. Optimizing Work Design with Activity Theory*, edited by G. Bedny and W. Karwowski, 407–31. Boca Raton, MA: CRC Press, Taylor & Francis Group.

McEwen, B. S., J. M. Weiss, and L. S. Schwartz. 1968. Selective retention of corticosterone by limbic structures in rat brain. *Letters to Nature* 220: 911–2.

McNab, F. and T. Klingberg. 2008. Prefrontal cortex and basal ganglia control access to working memory. *Nature Neuroscience* 11: 103–7.

Miller, E. K. and J. D. Cohen. 2001. An integrative theory of prefrontal cortex function. *Annual Review of Neuroscience* 24: 167–202.

Miltner, W. H. R., U. Lemke, T. Weiss, C. Holroyd, M. K. Scheffersand, and M. G. H. Coles. 2003. Implementation of error-processing in the human anterior cingulate cortex: A source analysis of the magnetic equivalent of the error-related negativity. *Biological Psychology* 64: 157–66.

Mitra, R., S. Jadhav, B. S. McEwen, A. Vyas, and S. Chattarji. 2005. Stress duration modulates the spatiotemporal patterns of spine formation in the basolateral amygdala. *Proceedings of the National Academy of Sciences of the United States of America* 102 (26): 9371–6.

Mitra, R. and R. M. Sapolsky. 2008. Acute corticosterone treatment is sufficient to induce anxiety and amygdaloid dendritic hypertrophy. *Proceedings of the National Academy of Sciences of the United States of America* 105 (14): 5573–8.

Mohanty, A., A. S. Engels, J. D. Herrington, W. Heller, M. Ringo Ho, M. T. Banich, A. G. Webb, S. L. Warren, and G. A. Miller. 2007. Differential engagement of anterior cingulate cortex subdivisions for cognitive and emotional function. *Psychophysiology* 44: 343–51.

Montague, P. R., S. E. Hyman, and J. D. Cohen. 2004. Computational roles for dopamine in behavioral control. *Nature* 431: 760–7.

Moustafa, A. A. and M. Gluck. 2011. Computational cognitive models of prefrontal-striatal-hippocampal interactions in Parkinson's disease and schizophrenia. *Neural Networks* 24 (6): 575–91.

Nitschke, J. B., I. Sarinopoulos, K. L. Mackiewicz, H. S. Schaefer, and R. J. Davidson. 2006. Functional neuroanatomy of aversion and its anticipation. *NeuroImage* 29: 106–16.

Ochsner, K. N., B. Hughes, E. R. Robertson, J. C. Cooper, and J. D. E. Gabrieli. 2009. Neural systems supporting the control of affective and cognitive conflict. *Journal of Cognitive Neuroscience* 12 (9): 1841–54.

O'Reilly, R. C. 2006. Biologically based computational model of high-level cognition. *Science* 314: 91–4.

O'Reilly, R. C. and M. J. Frank. 2006. Making working memory work: A computational model of learning in the prefrontal cortex and basal ganglia. *Neural Computation* 18: 283–328.

O'Reilly, R. C. and K. A. Norman. 2002. Hippocampal and neocortical contributions to memory: Advances in the complementary learning systems framework. *Trends in Cognitive Sciences* 6 (12): 505–10.

O'Reilly, R. C. and J. W. Rudy. 2001. Conjunctive representations in learning and memory: Principles of cortical and hippocampal function. *Psychological Review* 108 (2): 311–45.

Ortuño-Sahagún, D., M. C. Rivera-Cervantes, G. Gudiño-Cabrera, F. Junyent, E. Verdaguer, C. Auladell, M. Pallàs, A. Camins, and C. Beas-Zárate. 2012. Microarray analysis of rat hippocampus exposed to excitotoxicity: Reversal Na(+)/Ca(2+) exchanger NCX3 is overexpressed in glial cells. *Hippocampus* 22: 128–40.

Pacák, K. and M. Palkovitz. 2001. Stressor specificity of central neuroendocrine responses: Implications for stress-related disorders. *Endocrine Reviews* 22 (4): 502–48.

Packard, M. G. and B. J. Knowlton. 2002. Learning and memory functions of the basal ganglia. *Annual Review of Neuroscience* 25: 563–93.

Pessoa, L. 2010. Emotion and cognition and the amygdala: From "what is it?" to "what's to be done?". *Neuropsychologia* 48: 3416–29.

Phelps, E. A. 2004. Human emotion and memory: Interactions of the amygdala and hippocampal complex. *Current Opinion in Neurobiology* 14: 198–202.

Phelps, E. A. and J. E. LeDoux. 2005. Contributions of the amygdala to emotion processing: From animal models to human behavior. *Neuron* 48: 175–87.

Polli, F. E., J. J. S. Barton, M. S. Caln, K. N. Thakkar, S. L. Rauch, and D. S. Manoach. 2005. Rostral and dorsal anterior cingulate cortex make dissociable contributions during antisaccade error commission. *Proceedings of the National Academy of Sciences of the United States of America* 102 (43): 15700–5.

Redgrave, P., T. J. Prescott, and K. Gurney. 1999. The basal ganglia: A vertebrate solution to the selection problem? *Neuroscience* 89: 1009–23.

Roitman, J. D. and M. F. Roitman. 2010. Risk-preference differentiates orbitofrontal cortex responses to freely chosen reward outcomes. *European Journal of Neuroscience* 31: 1492–500.

Sapolsky, R. M. 2003. Stress and plasticity in the limbic system. *Neurochemical Research* 28 (11): 1735–42.

Satterthwaite, T. D., D. H. Wolf, A. E. Pinkham, K. Ruparel, M. A. Elliott, J. N. Valdez, E. Overton, J. Seubert, R. E. Gur, R. C. Gur, and J. Loughead, J. 2011. Opposing amygdala and ventral striatum connectivity during emotion identification. *Brain and Cognition* 76: 353–63.

Saunders, R. C., D. L. Rosene, and G. W. Van Hoesen. 1988. Comparison of the efferents of the amygdala and the hippocampal formation in the rhesus monkey: II. Reciprocal and non-reciprocal connections. *The Journal of Comparative Neurology* 271 (2): 185–207.

Schmidt, Ch., F. Collette, Ch. Cajochen, and P. Peigneux. 2007. A time to think: Circadian rhythms in human cognition. *Cognitive Nuropsychology* 24 (7): 755–89.

Schulz, K. P., A.-C. V. Bedard, R. Czarnecki, and J. Fan. 2011. Preparatory activity and connectivity in dorsal anterior cingulate cortex for cognitive control. *NeuroImage* 57: 242–50.

Shen, A. Y. and C. T. Tsai. 1995. Neural connection from hippocampus to the nucleus accumbens and the subpallidal area and their contribution to locomotor activity. *Chinese Journal of Physiology* 38 (2): 111–6.

Shima, K. and J. Tanji. 1998. Role for cingulate motor area cells in voluntary movement selection based on reward. *Science* 282: 1335–8.

Shin, L. M., P. J. Wahlen, R. K. Pitman, G. Bush, M. L. Macklin, N. B. Lasko, S. P. Orr, S. C. McInerney, and S. L. Rauch. 2001. An fMRI study of anterior cingulate function in posttraumatic stress disorder. *Biological Psychiatry* 50: 932–42.

Shors, T. J., G. Miesegaes, A. Beylin, M. Zhao, T. Rydel, and E. Gould. 2001. Neurogenesis in the adult is involved in the formation of trace memories. *Nature* 410: 372–6.

Simon, O., J. F. Mangin, L. Cohen, D. Le Bihan, and S. Dehaene. 2002. Topographical layout of hand, eye, calculation, and language-related areas in the human parietal lobe. *Neuron* 33: 475–87.

Squire, L. R. 1992. Memory and the hippocampus: A synthesis from findings with rats, monkeys, and humans. *Psychological Review* 99: 195–231.

Squire, L. R. and P. Alvarez. 1995. Retrograde amnesia and memory consolidation: A neurobiological perspective. *Current Opinion in Neurobiology* 5: 169–77.

Stefanacci, L. and D. G. Amaral. 2002. Some observations on cortical inputs to the Macaque monkey amygdala: An anterograde tracing study. *The Journal of Comparative Neurology* 451: 301–23.

Stocco, A., Ch. Lebiere, and J. R. Anderson. 2010. Conditional routing of information to the cortex: A model of the basal ganglia role in cognitive coordination. *Psychological Review* 117 (2): 541–74.

Stroop, J. R. 1935. Studies of interference in serial verbal reactions. *Journal of Experimental Psychology* 18: 643–62.

Tanji, J. and E. Hoshi. 2008. Role of the lateral prefrontal cortex in executive behavioral control. *Physiological Review* 88: 37–57.

Taylor, S. F., B. Martis, K. D. Fitzgerald, R. C. Welsh, J. L. Abelson, I. Liberzon, J. A. Himle, and W. Gehring. 2006. Medial frontal cortex activity and loss-related responses to errors. *The Journal of Neuroscience* 26 (15): 4063–70.

Tobler, P. N., C. D. Fiorillo, and W. Schultz. 2005. Adaptive coding of reward value by dopamine neurons. *Science* 307: 1642–5.

Tops, M., M. A. S. Boksem, P. Luu, and D. M. Tucker. 2010. Brain substrates of behavioral programs associated with self-regulation. *Frontiers in Psychology* 1 (152): 1–14.

Tsai, H. C., F. Zhang, A. Adamantidis, G. D. Stuber, A. Bonci, L. de Lecea, and K. Deisseroth. 2009. Phasic firing in dopaminergic neurons is sufficient for behavioral conditioning. *Science* 324 (5930): 1080–4.

Ulrich-Lai, Y. M. and J. P. Herman. 2009. Neural regulation of endocrine and autonomic stress responses. *Nature Reviews Neuroscience* 10: 397–409.

van Maanen, L., S. D. Brown, T. Eichele, E. J. Wagenmakers, T. Ho, J. Serences, and B. U. Forstmann. 2011. Neural correlates of trial-to-trial fluctuations in response caution. *The Journal of Neuroscience* 31 (48): 17488–95.

van Veen, V. and C. S. Carter. 2002a. The anterior cingulated as a conflict monitor: fMRI and ERP studies. *Physiology & Behavior* 77: 477–82.

van Veen, V. and C. S. Carter. 2002b. The timing of action-monitoring processes in the anterior cingulate cortex. *Journal of Cognitive Neuroscience* 14 (4): 593–602.

van Veen V. and C. S. Carter. 2006. Error detection, correction, and prevention in the brain: A brief review of data and theories. *Clinical EEG and Neuroscience* 37: 330–5.

Vermetten, E. and J. D. Bremner. 2002. Circuits and systems in stress. I. Preclinical studies. *Depression and Anxiety* 15: 126–47.

Vinogradova, O. S. 1995. Expression, control, and probable functional significance of the neuronal theta rhythm. *Progress in Neurobiology* 45: 523–83.

Vyas, A., R. Mitra, B. S. Shankaranarayana Rao, and S. Chattarji. 2002. Chronic stress induces contrasting patterns of dendritic remodeling in hippocampal and amygdaloid neurons. *The Journal of Neuroscience* 22 (15): 6810–8.

Wacker, J., D. G. Dillon, and D. A. Pizzagalli. 2009. The role of the nucleus accumbens and rostral anterior cingulated in anhedonia: Integration of resting EEG, fMRI and volumetric techniques. *NeuroImage* 46: 327–37.

Walker, D. L., D. J. Toufexis, and M. Davis, M. 2003. Role of the bed nucleus of the stria terminalis versus the amygdala in fear, stress, and anxiety. *European Journal of Pharmacology* 463: 199–216.

Weissman, D. H., A. S. Perkins, and M. G. Woldorff. 2007. Cognitive control in social situations: A role for the dorsolateral prefrontal cortex. *NeuroImage* 40: 955–62.

Whitlock, J., A. J. Heynen, M. G. Shuler, and M. F. Bear. 2006. Learning induces long-term potentiation in the hippocampus. *Science* 313: 1093–7.

Wood, J. N., S. G. Romero, K. M. Knutson, and J. Grafman. 2005. Representation of attitudinal knowledge: Role of prefrontal cortex, amygdala and parahippocampal gyrus. *Neuropsychologia* 43: 249–59.

Wood, G. E., L. T. Young, L. P. Ragan, B. Chen, and B. S. McEwen. 2004. Stress-induced structural remodeling in hippocampus: prevention by lithium treatment. *Proceedings of the National Academy of Sciences of the United States of America* 101 (11): 3973–8.

Yoo, S.-S., N. Gujar, P. Hu, F. A. Jolesz, and M. P. Walker. 2007. The human emotional brain without sleep—A prefrontal amygdala disconnect. *Current Biology* 17 (20): R877–8.

Yoshimura, S., Y. Okamoto, K. Onoda, M. Matsunaga, K. Ueda, S. Suzuki, and S. Yamawaki. 2010. Rostral anterior cingulate cortex activity mediates the relationship between the depressive symptoms and the medial prefrontal cortex activity. *Journal of Affective Disorders* 122: 76–85.

4

Object Perception versus Target-Directed Manual Actions

Gregory Króliczak, Cristiana Cavina-Pratesi, and Mary-Ellen Large

CONTENTS

4.1 Introduction

Imagine yourself picking up little stones during a relaxing walk on the seaside. Although pretty much effortless, grasping of a pebble on a sandy beach is quite a feat from the point of view of the neural processing involved. After all, even during such a simple visuomotor task the brain has to localize and identify the desired target, then align sensory information on the location and shape of the object with the initial position of the acting limb in order to generate specific motor programs encoding distance and direction, the required orientation and velocity of the arm, the proper positioning and preshaping of the hand, as well as opposing forces of the fingers to be applied at the object's center of mass (Goodale et al. 1991, 1994; Jakobson and Goodale 1991; Sakata et al. 1995). No matter how complex this processing might seem, however, the task is still quite trivial as the requirements for target selection are minimal in this case, and the object does not have any particular functional properties to be taken into account during action programming and execution. In fact, it stands to reason that a simple reach-to-grasp movement of this kind could be achieved by an online system sub-serving stimulus-driven (bottom-up) visuomotor transformations for action without any major input from perceptual modules of the brain (Goodale and Milner 1992). In other words, not only humans (or primates) but also many other animal species can and do deal with comparable visuomotor tasks even though their perceptual capabilities may not be nearly as sophisticated as ours.

It is not just the skill of picking up objects that is crucial for survival, but rather the ability to discriminate between and then recognize objects worth picking up and the expertise to decide how they should be handled. For example, a simple system for visuomotor hand guidance would be more than sufficient for carrying an edible item to the mouth, but it would be well beyond its capacity to make an informed selection of edible versus non-edible, or even preferred over other food items. Again, a specialized perceptual system, and its underlying memory, would be a key player in mediating this kind of object discrimination, recognition, and subsequent manual selection even though the proper action of grasping and then handling the target object (e.g., putting it into the mouth vs. putting into a trash bin, or on the shelf) could be successfully realized by an action system deprived of memory and conceptual knowledge (cf. Goodale and Humphrey 1998).

A different example of the pivotal role of perceptual processing in action guidance is the skill of using functional objects. The proper usage of common tools is almost a routine task for the majority of healthy adults. Indeed, for most of us using kitchen utensils seems easy, effortless, and safe. It is in fact remarkable how well matched in terms of grip size, strength, and arm and hand orientation our movements are when we reach for and then utilize functional objects. More importantly, unless there is some brain damage (Leiguarda 2005) or a competing cognitive task is involved (Creem and Proffitt 2001), these movements also reflect what we plan to do with them. Thus, we grasp scissors with our fingers already prepared for movements involving cutting paper or handle the shaft of a hammer with a grip already in position for pounding nails. Of course, we could equally well pick up these objects for other reasons: to remove them when they are not needed or to pass them, so that someone else could use them.

How do object properties become recognized visually so that relevant actions can take place later? Where in the brain do the physical properties of visual targets get encoded and then transformed for visually guided actions? Where are the functional aspects of objects recognized and where do function-appropriate hand and finger postures become integrated with the required metrical scaling of the grasp? It has been long postulated that the visual signals from the medial and polar parts of the occipital lobe, a structure receiving major neural projections from light-sensitive cells in the eye, diverge into separate cortical streams of information processing. At least one major projection runs ventro-laterally to the occipito-temporal regions, which are linked to object discrimination, semantic encoding, and visual cognition. Also a couple of major dorsal pathways run from the occipital lobe to the superior and inferior parietal lobules, which are in turn linked to different visuomotor interactions with the environment, spatial processing, as well as attention and action recognition (e.g., Culham and Kanwisher 2001; Goodale and Milner 1992; Rizzolatti and Matelli 2003; Ungerleider and Mishkin 1982). From the posterior parietal cortex (PPC) these pathways extend further to, and in fact most parietal regions have reciprocal connections with, the frontal and/or prefrontal cortex (e.g., Caminiti et al. 2005; Desmurget, Baraduc, and Guigon 2005), thus forming parieto-frontal networks for action planning and execution (e.g., Kroliczak et al. 2007, 2008; Kroliczak and Frey 2009; Schluter et al. 2001). These occipito-temporal and parieto-frontal networks are shown in Figure 4.1.

Within these broadly defined pathways, modern research on primates and humans has revealed the existence of numerous histologically and functionally distinct areas. Indeed,

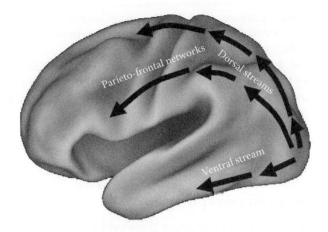

FIGURE 4.1
(**See color insert.**) A schematic diagram of different visual and visuomotor pathways in the brain. The diagram is mapped onto the inflated population-average, landmark, and surface-based (PALS) atlas implemented in CARET software.

both the perception-action model emphasizing the division of labor between the occipito-temporal and occipito-parieto-frontal cortices as well as the reports on different functional subdivisions of these relatively independent pathways can, arguably, be regarded as the most important legacies of the neuropsychological, neurophysiological, and functional magnetic resonance imaging (fMRI) research at the turn of the 21st century. To make these important distinctions, however, researchers must have studied different visual and action tasks in isolation. That is, the neural substrate of perceptual mechanisms have been typically investigated with no need for any overt manual responses (other than button presses when controlling for attention), and action has been studied either in the absence of perception (e.g., a case of patient D.F. tested first by Goodale et al. 1991) or with minimal demands on perceptual systems (e.g., reaching toward and grasping of simple and single objects). Moreover, in the action domain, the emphasis was typically put on disparate motor or visuomotor tasks (e.g., independent hand, eye, or head movements) rather than complex behavior involving numerous body parts. Therefore, it is still not clear how specific, versus codependent, the processing within the reported specialized modules and pathways is.

Although the performance of complex manual tasks no doubt requires that perceptual and motor processing is "inexorably linked at all levels, from the peripheral input to the higher cortical areas" (Guillery 2003, 546), the ideas of different informational requirements and disparate operating characteristics within the ventral and dorsal cortical pathways (Goodale and Milner 1992; Milner and Goodale 2006) are still enormously useful in describing functional divisions of the cerebral cortex. On the one hand, there is convincing evidence that visuomotor transformations for hand guidance are mediated by parieto-frontal representational systems. The subdivisions of these networks tend to be consistently activated by different goal-oriented actions. On the other hand, object-related areas within the occipito-temporal cortex do not necessarily get differentially activated during disparate visuomotor tasks. It is not to say, though, that conscious perception does not play a seminal role in adaptive motor behavior.

In our discussion of these topics, we will refer primarily to studies with the use of fMRI. Oftentimes, though, these investigations were guided by earlier neuropsychological research with patients and neurophysiological studies with macaque monkeys. Therefore, some references to patient literature, as well as interspecies comparisons will be inevitable. Within the past few years several excellent reviews of the cortical networks related to object perception (e.g., Grill-Spector and Malach 2004), action (e.g., Castiello and Begliomini 2008; Culham, Cavina Pratesi, and Singhal 2006; Culham and Valyear 2006), and tool use (Frey 2007, 2008; Lewis 2006) have been published. Our goal is to provide a unifying perspective on all of these topics in an up-to-date and concise review as well as to shed some new light on old findings.

4.2 Visual Processing and Perception

It makes a lot of sense that information about the world from early visual areas diverges immediately along different streams of processing. After all, the same visual input related to an external object is simultaneously made available for different purposes. These goals include, but are not limited to, closer perceptual inspection, which in part also depends on refining patterns of eye movements, as well as programming hand and head responses if they are immediately needed (e.g., either grasping and eating or just protection). In other words, this common starting point allows the many "unique" visual representations that might be simultaneously formed throughout the brain to be based on shared ground. (This argument also applies to direct subcortical projections to the cerebral cortex.) To be more specific, the shape of a knife and fork are represented in the ventral perceptual stream for their overt discrimination and identification. This representation is based on the same raw visual signals that are provided to the dorsal action stream for controlling the eye and subsequent hand movements necessary to grasp and properly use them. Although, the processing within the different visual and motor pathways typically takes place concurrently, and often in synchrony, for simplicity, we will first describe the functional divisions and the basic principles of visual processing within the ventral "vision for perception" pathway.

4.2.1 The Flow and Processing of Visual Information in the Occipital Cortex

The simplest approach to the organization of the ventral perceptual stream (also known as the "what pathway") is by adopting an anatomical postero-anterior perspective and tracing the flow and increased processing hierarchy of the visual input starting from the calcarine sulcus and the most posterior occipital pole toward the more anterior, ventro-lateral portions of the occipital and temporal cortex. Within this occipito-temporal stream of information flow, visual signals pass through progressively more complex processing stages resulting in global object representations, which are also linked to semantic memory. Depending on the location within the hierarchy, the sensitivity and response properties of neurons forming the pathway change quite substantially. That is, neural cells in early visual areas, for example the primary visual, striate cortex, or area V1, code merely local representations of the light striking the retina of the eye and, therefore, respond mainly to very fine details, such as edges and blobs. At the intermediate stages of the coding hierarchy, including processing within the extrastriate area V4 (especially in its ventral division or human V4v), there is already considerable sensitivity to more complex visual attributes, such as curvature or intersections between lines (Gallant, Shoup, and Mazer 2000). Finally, neurons in the lateral occipital and ventral temporal cortex respond to complex objects, such as letters, cars, faces, houses (Epstein and Kanwisher 1998; Grill-Spector et al. 1998; Kanwisher, McDermott, and Chun 1997; Moore and Price 1999).

One of the most striking features of neurons in the primary visual area is that they are arranged topographically, so that adjacent neural cells respond to neighboring regions in visual space (or their image projected onto the retina of the eye; hence the often-used term "retinotopic" organization). This means that early visual representations preserve the spatial layout of information present in a visual scene. Somewhat counterintuitive, but closely related to the optics of the eye and the orderly fashion in which retinal cells send their projections to V1, is the inversion of this layout. That is, objects in the upper visual field are represented by neurons located in the cortex below the calcarine sulcus and objects from the lower visual field are represented by neurons in the upper bank of the calcarine sulcus (see Figure 4.2). Similarly, information in the right visual field is represented by V1 neurons in the left hemisphere and vice versa for information in the left visual field. For the sake of completeness, it should be added that cells in the visual cortex are also ordered according to eccentricity maps. Indeed, these maps are distorted because more neurons represent foveal or central vision as compared to visual periphery. In the early visual areas, these foveal representations converge on the occipital pole and increasingly peripheral representations are found as one moves in an anterior direction from the pole.

Much of our understanding about the organization and functions of early retinotopic regions comes from studying the macaque monkey. More recently, however, this work has been also augmented by evidence from neuroimaging techniques such as positron emission tomography (PET) and fMRI (Sereno et al. 1995; Sereno, McDonald, and Allman 1994). Although there is general agreement that V1, V2, and MT/V5 (an early motion processing area) are regions that are homologous in monkeys and humans, it is important to keep in mind that comparisons between monkey and human brains are fraught with difficulties related to differences in both the size and structure of the brains (Sereno and Tootell 2005). These differences become quite marked when one starts comparing regions

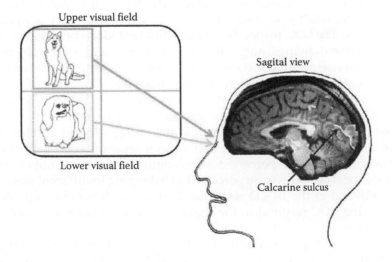

FIGURE 4.2

(See color insert.) An illustration of the retinotopic activation in V1 to upper and lower visual field stimulation. The percent blood oxygen level-dependent (BOLD) signal change (%BSC) for lower visual field displays (yellow/orange) is located along the upper bank of the calcarine sulcus (white line), and the %BSC for upper visual field displays (blue/green) is located along the lower bank.

involved in processing of color and more complex shapes. For example, the homology between human and monkey V4v is still in debate. That is, even though early fMRI studies in humans found an area with upper visual field representation that was similar to monkey V4 (Sereno et al. 1995), more recent studies have challenged this definition. One group argues that this region of the ventral visual cortex can be divided into a color selective area V8, and an upper visual field processing area called V4v (Hadjikhani et al. 1998). Another group argues that this region actually encodes a full hemifield, with a large lower visual field representation abutting V3 (Brewer et al. 2005; Wade et al. 2002; Wandell, Brewer, and Dougherty 2005).

4.2.2 Form Processing in the Lateral Occipital Complex

Retinotopic regions, such as V1, project to higher-order occipital and temporal visual areas selective to more complex visual features, including whole objects. In the macaque monkey, there are both sequential (or step-by-step; e.g., V1–V2–V4–TEO–TE) and skipping (omitting certain visual areas; e.g., V2–TEO) occipito-temporal projections of visual information from the striate and extrastriate cortex to the inferotemporal cortex. The integrity of these pathways has been shown to be essential for visual object recognition (Borra et al. 2010; Tanaka 1996). On the basis of its location, the macaque area TEO could be regarded a homolog of the human extrastriate ventro-lateral occipital area V8 (at least in the scheme proposed earlier by Ungerleider and Desimone [1986]) because V8 is just anterior to V4v. Although it has been argued that the visuotopic organization of V8 is quite disparate from that of TEO and making a homology case on those grounds is not plausible, it is important to note that area V8 sends its projections to the fusiform gyrus (Van Essen et al. 2001; Van Essen 2004), a cortical structure heavily involved in the processing of object properties in humans.

Using neuroimaging, it has been demonstrated that, in fact, there is quite a large swathe of occipital cortex called the lateral occipital complex (LOC) that responds preferentially to objects. Despite its name, though, this region extends from the lateral occipital lobe into its ventral parts and, notably, well into the fusiform gyrus and other temporal divisions of the visual cortex. The LOC responds to many different kinds of object images, including photographs, line drawings, and silhouettes of common everyday objects, as well as geometrical and nonsense shapes (Grill-Spector, Kourtzi, and Kanwisher 2001; Malach et al. 1995). The sensitivity of this region to object shape was shown in an elegant study by Kourtzi and Kanwisher (2001). They presented observers with novel stereoscopic images and manipulated the figure ground organization of these images, so that the same contour belonged to the figure in one display and the background in another display. The LOC showed a considerably reduced blood oxygen level-dependent (BOLD) response when identical contours were perceived as belonging to the same object. More importantly, when identical contours were perceived as belonging to different objects there was a significant rebound in the BOLD response. This research convincingly demonstrates that neurons in the LOC respond to the shape of objects rather than low-level features such as simple lines.

Another example of shape sensitivity of LOC neurons can be found in fMRI studies of "form from motion." In these displays, fragmented forms, which are invisible or rather unrecognizable when seen against a static background made up of similar fragments, are easily perceived when the object moves against the background (or the object and background move in different directions or speeds). Interestingly, though, when the target stimulus and background stop moving the percept of the object remains visible for a couple of seconds longer. This effect is called object persistence. Tutis Vilis and colleagues used this phenomenon to investigate the roles of the MT and LOC in processing object form derived from motion displays (Ferber, Humphrey, and Vilis 2003, 2005; Large, Aldcroft, and Vilis 2005). They presented pictures of fragmented objects against a background of randomly oriented lines. When the target display and its background were rotated in counter phase to each other the objects immediately popped out from among neighboring lines and became recognizable. After a short while, the motion was stopped and the participant was asked to press a button to indicate when they could no longer see the object. It was found that both the MT and LOC responded when the form was visible against the background. However, only activity in area LOC showed the effects of object persistence. This research demonstrates, then, that neurons in the LOC code for the actual shape of the object, not just the cues that segregate an object from its background.

4.2.3 LOC and Invariant Object Representations

Many other examples show that area LOC is responsive to object form but discerning form is not the only issue in recognizing objects. A quite striking feature of human visual cognition is that we are able to recognize objects even though their shapes and surface properties can vary considerably depending on the viewpoint of the observer, the lighting conditions, and the distance of the observer from the object in question. Take a moment to look at something in your environment. Perhaps you have a mug in front of you. Try looking down onto the mug. The shape that you see (a circle with a bar coming out of one side) is quite different from the shape you get from looking at the mug from a sideways point of view (a cylinder with another smaller curved cylinder attached to the side). However, from both viewpoints you know that it is a mug and you have a good idea where the handle is in case you want to pick it up. The kind of representation you need to recognize a mug from multiple viewpoints is called an invariant representation.

There is some evidence that area LOC supports invariant representations of objects. Certainly, LOC neurons demonstrate size invariance (Sawamura et al. 2005). This means that the neural activity in this region does not increase with changes in the size of objects. However, the evidence for position invariance is mixed. Early studies of the LOC did suggest that this region was non-retinotopic (Grill-Spector et al. 1999). However, more recently it has been shown that it has a contralateral preference, where the left LOC responds more strongly to objects presented in the right hemifield and the right LOC responds more strongly to objects presented in the left hemifield (Hemond, Kanwisher, and Op de Beeck 2007; Large et al. 2008; Niemeier et al. 2005). Similarly, the data on view-independent representations in the LOC are mixed. There is some evidence of viewpoint invariance in ventral parts of the LOC using long-lagged fMRI adaptation methods where there are many intervening stimuli between the test and adapting stimulus (James, Humphrey, Gati, Menon, et al. 2002; Vuilleumier et al. 2002). But this evidence is offset by other studies using short-lagged fMRI adaptation methods (where test stimulus is shortly followed by adapting stimulus) showing that neurons in the LOC code for view-dependent representations. The evidence from monkey neurophysiological studies is also mixed. A recent review by Tompa and Sary (2009) suggests that the current weight of evidence supports the claim that shape-selective cells in monkey inferotemporal cortex are viewpoint sensitive. So how is view-invariant object recognition accomplished? One possibility is that whilst single neurons, or subsets of neurons, may be tuned to particular viewpoints, activation of a population of neurons could hold a distributed representation of an object that would be robust to changes in viewpoint (Perrett, Oram, and Ashbridge 1998). Another possibility is that the ventral visual cortex codes for multiple viewpoints and other brain regions, such as the hippocampus, and the perirhinal cortex or prefrontal cortex codes for invariant representations (Andresen, Vinberg, and Grill-Spector 2009).

4.2.4 Coding of Geometric versus Material Properties of Objects

An important development in research on neural representations of object properties has been made recently by Goodale and coworkers (Cant and Goodale 2007; Cant, Arnott, and Goodale 2009) who suggested that there is an interesting division of labor within the visual ventral stream. Whereas the lateral occipital cortex was linked to discrimination of geometric properties of visually presented "nonsense" objects, the more medial activation loci were linked to processing of their material properties. Specifically, they have shown that while attention to geometric properties of objects (i.e., their shape) activated area LOC, attention to the material properties of the same objects (i.e., whether it was wood, tinfoil, marble, or other materials) activated more medial areas within the collateral sulcus, as well as the inferior occipital gyrus. This means that the antero-posterior perspective introduced earlier could now be supplemented with a new lateral–medial one. Indeed, this division of labor is particularly interesting if one takes into consideration the fact that surface features allow the brain to infer the material of which an object is composed of—a facility that is crucial for classifying objects in the natural world (Adelson 2001).

Interestingly, Cavina-Pratesi et al. (2010) provided evidence that areas activated either by geometrical (shape) or by surface (texture and color) properties of objects (see Figure 4.3) played a causally necessary role in the perceptual discrimination of these same features. In their study, it has been demonstrated that whereas one of their two patients with visual object agnosia (i.e., D.F.; Milner et al. 1991) performed well on texture and color discrimination but at chance on a shape discrimination task, the other (M.S.; Newcombe and Ratcliff 1975) showed the inverse pattern. This behavioral double dissociation was then matched by a parallel neuroimaging dissociation. Activation in medial occipito-temporal cortices was found only in patient D.F. during texture and color discrimination, whereas activation in the lateral occipito-temporal cortex was found only in patient M.S. during shape discrimination. Importantly, the location of feature-specific activations for shape, texture, and color that were identified in these two patients overlapped perfectly with activation loci found during performance of these same tasks in age-matched and young neurologically intact controls.

It is still a matter of debate whether information on structural and surface properties of objects processed in the ventral stream is also used by the dorsal action stream, when the perceiver is involved in motor behavior. Both structural and surface features of objects are indeed fundamental when we preshape our hands to pick up objects. Whereas geometrical features inform us about how much our fingers need to be opened to accommodate the object's dimensions, surface features provide hints about objects' weight and slipperiness. These pieces of information undoubtedly have an effect on the way the hand is guided during grasping and on how forces are applied to objects for lifting them (Eastough and Edwards 2007; Fikes, Klatzky, and Lederman 1994). It is well known, for example, that the distance between the index finger and the thumb during precision grip is proportional to the size of the object to be grasped (e.g., larger for an orange and smaller for a tangerine) and that the time to contact the object is longer when that same object is smooth and perceived as slippery, as compared to when it is rough and perceived as not slippery (Fikes, Klatzky, and Lederman 1994; Gentilucci 2002; Jakobson and Goodale 1991). Although it has been clearly shown that structural object features such as shape and size are in fact

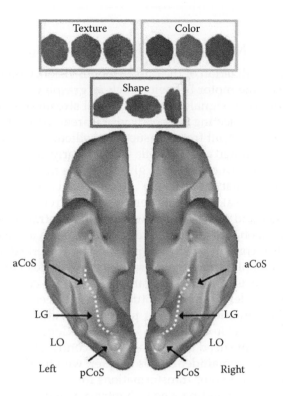

FIGURE 4.3

(See color insert.) A schematic representation of areas selective for geometrical and surface features of objects in the ventral perceptual stream. The left and the right hemispheres are shown from below. Brain areas are depicted accordingly to their stimulus preference: the lateral occipital (LO) area (marked in red) responded significantly more to shape than to texture and color stimuli. The posterior collateral sulcus (pCoS) responded more to texture than to shape and color stimuli. Finally, the anterior collateral sulcus (aCoS) and the lingual gyrus (LG) responded more to color than to shape and texture stimuli. It is quite clear that while the geometrical feature of shape is localized more laterally in the occipito-temporal cortex, surface features of texture and color reside more medially within the collateral sulcus (CoS) (depicted in dotted white lines) and the LG. Exemplars of the shape, color, and texture objects used in the experiment are shown in the upper portion of the figure.

computed primarily within the dorsal stream (e.g., in anterior parts of the intraparietal sulcus or aIPS) when the goal is grasping of an object, and within the ventral stream (LOC) when the goal is object discrimination (Cavina-Pratesi, Goodale, and Culham 2007), it is still not clear whether such a distinction is valid for surface properties. Of course, as will be discussed in the following sections, structural features of objects such as shape and size can be computed online in the dorsal stream even without any prior knowledge of the object to be grasped. Surface features such as texture, on the other hand, can indicate the weight and slipperiness of objects only when we have prior experience with these material properties (and this knowledge, as the current research indicates, is most likely stored in the ventro-medial parts of "the visual brain"). Given that recent tracing studies in the monkey (Borra et al. 2008) have highlighted the existence of a direct pathway connecting the ventral (temporal lobe) and the dorsal (anterior intraparietal sulcus or AIP) areas, it is quite possible that a homologous pathway might actually be able to carry prior object knowledge from occipito-temporal cortices to the human grasping area, namely the aIPS.

4.3 Cortical Circuitry Mediating Real-Time Grasping Movements

In their original conceptualization of the duplex model vision, Goodale and Milner (1992) hypothesized that real-time motor behavior, such as grasping, is mediated primarily by the transformations of visual signals along the dorsal stream of information processing, that is, along the pathway projecting from early visual areas to the PPC (which also receives considerable parallel visual input from the superior colliculus via the pulvinar nucleus of the thalamus) (see also Milner and Goodale 1995). Nearly 20 years ago, now, this proposal was an unexpected turn of thoughts given that the mainstream thinking was still highly influenced by the "what" and "where" account of visual processing by Ungerleider and Mishkin (1982). For the sake of completeness, we will reiterate here that in the model put forward by Goodale and Milner (1992), whereas the ventral stream provides detailed representations of visual objects for cognitive operations such as discrimination, recognition, identification (ideas consistent with the proposal by Ungerleider and Mishkin [1982]), as well as advance action planning, the dorsal stream provides flexible and real-time (or *online*) control of motor acts. Numerous examples of visual coding that quite nicely fit this simple and telling model on the perceptual side have been described in the previous sections. The potential limitations of object processing within the dorsal stream (rather than weaknesses of the model itself; see also Milner and Goodale 1995, 136–144), as well as situations when there is some need for ventral stream contributions to grasping have been also just alluded to. In the remainder of this chapter, we will discuss in more detail the cortical mechanisms of visuomotor transformations for action guidance. The most extensive review on these topics, including a new chapter devoted to recent fMRI, transcranial magnetic stimulation (TMS), and behavioral studies on perception and action, can still be found in the second edition of *The Visual Brain in Action* (Milner and Goodale 2006).

4.3.1 Grasping and Reaching in Monkeys and Humans

Performance of simple grasping movements with the upper limb, the ability common to monkeys and humans, depends largely on the brain's capacity to extract just three basic properties of external objects, namely, their shape, size, and orientation. Prehension would not be highly skilled, though, if these properties were not automatically transformed into programs specifying orchestrated patterns of distal muscle contractions and relaxations. It has been convincingly demonstrated that in monkeys the conversion of the two intrinsic object features (i.e., shape and size) to motor programs for the control of hand preshaping takes place in the pathway involving the inferior parietal lobule (IPL) and the ventral premotor (PMv) cortex (Rizzolatti et al. 1988; Sakata et al. 1995; Taira et al. 1990). Indeed, neurons in both these areas show substantial selectivity to shape and size of the to-be-grasped visual objects. Interestingly, it has been also suggested, and implemented in computational models of action guidance, that the automaticity of grasping behavior could be accounted for by the concept of motor schemas (Arbib 1981; Jeannerod et al. 1995). A schema in this context is understood as a rather abstract preset chain of highly automated computations (or algorithms) specifying a sequence of subcomponent movements evoked by the visual information projected along the parieto-frontal action networks.

Neuropsychological research in humans also shows that the basic intrinsic properties of objects for target-directed grasping are coded in the parietal lobes. This has been clearly evidenced by studies with patient D.F. Despite having visual form agnosia due to a rather large, though functionally focal (limited to ventro-lateral parts of the LOC) bilateral occipital lesions (James et al. 2003) and the resulting lack of explicit object form vision, she could still deftly grasp simple objects in her environment (Goodale et al. 1991). It has been demonstrated that this preserved skill is mediated by her almost-intact dorsal stream (James et al. 2003). There is also convincing evidence, exemplified by patient L.L. (with bilateral PPC hypometabolism; Sirigu et al. 1995), that the mechanisms (or schemas) transforming object shape information into more complex actions—for example, how to grasp a functional tool such as scissors, as well as higher-order action representations specifying the required pattern and range of movements—for example, sequences of finger movements necessary for effective use of scissors, are also stored in the parietal lobes. Patient L.L. can quite well direct her arm toward the objects she wants to grasp, which suggests that her behavior is indeed target directed. However, she can neither use precision grips skillfully nor spontaneously adopt functionally appropriate hand postures. If she does, she still cannot use the tool properly on the basis of visual information either because her visual action representations cannot be retrieved from within the parietal lobe or because her *hypoactive* parietal cortex (with inadequately engaged action schemas) does not have efficient access to supporting information stored elsewhere in the brain. It is important to emphasize that even in normal individuals, this "pragmatic" parietal processing of visual signals (Jeannerod et al. 1995) must often be supplemented with the perceptual or more "semantic" mode of analysis when action is planned ahead of time or after a delay period when the stimulus is not yet or no longer present. This is also the case when we need to deal with objects we have no experience with, and when quite complex objects or tools must be used in a particular sequence to achieve a desired goal (Arbib et al. 2009; Goodale and Westwood 2004; Goodale, Westwood, and Milner 2004; Jeannerod et al. 1995).

In contrast to patient L.L.'s problems (Sirigu et al. 1995), even the most accurately planned and executed finger movements for grasping would not lead to a competent behavior if the arm was not properly guided toward target objects located within a reachable distance. Both single-cell recording in the macaque monkey and neuropsychological research in humans suggest that PPC is also critically involved in visuomotor transformations for the control of the arm and in representing spatial relationships between the acting limb and the desired target. It has been shown, for example, that within the monkey parietal cortex numerous areas are involved in coding the upper arm position and the desired movements, the most important being the medial intraparietal area (MIP) and the more medially located visual area V6A (Colby and Duhamel 1991; Evangeliou et al. 2009; Galletti et al. 1996; Galletti et al. 2003). In humans, there is also some evidence that the superior parietal lobule (SPL), and the superior parieto-occipital cortex (SPOC), in addition to preferentially representing near space (Quinlan and Culham 2007) and objects located within a hand-reachable distance (Gallivan, Cavina-Pratesi, and Culham 2009), is also directly involved in the control of reaching (Connolly, Anderson, and Goodale 2003; de Jong, van der Graaf, and Paans 2001; Prado et al. 2005) and pointing movements (Astafiev et al. 2003). Similarly to IPL, which sends projections to the premotor cortex (here PMv), SPL coding of visuomotor signals related to arm movements is also projected to the premotor cortex, but in this case, to its more superior division, namely the dorsal premotor (PMd) cortex (Rizzolatti, Luppino, and Matelli 1998).

The two major, relatively independent parieto-frontal pathways devoted to specific sensorimotor transformations for grasping and reaching will be now discussed in turn. It should be emphasized, however, that in more complex behavior than the tasks studied in well-controlled laboratory experiments on very specific aspects of motor behavior (i.e., grasping vs. reaching, precision grasping vs. power grips, etc.), these pathways would be expected to closely collaborate.

4.3.2 IPL–PMv Grasp Network in Monkeys

Although the final stages of grasp execution critically depend on the primary motor (M1) cortex (also known as Brodmann area 4 or field F1; Matelli, Luppino, and Rizzolatti 1985), the integrity of M1 would not suffice for target-directed grip formation. The main reason is that visually selective neurons, whose responses are independent of eye movements and finger muscle contractions, are only sparsely scattered throughout the depth of the motor cortex (Wannier, Maier, and Hepp-Reymond 1989). In other words, a disorder of normal grasping caused by M1 lesions is primarily due a loss of the (stimulus independent) basic ability to move individual fingers (Passingham, Perry, and Wilkinson 1978) rather than a disruption of the last phase of visual or somatosensory processing that mediates grasping. Thus, the actual planning, programming, and the control of the ongoing movements based on visual signals have to take place in the premotor and parietal areas.

As we mentioned earlier, the most basic target-directed grasping depends critically on the brain's ability to extract such intrinsic object properties as shape and size. Following the initial stage of purely visual processing, this information must be transformed into programs defining specific patterns of finger movements and the required configuration of the hand. In the macaque monkey, these transformations take place in a pathway connecting the anterior intraparietal (AIP) area and the ventral premotor cortex or PMv. The AIP, as the name implies, is located anteriorly within the major parietal sulcus—the intraparietal sulcus (IPS)—dividing the PPC into the IPL and SPL. Notably, because AIP is actually found on the ventro-lateral bank of the IPS, in terms of cortical anatomy it belongs to the IPL. Its frontal target, area PMv, consists of two regions the more posterior area F4 and anterior to it area F5. The AIP sends its major projections to frontal area F5 (Rizzolatti, Luppino, and Matelli 1998).

AIP neurons can be classified into three groups of "manipulation" cells: (1) motor-dominant, (2) visuomotor, and (3) visual-dominant (Sakata et al. 1995; Taira et al. 1990). *Motor-dominant* cells show significant activation during grasping movements irrespective of whether tested in darkness or light, and the majority of neurons belonging to this category preferentially code different grasp types. *Visuomotor* cells respond more strongly in light, and even though they are also active in darkness their responses are less vigorous than in the presence of visible targets. Importantly, the intrinsic visual properties of the targets that are most effective in triggering a neuron, and the most effective type of grasp that is required for generating a similar response are clearly related. Finally, *visual-dominant* cells show selective activation only when the stimulus is visible. This is the case even when the monkey is not required to respond following the presentation of the object. Indeed, there is convincing evidence that these neurons can selectively represent the three-dimensional shapes of the potential action targets (see also Sakata et al. 1998).

As the AIP sends predominant projections to the premotor area F5, both areas are expected to have similar functional properties. However, in addition to coding disparate finger movements and different configurations of the acting hand, there is some evidence that area F5 codes both hand and mouth responses (Rizzolatti, Luppino, and Matelli 1998). Nevertheless, the hand manipulation F5 neurons can also be classified into distinctive groups, such as visual-dominant and visuomotor. Similarly to area AIP, it has been observed that many F5 units fire during the presentation of three-dimensional objects even when the monkey is not allowed to respond to targets on given trials (Murata et al. 1997). Visuomotor cells, activated best during actions performed in light, can be further subdivided on the basis of the task that is most efficient in triggering their responses. The most widely represented actions in the visuomotor cells of the PMv are grasping, holding, tearing, and manipulating. As to "prehension cells," F5 seems to code hand movements during both the programming and the execution phase of visually guided grasping (Rizzolatti et al. 1988). More specifically, while some neurons respond quite vigorously in advance of the onset of specific hand movements, others seem to be involved primarily in the control of grasp aperture, and yet another group of cells responds mainly during the final stages of grasping (most likely controlling finger adjustments after their contact with an object). Notably, the majority of neurons that seem to mediate grasp responses are in fact very selective for types of prehension movements, such as different configurations of fingers during precision versus power grip. Again, cells coding specific hand configurations can also be effectively triggered by shapes most compatible with a cell's preferred hand/finger postures (Rizzolatti et al. 1996). This also suggests that such neurons might be involved in the process of selecting appropriate grasp and manipulation movements (Luppino et al. 1999).

All in all, the parieto-frontal network whose main nodes are areas AIP and F5 seems to play a major role in transforming intrinsic object properties into suitable hand movements (Jeannerod et al. 1995). The pragmatic processing of the target object's shape and its other affordances seems to take place in the AIP. The conversion of these representations into sets of specific movement parameters, including selection of different types of grasps, seems to be mediated by the PMv. These hypotheses gain some support from inactivation studies which also suggest that it is not the ability to perform or control the actual finger movements that is interrupted by selective inactivation of the AIP or PMv, but rather the conversion of three-dimensional object information into appropriate patterns of hand/finger configurations (Gallese et al. 1994, 1997).

It also should be mentioned that F5 and AIP neurons show yet another important property, that is, mirror responses: they show selective activation both when the monkey performs a particular action and when it observes another individual (either monkey or human) performing a similar action (di Pellegrino et al. 1992; Gallese et al. 1996; Rizzolatti et al. 1996). In this context, PMv and IPL neurons form two broader classes of cells: *canonical neurons*—coding primarily the properties of presented objects, and *mirror neurons*—coding performed and observed target-directed actions (Rizzolatti and Luppino 2001). Indeed, the mirror neurons are not only sensitive to interactions between a hand or mouth and an object (whether these interactions are performed or observed), but they also are quite selective to the context in which the same movements take place (Fogassi et al. 2005). For example, most IPL visuomotor neurons tuned to grasping will show diametrically different responses depending on the goal of the act, that is, whether the movement is performed with an intention to eat versus an intention to place a grasped item in a container (even when it is near the mouth). As these cells discharge before an observed act can be unambiguously recognized as a specific ongoing motor behavior, it has been argued that these neurons also allow the observer to understand the agent's intentions (Fogassi et al. 2005).

4.3.3 SPL–PMd Reach Network in Monkeys

As the success of grasping clearly depends on the proper guidance of the arm toward targets located within a reachable distance, it might be expected that reaching and grasping are inseparable and, therefore, are represented within the same cortical pathways. Quite the contrary, neither neurophysiological nor neuropsychological studies support this intuition. Whereas the control of grasping is primarily mediated by the "ventro-dorsal" IPL–PMv pathway, the visuomotor transformations for reaching movements seem to take place mainly in the "dorso-dorsal" SPL–PMd pathway (Rizzolatti and Matelli 2003). Some SPL areas that are involved in the control of upper limb movements do so on the basis of trans- formations of somatosensory stimuli; however, there are two areas, namely V6A and the MIP area, that to a large extent guide the arm on the basis of visual information (Colby et al. 1988; Galletti et al. 1996; see also Kalaska 1996).

The visual input to the SPL comes from striate and extrastriate visual areas such as V1, V2, V3, and V3A, via the parieto-occipital (PO) area, which has been recently subdivided into V6 and V6A (Galletti et al. 1996, 1999). While area V6 belongs to the occipital lobe and seems to be involved in purely visual analyses, V6A already belongs to the parietal cortex and these neurons show more complex response properties (Rizzolatti and Matelli 2003). Indeed, about half of the V6A neurons respond to visual stimuli and the remaining units discharge in association with either arm or eye movements (Galletti et al. 1996, 1997). Area MIP, found on the dorso-medial bank of the intraparietal sulcus, is located just anteriorly to area V6A and, therefore, both occupy caudal parts of monkey SPL. The visual information from V6 is in fact transferred both to V6A and to MIP. Perhaps following some combinato- rial processing with somatosensory signals, both V6A and MIP send this information to the dorsal premotor cortex, primarily area F2. This frontal area seems to have a clear somato- topic organization and represents both proximal arm and leg movements (Dum and Strick 1991; Kurata 1989); there is some evidence that it may control distal arm movements as well (He, Dum, and Strick 1993). Notably, F2 contains cells that show activity in advance of action onset as well as cells whose responses clearly coincide with the ongoing arm move- ments. More specifically, some "set-related" neurons in F2 respond to visual instructional cues informing the monkey what movement it is expected to perform (Caminiti, Ferraina, and Johnson 1996; Johnson et al. 1996). It is thought that this anticipatory discharge may play an important role in motor preparation (Wise et al. 1997).

In sum, one of the most important functions of the V6A/MIP-F2 circuit seems to be mon- itoring and controlling arm position during the transport phase of target-directed grasp- ing. Within the areas that form this parieto-frontal *reach network*, there are neurons with quite selective properties: some process visuo-spatial signals associated with movement, others the related set (e.g., they show evidence of preparatory activity), yet others code arm movements or just limb position. In F2, there is some evidence for a rostral to caudal gradi- ent of this neural selectivity, from visuo-spatial to movement related, respectively. A simi- lar gradient-like distribution of functional properties has been also observed in the SPL, with set-related activation encountered more often within the IPS, namely MIP (Johnson et al. 1996), rather than in V6A. A close proximity of SPL areas involved in somatosensory perception makes the V6A/MIP-F2 parieto-frontal network for visual reaching an ideal place for combining visual and somatic information.

4.3.4 Evidence for Grasp, Object, and Reach-Related Processing within the Human Dorsal Action Stream

Grafton and colleagues were among the first to investigate a putative homologue of the AIP-F5 network in humans (Grafton, Arbib et al. 1996; Grafton, Fagg et al. 1996). Using PET in right-handed individuals, they demonstrated that grasp observation was associ- ated with contralateral, left-hemispheric activation in *pars triangularis* of the inferior fron- tal gyrus (IFG; Brodmann's area [BA] 45), rostral parts of the left supramarginal gyrus (anterior SMG; BA 40), and right PMd (BA 6), which is a putative homolog of F2 in the monkey. Somewhat surprising, however, was that real reach-to-grasp movements with the right dominant hand were mediated largely by neural activity in caudal parts of the left superior frontal gyrus (SFG, BA 6; that is a putative homolog of F2 in the monkey), and the left SPL. Although this difficulty with identifying the expected grasp network could have been caused by the use of a relatively undemanding task, and a limited spatiotemporal resolution of PET, Grafton and colleagues have also put forward an interesting hypothesis that this more superior (SPL–PMd) activation pattern reflects an engagement of the cortical system for "pragmatic" manipulation of simple objects, also referred to as the circuit for *acting on objects* (Grafton, Fagg, et al. 1996; Johnson and Grafton 2003).

It was only a couple of years later that, in an excellent combined fMRI and lesion study, Binkofski et al. (1998) convincingly demonstrated that grasping, contrasted with pointing movements, did lead to activation within the anterior intraparietal sulcus (with the aIPS being a putative homolog of monkey AIP). Similarly, lesions in and around the aIPS were shown to produce deficits in hand preshaping during object prehension. Yet another important piece of information about the human "grasp network" came a year later when Binkofski and colleagues showed evidence that, even when vision is not available, manual exploration of complex versus simple shapes leads to activation in the PMv, aIPS, and SPL (Binkofski, Buccino, Posse et al. 1999; Binkofski, Buccino, Stephan et al. 1999). On the basis of these data, it was argued that in humans there are parieto-frontal circuits engaged in object manipulation (and most likely grasping) that are homologs of the same pathways in the monkey. Notably, the observation that these putative homologs are involved in the control of hand manipulation even in the absence of vision suggests that within this network in humans and monkeys not only are there similar cell types (including motor-dominant neurons) but that also motor representations (or schemas) for grasping may extensively utilize input from bimodal (or even polymodal) cells.

Although within the past 14 years researchers have utilized different approaches to studying target-directed grasping in humans, including neuroimaging (Begliomini et al. 2007; Binkofski et al. 1998; Cavina-Pratesi, Goodale, and Culham 2007; Culham et al. 2003; Faillenot et al. 1997; Frey et al. 2005; Grafton et al. 1996; James et al. 2003; Simon et al. 2002), a TMS technique (Glover, Miall, and Rushworth 2005; Tunik, Frey, and Grafton 2005; Rice, Tunik, and Grafton 2006) or high-density electroencephalography (Tunik et al. 2008), the majority of these studies invariably point to the IPL—aIPS in particular, but also SMG—as a brain region critically involved in the programming, execution, and online corrections of these movements. There is also some evidence that aIPS activity during real grasping is typically bilateral (e.g., Culham et al. 2003; Kroliczak et al. 2007), and this effect may be independent of the hand used (Begliomini et al. 2008). In contrast, pantomimed grasping with the right hand (when compared with pantomimed reaching) seems to be associated predominantly with right-hemispheric processing, consisting of the mid-IPS, SMG, and SPL rather than the aIPS (Kroliczak et al. 2007). This latter finding suggests that fake grasping, performed away from the target object, relies more on visuo-spatial processing necessary for reprogramming of movement kinematics, and that these transformations might be characteristic of the right hemisphere.

Notably, the bilateral engagement of the aIPS during real grasping seems to be independent not only of the hand but also of handedness. Nevertheless, some important hand- and handedness-related differences in the level of activation are associated with prehension movements. While right-handers do show greater involvement of the contralateral left aIPS when using their dominant hand (Begliomini et al. 2008; see also Kroliczak et al. 2007), the opposite pattern is not found when they make use of their non-dominant left hand. Indeed, similar activation levels have been observed during left-hand prehension both in right- and left-handers. In addition, the latter group also seems to show comparable bilateral aIPS signal changes for both hands (Begliomini et al. 2008).

Human neuroimaging studies have been less successful in showing the contribution of the PMv to real target-directed grasping. As already suggested elsewhere (Castiello and Begliomini 2008), the primary reason for this might be a combination of somewhat different processing characteristics within human aIPS and PMv, and the use of subtraction methods in fMRI studies. Although the removal of fMRI signal related to the *reach component* from the overall signal detected during the reach-to-grasp movement makes an excellent *aIPS localizer* (Cavina-Pratesi, Goodale, and Culham 2007; Culham et al. 2003; Kroliczak et al. 2007), the process of selection and coding hand actions in the PMv might be more sensitive to both visual and somatosensory activity related to the required hand and arm movements. Therefore, the subtraction may result in a failure to demonstrate PMv involvement in prehension even if this area does play a major role in guiding the hand toward the desired target.

In our opinion, if the aIPS is trully concerned with pragmatic processing of a target object's shape and its other affordances then it would not have cells coding reaching movements nor would it rely on neural responses coding the arm and hand displacement. Indeed, there is now clear evidence that the aIPS in not involved in the control of reaching for accurate grasping in peripersonal space; it is the superior parieto-occipital cortex (SPOC) which is a putative homolog of monkey area V6A (see also Connolly, Anderson, and Goodale 2003; Gallivan, Cavina-Pratesi, and Culham 2009). In other words, running an fMRI contrast of "Grasping–Reaching" makes a lot of sense when one wants to localize the aIPS. However, if the PMv is engaged more in the conversion of object shape and other affordances into appropriate patterns of hand/finger configurations, then the removal of signal associated with the reach component would result in taking away a large chunk of PMv processing. Depending on the specifics of the task, keeping such signals might be quite important in avoiding a null result.

As to the putative human homolog of monkey area MIP, Simon et al. (2002; see also Hinkley et al. 2009) have found a cluster of activation in the left middle IPS which is involved in the control of reach-to-grasp movements, and pointing. Other studies have also demonstrated that activation in this same vicinity contributes to the updating of spatial information for pointing (Medendorp et al. 2003), and seems to be involved in the adjustment of reaching movements to a dynamic environment (Della-Maggiore et al. 2004). It is interesting to note that some earlier studies investigating the neural correlates of reaching and pointing identified signal increases outside the IPS, either close to the superior parieto-occipital cortex (already referred to as SPOC) or near the posterior cingulate gyrus (Astafiev et al. 2003; Connolly, Anderson, and Goodale 2003). Moreover, in a recent study by Cavina-Pratesi et al. (2006) it has been found that area SPOC is indeed more active for hand grasping (including the transport of the arm), as compared to when the same object is located close to the hand and no reaching action is required.

4.4 Differential Selectivity to Grasp and Object Properties within the Dorsal and Ventral Stream

To examine the selectivity of neurons involved in visuomotor control within a human parietal and premotor cortex, Kroliczak et al. (2008) have recently used an fMRI adaptation paradigm (cf. Grill-Spector et al. 1999) in which participants repeatedly grasped either the same or different objects, using the same or different grasp types. As mentioned earlier, in such a paradigm inferences about neural properties are made on the basis of decreases or rebounds of activation following back-to-back trials (Grill-Spector, Henson, and Martin 2006). Given the neurophysiological evidence that AIP "manipulation cells" encode both the grasp type and the object shape (Murata et al. 2000), Kroliczak et al. (2008) hypothesized that human aIPS and PMv would show reduced fMRI activity when both the grip and the object shape is repeated, relative to trials in which both of these attributes get changed.

The most relevant anatomical landmarks related to all outcomes from this study are shown in Figure 4.4a. To give the whole picture, a conventional subtraction method has been also used and we will start with describing these results. As can be seen in Figure 4.4b, a traditional contrast of grasping versus reaching revealed the expected bilateral activation within and along the rostral and caudal banks of the IPS, including area aIPS on both sides. In the right hemisphere, IPS activation extended onto the lateral convexity of the supramarginal gyrus (SMG) and there was a cluster of activation in the right PMv. A distinct focus of activation was also observed in the SPL, bilaterally, namely in the mid-SPL. In addition, there was pronounced bilateral activity at the junction of the superior frontal sulcus (SFS) and precentral sulcus, which likely corresponds to the dorsal premotor (PMd) cortex. Of course, these activation foci were accompanied by motor, somatosensory, and supplementary motor area (mainly pre-SMA) activity that would be revealed by the execution of any other action tasks. These results are quite consistent with all earlier studies on neural bases of target-directed grasping and in good agreement with the division of labor proposed for the parieto-frontal pathways of the dorsal action stream. The only exception seems to be a large cluster of ventral stream activation located primarily in the right caudal inferior temporal gyrus (cITG). Such activation would not be expected during real grasping after the subtraction of activation related to target-directed reaching.

More interesting, however, are the results from the adaptation contrasts. Although, as can be seen in Figure 4.4c, a similar pattern of parietal and dorsal premotor activation was observed when performance of different grasping movements was contrasted with the same grasping movements, there were some important differences as well. The most obvious was the absence of activation in the cITG and right PMv, which immediately suggests that these signal foci were more involved in object rather than grasp processing. Notably, there was now a small cluster of activation in the left PMv, as well as a larger anterior cluster in the left middle frontal gyrus (MFG). Grasp adaptation was also observed in the left central sulcus and this activation focus most likely corresponds to the hand area of the primary motor cortex (M1). On the basis of what is known about these areas and their mutual connections, the pattern of activity revealed by the grasp adaptation contrast suggests that both the ventro-dorsal and dorso-dorsal streams contribute to complex target-directed grasping. Given that the task was quite demanding from the kinematic point of view, and also involved the maintenance of instructional cues, an additional engagement of MFG is not surprising either.

Areas that showed decreases of activation following repeated presentations of the objects, and, therefore, sensitive to object perception (see Figure 4.4d), were found both in temporal and parieto-frontal regions. Within the ventral stream, adaptation to object properties was observed bilaterally in the occipito-temporal sulci (OTS). In both hemispheres, this activation extended medially onto the posterior fusiform gyrus (pFus), a region discussed earlier in the context of object perception. In the right hemisphere, this OTS activation extended also superiorly onto cITG and the whole cluster pretty much overlapped with a ventral activation focus revealed in a contrast of grasping versus reaching. This is why we emphasized its role in object rather than grasp processing. It is quite possible, though, that this information is sent to the aIPS for better control of visuomotor transformations that

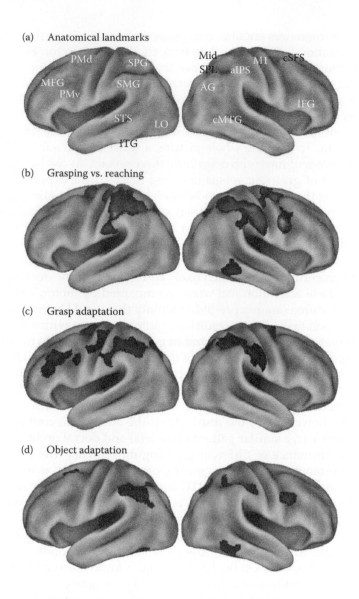

FIGURE 4.4

Activation in three contrasts of the study by Kroliczak et al. (2008) represented as dark blobs on surface render-ings. (a) Anatomical landmarks. (b) The grasp network from a contrast of "grasping versus reaching"; neural activity was found primarily in the dorsal stream, and there was a single cluster of activation in the ventral stream. (c) The *grasp adaptation network* revealed by a contrast of "different grasp versus same grasp"; grasp selectivity evidenced by lower activation (i.e., adaptation) during repeated grasping was observed in the same parietal areas as in b, but was smaller in its extent. Activation in the PMv was now on the left and there was also activation in the MFG and left M1. (d) The *object adaptation network* revealed by a contrast of "different object versus same object"; object selectivity evidenced by lower activation during object repetition was observed bilaterally in the IPS (including the aIPS), the left SMG, and the right mid-SPL. The PMv was activated on the right, the cSFS on the left, and the occipito-temporal sulcus/posterior fusiform gyrus (on the more ventral surfaces) bilaterally. aIPS, anterior intraparietal sulcus; SMG, supramarginal gyrus; AG, angular gyrus; M1, primary motor cortex; mid-SPL, middle superior parietal gyrus; cMTG, caudal middle temporal gyrus; LO, the lateral occipital area; STS, superior temporal sulcus; ITG, inferior temporal gyrus; PMv, ventral premotor cortex; PMd, dorsal premotor cortex; MFG, middle frontal gyrus; IFG, inferior frontal gyrus; cSFS, caudal superior frontal sulcus.

take place there. These results indicate that both the ventral and dorsal stream pathways are very sensitive to object properties, in particular when real three-dimensional objects are presented. Indeed, they must be; otherwise skilled visuomotor behavior would not be possible. The repetition suppression or fMRI adaptation to both repeated grasps and repeated objects that was observed in the study by Kroliczak et al. (2008) within the aIPS is consistent with the grasp and object tuning reported earlier in macaque AIP (e.g., Murata et al. 2000).

Of special note are the observed two types of adaptation in three frontal lobe areas, namely: (1) the ventral premotor cortex, with grasp adaptation observed in the left PMv and object adaptation in the right PMv; (2) the bilateral dorsal premotor cortex, with its grasp adaptation; and (3) the left middle frontal gyrus, where similarly to the PMd, only grasp adaptation was found in the whole brain analysis. Within the left-lateralized network, all the frontal areas selective for grasp type also showed substantial object selectivity within the confines of their respective regions of interest (ROIs). However, neither of the two frontal areas selective to object properties was at the same time sensitive to grasp type. In other words, it seems that neural populations with grasp selectivity (e.g., within the left PMv and MFG) also have some degree of sensitivity to different object features (such as shape), whereas populations demonstrating object selectivity are not necessarily selective for different kinds of grasp.

In contrast to the bilateral aIPS and left PMv, the left PMd showed less and the right PMd showed no sensitivity to object shape, although grasp selectivity was quite robust on both sides. A recent TMS study by Davare et al. (2006) reported a strikingly similar dissociation between the PMv and PMd. Specifically, when applied to the PMv, TMS disrupted the positioning of the fingers on the object, whereas when applied to the PMd, it disrupted the subsequent lifting phase of the movement. Presumably the earlier grasping phase relies more on object shape information than the later lifting phase. Thus, their results are consistent with the findings reported by Kroliczak et al. (2008), suggesting that object shape selectivity and shape-to-grasp matching is more important in the PMv than in the PMd.

Finally, Kroliczak et al. (2008) also reported bilateral foci of object adaptation in the ventral perceptual stream, where the activity in the occipito-temporal sulcus also extended onto the posterior fusiform gyrus. This OTS/pFus activity was not in the classic region of the lateral occipital area (LO, within the lateral occipital complex or LOC described earlier; see also Grill-Spector, Kourtzi, and Kanwisher 2001). It was located more ventrally and anteriorly even with respect to the tactile–visual division of the LOC (LOtv) described by Amedi et al. (2001). Its location seemed quite similar, however, to the ventral temporal cortex activity observed by James, Humphrey, Gati, Servos et al. (2002) during haptic exploration of three-dimensional objects. Taken together, these results suggest that the OTS/pFus may be involved in visual and haptic form analyses of three-dimensional objects and that this information might be passed to the dorsal stream in order to support visuomotor processing for accurate grasping.

4.4.1 Grasping as a Prerequisite of Tool Use

The ability to skillfully use tools and other utensils critically depends on at least four types of neural representations: (1) providing intact semantic knowledge of tools; (2) coding possible functions from object structure; (3) guiding reach-to-grasp movements directed at an already recognized object; and (4) sequencing functionally adequate actions. Of course, it is not enough that these different sets of representations (or schemas) are intact; they need to interact flawlessly (cf. Leiguarda 2005).

As can be inferred from the discussion so far, the two major parieto-frontal networks mediating visuomotor coding for target-directed grasping may also play quite important, complementary roles in tool use tasks. The SPL–PMd pathway may be critical in guiding the arm toward a tool and in controlling the most basic manipulation of an object such as whole-hand prehension ("acting on" objects). The IPL–PMv pathway, on the other hand, may be critical in extracting object shape information for precision grips and the necessary hand/finger configurations (which can be engaged for "acting with" objects; Johnson and Grafton 2003). Indeed, there is convincing evidence that both of these pathways may quite automatically guide skillful complex actions even when some cognitive functions are impaired.

Many apraxic patients (who, as a result of selective left-hemispheric lesions, are unable to skillfully demonstrate the use of tools in the absence of language comprehension disorders and basic sensorimotor impairments) often show the so-called voluntary–automatic dissociation. That is, they execute well-preserved and functionally accurate grasping movements in a natural context (Goldenberg and Hagmann 1998; Leiguarda 2005). It is only in the clinical setting, when the actions need to be invoked outside this natural context (e.g., pantomimed to verbal commands, or in the absence of the "recipient" object), that tool-use deficits become apparent. In other words, it is the tool-use knowledge, or information necessary for sequencing functionally adequate actions (e.g., Hodges et al. 2000), and/or an inability to implement this knowledge into action (e.g., Moreaud, Charnallet, and Pellat 1998) that is most often impaired in apraxia. It is not the skill of performing functionally appropriate initial grasps—which even in apraxic patients are almost always correct—when the task is to use a tool (Randerath et al. 2009). This suggests that the ability to infer "function from structure," at least for grasping (not necessarily for using) objects might be also "encapsulated" in the dorsal stream (cf. Goodale, Kroliczak, and Westwood 2005).

If the abilities such as inferring function from structure, transforming visuomotor signals into appropriate target-directed grasping, as well as implementing object knowledge into appropriate sequences of functional movements were all mediated by the dorsal stream, then it could turn out that at the very core of any purposeful hand actions there is a shared parieto-frontal representational system. In its most basic form, this system may involve primarily the intraparietal sulcus and the superior frontal cortices, including the bilateral dorsal premotor cortex. The subdivisions of this network tend to be consistently activated by different goal-oriented actions, such as object grasping or execution of tool use, which in its fullest form also consists of the grasp component. The more complex and demanding the task the more additional extensions of this network will get recruited, including the ventral premotor cortex, the supramarginal and middle frontal gyri, as well as the caudal middle temporal (coding category-specific knowledge; Martin et al. 1996), and inferior temporal gyri (supporting aIPS in its object processing; Kroliczak et al. 2008). These hypotheses gain support from a recent study by Kroliczak and Frey (2009). Unlike action execution, though, the retrieval of object and/or action knowledge and their integration into actions plans is still expected to be strongly left-lateralized irrespective of the manual task to be performed.

4.4.2 Conclusions

In the past 15 years, enormous progress has been made in our understanding of the neural substrates of perception and action. Much of this development has been made with the use of fMRI. Thanks to tremendous advances in this technology, we learned not only about the topographical organization of human visual areas in the cerebral cortex, but also about how we perceive objects, learn and store knowledge of object functions, and use this information in action planning. Although mapping of the human dorsal stream has initially made smaller strides, it gained some momentum more recently. It turns out that a relatively large and "superior" chunk of our brain seems to be devoted to action guidance. It is not that surprising because "the ultimate reason we have brains is not so much to perceive the world as it is to act upon it" (Goodale, Kroliczak, and Westwood 2005, 269). Evidence from numerous studies, including those reviewed in this chapter, support and extend the idea that the ventral and dorsal streams of visual processing play different but complementary roles in guiding our behavior. Although at the very core of any purposeful hand actions there might be a shared parieto-frontal representational system, we expect that the more complex the task the more ventral engagement would be present. Of course, more research on the contributions of the dorsal and ventral streams to adaptive behavior, and the broader principles by which they might be organized, is needed.

References

Adelson, E. H. 2001. On seeing stuff: The perception of materials by humans and machines. In *Proceedings of the SPIE. Human Vision and Electronic Imaging VI*, Vol. 4299, edited by B. E. Rogowitz and T. N. Pappas, 1–12. Bellingham, WA: International Society for Optical Engineering.

Amedi, A., R. Malach, T. Hendler, S. Peled, and E. Zohary. 2001. Visuo-haptic object-related activation in the ventral visual pathway. *Nature Neuroscience* 4 (3): 324–30.

Andresen, D. R., J. Vinberg, and K. Grill-Spector. 2009. The representation of object viewpoint in human visual cortex. *NeuroImage* 45 (2): 522–36.

Arbib, M. A. 1981. Perceptual structures and distributed motor control. In *Handbook of Physiology. Section 2: The Nervous System. Volume II, Motor Control, Part 1*, edited by V. B. Brooks, 1449–80. Bethesda, MD: American Physiological Society.

Arbib, M. A., J. B. Bonaiuto, S. Jacobs, and S. H. Frey. 2009. Tool use and the distalization of the end-effector. *Psychological Research* 73 (4): 441–62.

Astafiev, S. V., G. L. Shulman, C. M. Stanley, A. Z. Snyder, D. C. Van Essen, and M. Corbetta. 2003. Functional organization of human intraparietal and frontal cortex for attending, looking, and pointing. *Journal of Neuroscience* 23 (11): 4689–99.

Begliomini, C., C. Nelini, A. Caria, W. Grodd, and U. Castiello. 2008. Cortical activations in humans grasp-related areas depend on hand used and handedness. *PLoS One* 3 (10): e3388.

Begliomini, C., M. B. Wall, A. T. Smith, and U. Castiello. 2007. Differential cortical activity for precision and whole-hand visually guided grasping in humans. *European Journal of Neuroscience* 25 (4): 1245–52.

Binkofski, F., G. Buccino, S. Posse, R. J. Seitz, G. Rizzolatti, and H. Freund. 1999a. A fronto-parietal circuit for object manipulation in man: Evidence from an fMRI-study. *European Journal of Neuroscience* 11 (9): 3276–86

Binkofski, F., G. Buccino, K. M. Stephan, G. Rizzolatti, R. J. Seitz, and H. J. Freund. 1999b. A parieto-premotor network for object manipulation: Evidence from neuroimaging. *Experimental Brain Research* 128 (1–2): 210–3.

Binkofski, F., C. Dohle, S. Posse, K. M. Stephan, H. Hefter, R. J. Seitz, and H. J. Freund. 1998. Human anterior intraparietal area subserves prehension: A combined lesion and functional MRI activation study. *Neurology* 50 (5): 1253–9.

Borra, E., A. Belmalih, R. Calzavara, M. Gerbella, A. Murata, S. Rozzi, and G. Luppino. 2008. Cortical connections of the macaque anterior intraparietal (AIP) area. *Cerebral Cortex* 18 (5): 1094–111.

Borra, E., N. Ichinohe, T. Sato, M. Tanifuji, and K. S. Rockland. 2010. Cortical connections to area TE in monkey: Hybrid modular and distributed organization. *Cerebral Cortex* 20 (2): 257–70.

Brewer, A. A., J. Liu, A. R. Wade, and B. A. Wandell. 2005. Visual field maps and stimulus selectivity in human ventral occipital cortex. *Nature Neuroscience* 8 (8): 1102–9.

Caminiti, R., S. Ferraina, A. Battaglia-Mayer, M. Mascaro, and Y. Burnod. 2005. Parallel parietofrontal circuits for sensorimotor transformations. In *Higher-Order Motor Disorders. From Neuroanatomy and Neurobiology to Clinical Neurology*, edited by H.-J. Freund, M. Jeannerod, M. Hallett, and R. Leiguarda, 23–42. Oxford: Oxford University Press.

Caminiti, R., S. Ferraina, and P. B. Johnson. 1996. The sources of visual information to the primate frontal lobe: A novel role for the superior parietal lobule. *Cerebral Cortex* 6: 319–328.

Cant, J. S., S. R. Arnott, and M. A. Goodale. 2009. fMR-adaptation reveals separate processing regions for the perception of form and texture in the human ventral stream. *Experimental Brain Research* 192 (3): 391–405.

Cant, J. S. and M. A. Goodale. 2007. Attention to form or surface properties modulates different regions of human occipitotemporal cortex. *Cerebral Cortex* 17 (3): 713–31.

Castiello, U. and C. Begliomini. 2008. The cortical control of visually guided grasping. *Neuroscientist* 14 (2): 157–70.

Cavina-Pratesi, C., P. Fattori, C. Galletti, D. Quinlan, M. A. Goodale, and J. Culham. 2006. Event-related fMRI reveals a dissociation in the parietal lobe between transport and grip components in reach-to-grasp movements. In *Society for Neuroscience (SFN)*, Atlanta, Georgia.

Cavina-Pratesi, C., M. A. Goodale, and J. C. Culham. 2007. FMRI reveals a dissociation between grasping and perceiving the size of real 3D objects. *PLoS One* 2: e424.

Cavina-Pratesi, C., R. W. Kentridge, C. A. Heywood, and A. D. Milner. 2010. Separate processing of texture and form in the ventral stream: Evidence from fMRI and visual agnosia. *Cerebral Cortex* 20 (2): 433–46.

Colby, C. L. and J. R. Duhamel. 1991. Heterogeneity of extrastriate visual areas and multiple parietal areas in the macaque monkey. *Neuropsychologia* 29 (6): 517–37.

Colby, C. L., R. Gattass, C. R. Olson, and C. G. Gross. 1988. Topographical organization of cortical afferents to extrastriate visual area PO in the macaque: A dual tracer study. *Journal of Comparative Neurology* 269: 392–413.

Connolly, J. D., R. A. Andersen, and M. A. Goodale. 2003. FMRI evidence for a "parietal reach region" in the human brain. *Experimental Brain Research* 153 (2): 140–5.

Creem, S. H. and D. R. Proffitt. 2001. Grasping objects by their handles: A necessary interaction between cognition and action. *Journal of Experimental Psychology: Human Perception and Performance* 27 (1): 218–28.

Culham, J. C., C. Cavina-Pratesi, and A. Singhal. 2006. The role of parietal cortex in visuomotor control: What have we learned from neuroimaging? *Neuropsychologia* 44 (13): 2668–84.

Culham, J. C., S. L. Danckert, J. F. DeSouza, J. S. Gati, R. S. Menon, and M. A. Goodale. 2003. Visually guided grasping produces fMRI activation in dorsal but not ventral stream brain areas. *Experimental Brain Research* 153 (2): 180–9.

Culham, J. C. and N. G. Kanwisher. 2001. Neuroimaging of cognitive functions in human parietal cortex. *Current Opinion in Neurobiology* 11 (2): 157–63.

Culham, J. C. and K. F. Valyear. 2006. Human parietal cortex in action. *Current Opinion in Neurobiology* 16 (2): 205–12.

Davare, M., M. Andres, G. Cosnard, J. L. Thonnard, and E. Olivier. 2006. Dissociating the role of ventral and dorsal premotor cortex in precision grasping. *Journal of Neuroscience* 26 (8): 2260–8.

de Jong, B. M., F. H. van der Graaf, and A. M. Paans. 2001. Brain activation related to the representations of external space and body scheme in visuomotor control. *NeuroImage* 14 (5): 1128–35.

Della-Maggiore, V., N. Malfait, D. J. Ostry, and T. Paus. 2004. Stimulation of the posterior parietal cortex interferes with arm trajectory adjustments during the learning of new dynamics. *Journal of Neuroscience* 24 (44): 9971–6.

Desmurget, M., P. Baraduc, and E. Guigon. 2005. The planning and control of reaching and grasping movements. In *Higher-Order Motor Disorders. From Neuroanatomy and Neurobiology to Clinical Neurology*, edited by H.-J. Freund, M. Jeannerod, M. Hallett, and R. Leiguarda, 43–55. Oxford: Oxford University Press.

di Pellegrino, G., L. Fadiga, L. Fogassi, V. Gallese, and G. Rizzolatti. 1992. Understanding motor events: A neurophysiological study. *Experimental Brain Research* 91 (1): 176–80.

Dum, R. P. and P. L. Strick. 1991. The origin of corticospinal projections from the premotor areas in the frontal lobe. *Journal of Neuroscience* 11 (3): 667–89.

Eastough, D. and M. G. Edwards. 2007. Movement kinematics in prehension are affected by grasping objects of different mass. *Experimental Brain Research* 176 (1): 193–8.

Epstein, R. and N. Kanwisher. 1998. A cortical representation of the local visual environment. *Nature* 392: 598–601.

Evangeliou, M. N., V. Raos, C. Galletti, and H. E. Savaki. 2009. Functional imaging of the parietal cortex during action execution and observation. *Cerebral Cortex* 19 (3): 624–39.

Faillenot, I., I. Toni, J. Decety, M. C. Gregoire, and M. Jeannerod. 1997. Visual pathways for object-oriented action and object recognition: Functional anatomy with PET. *Cerebral Cortex* 7 (1): 77–85.

Ferber, S., G. K. Humphrey, and T. Vilis. 2003. The lateral occipital complex subserves the perceptual persistence of motion-defined groupings. *Cerebral Cortex* 13 (7): 716–21.

Ferber, S., G. K. Humphrey, and T. Vilis. 2005. Segregation and persistence of form in the lateral occipital complex. *Neuropsychologia* 43 (1): 41–51.

Fikes, T. G., R. L. Klatzky, and S. J. Lederman. 1994. Effects of object texture on precontact movement time in human prehension. *Journal of Motivational Behavior* 26 (4): 325–32.

Fogassi, L., P. F. Ferrari, B. Gesierich, S. Rozzi, F. Chersi, and G. Rizzolatti. 2005. Parietal lobe: From action organization to intention understanding. *Science* 308 (5722): 662–7.

Frey, S. H. 2007. What puts the how in where? Tool use and the divided visual streams hypothesis. *Cortex* 43 (3): 368–75.

Frey, S. H. 2008. Tool use, communicative gesture and cerebral asymmetries in the modern human brain. *Philosophical Transactions of the Royal Society of London B: Biological Science* 363: 1951–1957.

Frey, S. H., D. Vinton, R. Norlund, and S. T. Grafton. 2005. Cortical topography of human anterior intraparietal cortex active during visually guided grasping. *Cognitive Brain Research* 23 (2–3): 397–405.

Gallant, J. L., R. E. Shoup, and J. A. Mazer. 2000. A human extrastriate area functionally homologous to macaque V4. *Neuron* 27 (2): 227–35.

Gallese, V., L. Fadiga, L. Fogassi, G. Luppino, and A. Murata. 1997. A parietal-frontal circuit for hand grasping movements in the monkey: Evidence from reversible inactivation experiments. In *Parietal Lobe Contributions to Orientation in 3D Space*, edited by P. Thier and H. O. Karnath, 255–70. Heidelberg: Springer.

Gallese, V., L. Fadiga, L. Fogassi, and G. Rizzolatti. 1996. Action recognition in the premotor cortex. *Brain* 119: 593–609.

Gallese, V., A. Murata, M. Kaseda, N. Niki, and H. Sakata. 1994. Deficit of hand preshaping after muscimol injection in monkey parietal cortex. *NeuroReport* 5 (12): 1525–9.

Galletti, C., P. Fattori, P. P. Battaglini, S. Shipp, and S. Zeki. 1996. Functional demarcation of a border between areas V6 and V6A in the superior parietal gyrus of the macaque monkey. *European Journal of Neuroscience* 8 (1): 30–52.

Galletti, C., P. Fattori, M. Gamberini, and D. F. Kutz. 1999. The cortical visual area V6: Brain location and visual topography. *European Journal of Neuroscience* 11 (11): 3922–36.

Galletti, C., P. Fattori, D. F. Kutz, and P. P. Battaglini. 1997. Arm movement-related neurons in the visual area V6A of the macaque superior parietal lobule. *European Journal of Neuroscience* 9 (2): 410–3.

Galletti, C., D. F. Kutz, M. Gamberini, R. Breveglieri, and P. Fattori. 2003. Role of the medial parieto-occipital cortex in the control of reaching and grasping movements. *Experimental Brain Research* 153 (2): 158–70.

Gallivan, J. P., C. Cavina-Pratesi, and J. C. Culham. 2009. Is that within reach? fMRI reveals that the human superior parieto-occipital cortex encodes objects reachable by the hand. *Journal of Neuroscience* 29 (14): 4381–91.

Gentilucci, M. 2002. Object motor representation and reaching-grasping control. *Neuropsychologia* 40 (8): 1139–53.

Glover, S., R. C. Miall, and M. F. Rushworth. 2005. Parietal rTMS disrupts the initiation but not the execution of on-line adjustments to a perturbation of object size. *Journal of Cognitive Neuroscience* 17 (1): 124–36.

Goldenberg, G. and S. Hagmann. 1998. Tool use and mechanical problem solving in apraxia. *Neuropsychologia* 36 (7): 581–9.

Goodale, M. A. and G. K. Humphrey. 1998. The objects of action and perception. *Cognition* 67 (1–2): 181–207.

Goodale, M. A., G. Kroliczak, and D. A. Westwood. 2005. Dual routes to action: Contributions of the dorsal and ventral streams to adaptive behavior. *Progress in Brain Research* 149: 269–83.

Goodale, M. A. and A. D. Milner. 1992. Separate visual pathways for perception and action. *Trends in Neuroscience* 15 (1): 20–25.

Goodale, M. A., A. D. Milner, L. S. Jakobson, and D. P. Carey. 1991. A neurological dissociation between perceiving objects and grasping them. *Nature* 349 (6305): 154–6.

Goodale, M. A., J. P. Meenan, H. H. Bulthoff, D. A. Nicolle, K. J. Murphy, and C. I. Racicot. 1994. Separate neural pathways for the visual analysis of object shape in perception and prehension. *Current Biology* 4 (7): 604–10.

Goodale, M. A. and D. A. Westwood. 2004. An evolving view of duplex vision: Separate but interacting cortical pathways for perception and action. *Current Opinion in Neurobiology* 14 (2): 203–11.

Goodale, M. A., D. A. Westwood, and A. D. Milner. 2004. Two distinct modes of control for object-directed action. *Progress in Brain Research* 144: 131–44.

Grafton, S. T., M. A. Arbib, L. Fadiga, and G. Rizzolatti. 1996. Localization of grasp representations in humans by positron emission tomography. 2. Observation compared with imagination. *Experimental Brain Research* 112 (1): 103–11.

Grafton, S. T., A. H. Fagg, R. P. Woods, and M. A. Arbib. 1996. Functional anatomy of pointing and grasping in humans. *Cerebral Cortex* 6 (2): 226–37.

Grill-Spector, K., R. Henson, and A. Martin. 2006. Repetition and the brain: Neural models of stimulus-specific effects. *Trends in Cognitive Science* 10 (1): 14–23.

Grill-Spector, K., T. Kushnir, S. Edelman, G. Avidan, Y. Itzchak, and R. Malach. 1999. Differential processing of objects under various viewing conditions in the human lateral occipital complex. *Neuron* 24 (1): 187–203.

Grill-Spector, K., T. Kushnir, T. Hendler, S. Edelman, Y. Itzchak, and R. Malach. 1998. A sequence of object-processing stages revealed by fMRI in the human occipital lobe. *Human Brain Mapping* 6 (4): 316–28.

Grill-Spector, K., Z. Kourtzi, and N. Kanwisher. 2001. The lateral occipital complex and its role in object recognition. *Vision Research* 41 (10–11): 1409–22.

Grill-Spector, K. and R. Malach. 2004. The human visual cortex. *Annual Review of Neuroscience* 27: 649–77.

Guillery, R. W. 2003. Branching thalamic afferents link action and perception. *Journal of Neurophysiology* 90 (2): 539–48.

Hadjikhani, N., A. K. Liu, A. M. Dale, P. Cavanagh, and R. B. Tootell. 1998. Retinotopy and color sensitivity in human visual cortical area V8. *Nature Neuroscience* 1 (3): 235–41.

He, S. Q., R. P. Dum, and P. L. Strick. 1993. Topographic organization of corticospinal projections from the frontal lobe: Motor areas on the lateral surface of the hemisphere. *Journal of Neuroscience* 13 (3): 952–80.

Hemond, C. C., N. G. Kanwisher, and H. P. Op de Beeck. 2007. A preference for contralateral stimuli in human object- and face-selective cortex. *PLoS One* 2 (6): e574.

Hinkley, L. B., L. A. Krubitzer, J. Padberg, and E. A. Disbrow. 2009. Visual-manual exploration and posterior parietal cortex in humans. *Journal of Neurophysiology* 102 (6): 3433–46.

Hodges, J. R., S. Bozeat, M. A. Lambon Ralph, K. Patterson, and J. Spatt. 2000. The role of conceptual knowledge in object use evidence from semantic dementia. *Brain* 123 (Pt 9): 1913–25.

Jakobson, L. S. and M. A. Goodale. 1991. Factors affecting higher-order movement planning: A kinematic analysis of human prehension. *Experimental Brain Research* 86 (1): 199–208.

James, T. W., J. Culham, G. K. Humphrey, A. D. Milner, and M. A. Goodale. 2003. Ventral occipital lesions impair object recognition but not object-directed grasping: An fMRI study. *Brain* 126 (Pt 11): 2463–75.

James, T., G. Humphrey, J. Gati, R. Menon, and M. Goodale. 2002. Differential effects of viewpoint on object-driven activation in dorsal and ventral streams. *Neuron* 35 (4): 793.

James, T. W., G. K. Humphrey, J. S. Gati, P. Servos, R. S. Menon, and M. A. Goodale. 2002. Haptic study of three-dimensional objects activates extrastriate visual areas. *Neuropsychologia* 40 (10): 1706–14.

Jeannerod, M., M. A. Arbib, G. Rizzolatti, and H. Sakata. 1995. Grasping objects: The cortical mechanisms of visuomotor transformation. *Trends in Cognitive Sciences* 18 (7): 314–20.

Johnson, P. B., S. Ferraina, L. Bianchi, and R. Caminiti. 1996. Cortical networks for visual reaching: Physiological and anatomical organization of frontal and parietal lobe arm regions. *Cerebral Cortex* 6 (2): 102–19.

Johnson, S. H. and S. T. Grafton. 2003. From "acting on" to "acting with": The functional anatomy of object-oriented action schemata. *Progress in Brain Research* 142: 127–39.

Kalaska, J. F. 1996. Parietal cortex area 5 and visuomotor behavior. *Canadian Journal of Physiology and Pharmacology* 74 (4): 483–98.

Kanwisher, N., J. McDermott, and M. M. Chun. 1997. The fusiform face area: A module in human extrastriate cortex specialized for face perception. *Journal of Neuroscience* 17 (11): 4302–4311.

Kourtzi, Z. and N. Kanwisher. 2001. Representation of perceived object shape by the human lateral occipital complex. *Science* 293 (5534): 1506–9.

Kroliczak, G., C. Cavina-Pratesi, D. A. Goodman, and J. C. Culham. 2007. What does the brain do when you fake it? An FMRI study of pantomimed and real grasping. *Journal of Neurophysiology* 97 (3): 2410–22.

Kroliczak, G. and S. H. Frey. 2009. A common network in the left cerebral hemisphere represents planning of tool use pantomimes and familiar intransitive gestures at the hand-independent level. *Cerebral Cortex* 19 (10): 2396–410.

Kroliczak, G., T. D. McAdam, D. J. Quinlan, and J. C. Culham. 2008. The human dorsal stream adapts to real actions and 3D shape processing: A functional magnetic resonance imaging study. *Journal of Neurophysiology* 100: 2627–39.

Kurata, K. 1989. Distribution of neurons with set- and movement-related activity before hand and foot movements in the premotor cortex of rhesus monkeys. *Experimental Brain Research* 77 (2): 245–56.

Large, M. E., A. Aldcroft, and T. Vilis. 2005. Perceptual continuity and the emergence of perceptual persistence in the ventral visual pathway. *Journal of Neurophysiology* 93 (6): 3453–62.

Large, M. E., J. Culham, A. Kuchinad, A. Aldcroft, and T. Vilis. 2008. fMRI reveals greater within- than between-hemifield integration in the human lateral occipital cortex. *European Journal of Neuroscience* 27 (12): 3299–309.

Leiguarda, R. 2005. Apraxias as traditionally defined. In *Higher-Order Motor Disorders: From Neuroanatomy and Neurobiology to Clinical Neurology*, edited by H.-J. Freund, M. Jeannerod, M. Hallett, and R. Leiguarda, 303–38. Oxford: Oxford University Press.

Lewis, J. W. 2006. Cortical networks related to human use of tools. *Neuroscientist* 12 (3): 211–31.

Luppino, G., A. Murata, P. Govoni, and M. Matelli. 1999. Largely segregated parietofrontal connections linking rostral intraparietal cortex (areas AIP and VIP) and the ventral premotor cortex (areas F5 and F4). *Experimental Brain Research* 128 (1–2): 181–7.

Malach, R., J. B. Reppas, R. R. Benson, K. K. Kwong, H. Jiang, W. A. Kennedy, P. J. Ledden, T. J. Brady, B. R. Rosen, and R. B. Tootell. 1995. Object-related activity revealed by functional magnetic resonance imaging in human occipital cortex. *Proceedings of the National Academy of Sciences of the United States of America* 92 (18): 8135–9.

Martin, A., C. L. Wiggs, L. G. Ungerleider, and J. V. Haxby. 1996. Neural correlates of category-specific knowledge. *Nature* 379 (6566): 649–52.

Matelli, M., G. Luppino, and G. Rizzolatti. 1985. Patterns of cytochrome oxidase activity in the frontal agranular cortex of the macaque monkey. *Behavioural Brain Research* 18 (2): 125–36.

Medendorp, W. P., H. C. Goltz, T. Vilis, and J. D. Crawford. 2003. Gaze-centered updating of visual space in human parietal cortex. *Journal of Neuroscience* 23 (15): 6209–14.

Milner, A. D. and M. A. Goodale. 1995. *The Visual Brain in Action.* Oxford, England: Oxford University Press.

Milner, A. D. and M. A. Goodale. 2006. *The Visual Brain in Action*, 2nd ed., Oxford Psychology Series. Oxford: Oxford Uiversity Press.

Milner, A. D., D. I. Perrett, R. S. Johnston, P. J. Benson, T. R. Jordan, D. W. Heeley, D. Bettucci et al. 1991. Perception and action in "visual form agnosia". *Brain* 114 (Pt 1B): 405–28.

Moore, C. J. and C. J. Price. 1999. Three distinct ventral occipitotemporal regions for reading and object naming. *NeuroImage* 10 (2): 181–92.

Moreaud, O., A. Charnallet, and J. Pellat. 1998. Identification without manipulation: A study of the relations between object use and semantic memory. *Neuropsychologia* 36 (12): 1295–301.

Murata, A., L. Fadiga, L. Fogassi, V. Gallese, V. Raos, and G. Rizzolatti. 1997. Object representation in the ventral premotor cortex (area F5) of the monkey. *Journal of Neurophysiology* 78 (4): 2226–30.

Murata, A., V. Gallese, G. Luppino, M. Kaseda, and H. Sakata. 2000. Selectivity for the shape, size, and orientation of objects for grasping in neurons of monkey parietal area AIP. *Journal of Neurophysiology* 83 (5): 2580–601.

Newcombe, F. and G. Ratcliff. 1975. Agnosia: A disorder of object recognition. In *Les Syndromes de disconnexion calleuse chez l'homme*, edited by F. Michel and B. Schott, 317–41. Lyon, France: Hôpital Neurologique.

Niemeier, M., H. C. Goltz, A. Kuchinad, D. B. Tweed, and T. Vilis. 2005. A contralateral preference in the lateral occipital area: Sensory and attentional mechanisms. *Cerebral Cortex* 15 (3): 325–31.

Passingham, R., H. Perry, and F. Wilkinson. 1978. Failure to develop a precision grip in monkeys with unilateral neocortical lesions made in infancy. *Brain Research* 145 (2): 410–4.

Perrett, D. I., M. W. Oram, and E. Ashbridge. 1998. Evidence accumulation in cell populations responsive to faces: An account of generalisation of recognition without mental transformations. *Cognition* 67 (1–2): 111–45.

Prado, J., S. Clavagnier, H. Otzenberger, C. Scheiber, H. Kennedy, and M. T. Perenin. 2005. Two cortical systems for reaching in central and peripheral vision. *Neuron* 48 (5): 849–58.

Quinlan, D. J. and J. C. Culham. 2007. fMRI reveals a preference for near viewing in the human parieto-occipital cortex. *NeuroImage* 36 (1): 167–87.

Randerath, J., Y. Li, G. Goldenberg, and J. Hermsdorfer. 2009. Grasping tools: Effects of task and apraxia. *Neuropsychologia* 47 (2): 497–505.

Rice, N. J., E. Tunik, and S. T. Grafton. 2006. The anterior intraparietal sulcus mediates grasp execution, independent of requirement to update: New insights from transcranial magnetic stimulation. *Journal of Neuroscience* 26 (31): 8176–82.

Rizzolatti, G., R. Camarda, L. Fogassi, M. Gentilucci, G. Luppino, and M. Matelli. 1988. Functional organization of inferior area 6 in the macaque monkey. II. Area F5 and the control of distal movements. *Experimental Brain Research* 71 (3): 491–507.

Rizzolatti, G., L. Fadiga, V. Gallese, and L. Fogassi. 1996. Premotor cortex and the recognition of motor actions. *Cognitive Brain Research* 3 (2): 131–41.

Rizzolatti, G. and G. Luppino. 2001. The cortical motor system. *Neuron* 31 (6): 889–901.

Rizzolatti, G., G. Luppino, and M. Matelli. 1998. The organization of the cortical motor system: New concepts. *Electroencephalography and Clin Neurophysiology* 106 (4): 283–96.

Rizzolatti, G. and M. Matelli. 2003. Two different streams form the dorsal visual system: Anatomy and functions. *Experimental Brain Research* 153 (2): 146–57.

Sakata, H., M. Taira, A. Murata, and S. Mine. 1995. Neural mechanisms of visual guidance of hand action in the parietal cortex of the monkey. *Cerebral Cortex* 5 (5): 429–38.

Sakata, H., M. Taira, M. Kusunoki, A. Murata, Y. Tanaka, and K. Tsutsui. 1998. Neural coding of 3D features of objects for hand action in the parietal cortex of the monkey. *Philosophical Transactions of the Royal Society of London B: Biological Sciences* 353 (1373): 1363–73.

Sawamura, H., S. Georgieva, R. Vogels, W. Vanduffel, and G. A. Orban. 2005. Using functional magnetic resonance imaging to assess adaptation and size invariance of shape processing by humans and monkeys. *Journal of Neuroscience* 25 (17): 4294–306.

Schluter, N. D., M. Krams, M. F. Rushworth, and R. E. Passingham. 2001. Cerebral dominance for action in the human brain: The selection of actions. *Neuropsychologia* 39 (2): 105–13.

Sereno, M. I., A. M. Dale, J. B. Reppas, K. K. Kwong, J. W. Belliveau, T. J. Brady, B. R. Rosen, and R. B. Tootell. 1995. Borders of multiple visual areas in humans revealed by functional magnetic resonance imaging. *Science* 268 (5212): 889–93.

Sereno, M. I., C. T. McDonald, and J. M. Allman. 1994. Analysis of retinotopic maps in extrastriate cortex. *Cerebral Cortex* 4 (6): 601–20.

Sereno, M. I. and R. B. Tootell. 2005. From monkeys to humans: What do we now know about brain homologies? *Current Opinion in Neurobiology* 15 (2): 135–44.

Simon, O., J. F. Mangin, L. Cohen, D. Le Bihan, and S. Dehaene. 2002. Topographical layout of hand, eye, calculation, and language-related areas in the human parietal lobe. *Neuron* 33 (3): 475–87.

Sirigu, A., L. Cohen, J. R. Duhamel, B. Pillon, B. Dubois, and Y. Agid. 1995. A selective impairment of hand posture for object utilization in apraxia. *Cortex* 31 (1): 41–55.

Taira, M., S. Mine, A. P. Georgopoulos, A. Murata, and H. Sakata. 1990. Parietal cortex neurons of the monkey related to the visual guidance of hand movement. *Experimental Brain Research* 83 (1): 29–36.

Tanaka, K. 1996. Representation of visual features of objects in the inferotemporal cortex. *Neural Networks* 9 (8): 1459–75.

Tompa, T. and G. Sary. 2009. A review on the inferior temporal cortex of the macaque. *Brain Research Reviews* 62 (2): 165–82.

Tunik, E., S. H. Frey, and S. T. Grafton. 2005. Virtual lesions of the anterior intraparietal area disrupt goal-dependent on-line adjustments of grasp. *Nature Neuroscience* 8 (4): 505–11.

Tunik, E., S. Ortigue, S. V. Adamovich, and S. T. Grafton. 2008. Differential recruitment of anterior intraparietal sulcus and superior parietal lobule during visually guided grasping revealed by electrical neuroimaging. *Journal of Neuroscience* 28 (50): 13615–20.

Ungerleider, L. G. and R. Desimone. 1986. Cortical connections of visual area MT in the macaque. *Journal of Comparative Neurology* 248 (2): 190–222.

Ungerleider, L. G. and M. Mishkin. 1982. Two cortical visual systems. In *Analysis of Visual Behavior*, edited by D. J. Ingle, M. A. Goodale, and R. J. W. Mansfield, 549–86. Cambridge, MA: MIT Press.

Van Essen, D. C. 2004. Organization of visual areas in Macaque and human cerebral cortex. In *The Visual Neurosciences*, edited by L. Chalupa and J. S. Werner, 507–21. Cambridge, MA: MIT Press.

Van Essen, D. C., J. W. Lewis, H. A. Drury, N. Hadjikhani, R. B. Tootell, M. Bakircioglu, and M. I. Miller. 2001. Mapping visual cortex in monkeys and humans using surface-based atlases. *Vision Research* 41 (10–11): 1359–78.

Vuilleumier, P., R. N. Henson, J. Driver, and R. J. Dolan. 2002. Multiple levels of visual object constancy revealed by event-related fMRI of repetition priming. *Nature Neuroscience* 5 (5): 491–9.

Wade, A. R., A. A. Brewer, J. W. Rieger, and B. A. Wandell. 2002. Functional measurements of human ventral occipital cortex: Retinotopy and colour. *Philosophical Transactions of the Royal Society of London B: Biological Science* 357 (1424): 963–73.

Wandell, B. A., A. A. Brewer, and R. F. Dougherty. 2005. Visual field map clusters in human cortex. *Philosophical Transactions of the Royal Society of London B: Biological Science* 360 (1456): 693–707.

Wannier, T. M., M. A. Maier, and M. C. Hepp-Reymond. 1989. Responses of motor cortex neurons to visual stimulation in the alert monkey. *Neuroscience Letters* 98 (1): 63–8.

Wise, S. P., D. Boussaoud, P. B. Johnson, and R. Caminiti. 1997. Premotor and parietal cortex: Corticocortical connectivity and combinatorial computations. *Annual Reviews in Neuroscience* 20: 25–42.

5

Neural Control of Visually Guided Eye Movements

Peter H. Schiller

CONTENTS

5.1 Introduction

In the course of evolution, along with the emergence of the eyes arose the extraocular muscles to move them about. Initially, the retina itself was not highly specialized; the density of photoreceptors was similar throughout the eye. Subsequently, a major specialization has occurred in numerous species: To improve acuity, rather than increasing the density of photoreceptors throughout the eye, which would have required an inordinately large number of neurons, the increase in density was limited to just a small region that we call the fovea. As the basic mechanisms were already present to move the eyes about, their capacity was increased to extend the range and velocity of eye movements, thereby enabling organisms to shift their center of gaze rapidly from location to location and to maintain the center of gaze on objects when there is motion. The two distinct systems that have emerged are saccadic eye movements that rapidly shift the center of gaze from one location to another and tracking eye movements that can stabilize the eye on the visual scene, keep the two eyes in register, and allow for keeping the center of gaze on selected targets when there is movement. One may pose the question then as to why the extraocular muscles have evolved in the first place in animals that have photoreceptors of similar density throughout the eye. The prime reason seems to be that movement of living organisms is pervasive; unless the eyes can be stabilized on the visual scene, images would become blurred. Two major systems have evolved to combat such blurring: a specialized set of retinal ganglion cells selective for direction of motion called the cells of Dogiel, and the vestibular system that makes extensive connections with the eye muscles through the brainstem oculomotor complex. Any movement made results in compensatory counter-rotation of the eyes, thereby stabilizing them with respect to the visual scene. The major neural mechanism involved in this stabilization process is the accessory optic system that will be discussed in Section 5.7 of this review.

During the evolutionary process, problems have been solved in numerous different ways. This is also true for the emergence of the eyes. Some species have eyes that actually do not move. In fact in some of these animals, such as the owl, have eyes that are conically shaped and are thereby fixed in the head. So, how do such animals prevent image blurring? They typically have small and lightly weighted heads that they can move about quite rapidly thereby preventing blurring.

The eyes of most species are in motion most of the time during their waking hours. Humans make about 3 saccadic eye movements per second, some 170,000 a day, and about 5 billion in an average lifetime. During the intervening fixations, each of which lasts 200–500 milliseconds, the eyes are stationary in the orbit only when neither the head nor the object viewed is in motion. If there is motion, the object remains on the fovea by virtue of the fact that the eyes track it.

The neural systems involved in the control of visually guided eye movements are numerous and complex yet are tremendously robust. Seldom does one hear about individuals complaining at the end of the day of having become tired of making those 170,000 saccades and endless pursuit eye movements.

That saccadic and tracking eye movements for the most part are controlled by different neural systems at higher levels in the nervous system has been known for a long time. When the velocity of an object to be tracked is gradually increased, a sudden break in performance occurs when tracking breaks down; the eye can no longer keep up with the moving object. When this happens, the saccadic system kicks in and moves the eyes to catch up with the object. Thus, there is a clear velocity discontinuum between tracking and saccadic eye movements. The two systems also have dramatically different latency responses for the initiation of tracking and saccadic eye movements. This was first shown by Rashbass (1961). He introduced the so-called step-ramp paradigm: A fixation spot is turned on first. A little while after, subjects look at this spot; it is turned off and a moving spot is presented in the periphery. The task of the subject is to make a saccade to the target and to track it.

An example of this is shown in Figure 5.1. The data in this case were collected from a monkey (Schiller and Logothetis 1987). Examination of the eye traces shows something quite remarkable: the eyes begin to track the peripheral spot with a latency of 75–100 milliseconds, and do so before the saccade is initiated to it with a latency of 125–150 milliseconds. In fact, it has been shown that when a large portion of the visual field is set in motion pursuit movements can be initiated in less time than 50 milliseconds, provided the stimuli have high contrast (Miles, Kawano, and Optican 1986). High contrast assures rapid conduction velocities through the retina.

These observations have established that there are largely different neural mechanisms involved in the control of saccadic and tracking eye movements. In what follows, I will first discuss the various neural systems of saccadic eye-movement generation. Both the

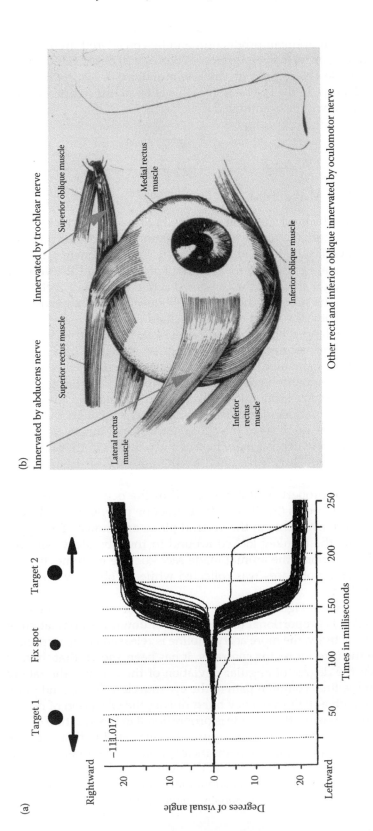

FIGURE 5.1

(See color insert.) (a) Horizontal eye-movement traces obtained while a monkey performed on a step-ramp task. Following fixation of a central spot it was doused; at the same time, a similar spot appeared either to the right or the left of fixation at an 18-degree eccentricity and was moved peripherally along the horizontal axis at 20 degrees per second. Eye-movement trace collection began when the target was turned on in the periphery. The shorter latencies involved in activating the pursuit system are made evident by the fact that pursuit eye movements for the moving target actually began before the monkey acquired it for foveal viewing with a saccadic eye movement. Pursuit eye movements in this situation began between 75 and 100 milliseconds whereas the saccades were initiated between 125 and 150 milliseconds. (Adapted from Schiller, P. H. and Logothetis, N. K. *Association for Research in Vision and Ophthalmology, 303,* 1987.) (b) The human eye and the six extraocular muscles. As indicated, the lateral rectus is innervated by the abducens nerve, the superior oblique by the trochlear nerve, and the rest by the oculomotor nerve (the sixth, fourth, and third cranial nerves, respectively). (From Sekuler, R. and R. Blake. 1990. In *Perception,* 2nd ed., edited by B. R. Fetterolf and T. Holton, 23–60. New York: McGraw-Hill Publishing.)

sensory and motor aspects of eye-movement production will be considered. In doing so, the functions of neural systems involved in eye-movement control will be examined using several different techniques: single-cell recordings, microstimulation, tissue inactivation, and pharmacological manipulations. In the last section of this chapter, the neural systems involved in pursuit eye movement will be examined.

5.2 Brainstem Control of Eye Movement

Each eye is moved around in the orbit by extraocular muscles. Figure 5.1b provides a schematic of this arrangement in the human. Each eye has six distinct extraocular muscles. Four of these are the medial, lateral, superior, and inferior recti. Each opponent pair may be thought of as moving the eyes along two prime axes, the horizontal and the vertical. Diagonal eye movements are brought about by the combined action of the four recti muscles. The remaining two muscles, the superior and inferior obliques, participate mostly in inducing eye rotation that comes into play when the head is tilted.

The eye is a nearly perfectly balanced ball that is nicely viscous damped in its orbit. Unlike other muscle systems, it was not necessary to design the system to carry loads. The fibers of each muscle are not segmented; they run the entire length of the muscle. These facts make the analysis of eye motion readily amenable to study. Figure 5.1b also shows how the extraocular muscles are innervated. Three sets of cranial nuclei contain the neurons that innervate the six extraocular muscles of each eye through the third, fourth, and sixth cranial nerves: The neurons of the oculomotor nuclei innervate all the muscles except for the lateral rectus which is innervated by the neurons in the abducens nucleus and the superior oblique which is innervated by the neurons of the trochlear nucleus.

Figure 5.2a shows the response properties of a single cell in the oculomotor nucleus whose axon innervates the inferior rectus (Schiller 1970). The action potentials for the cell over time and the monkey's eye movements in the vertical plane are shown. The upper set of traces was collected while the monkey looked around in the laboratory with his head restrained. Under such conditions, the animal made saccadic eye movements with intervening fixations. The lower set of traces was collected while an object was moved downward in front of the monkey.

Three points should be noted about Figure 5.1a. The first is that the rate of maintained activity exhibited by this neuron is proportional to the degree of downward deviation of the eye in orbit. The higher the activity, the more acetylcholine is released at the terminals and, consequently, the more the inferior rectus contracts. It has been shown that there is a linear relationship between the degree of angular deviation of the eye and the rate of activity in neurons that form the final common path to the eye muscles. The second point is that the neuron discharges with a high frequency burst during the execution of downward saccadic eye movements; the size of the saccade is proportional to the duration of this high frequency burst. Upward saccades seen in the figure are associated with a pause of activity during which it is safe to assume that the neurons innervating the superior rectus discharge with high frequencies. The third point is that the neuron discharges in association with pursuit eye movements in a similar proportional fashion as was revealed when the monkey was fixating various objects in the stationary visual scene. This can be seen in the lower set of traces of Figure 5.2a.

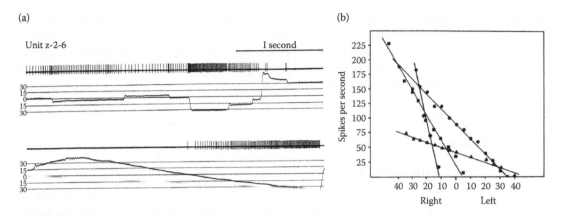

FIGURE 5.2
(a) Action potentials obtained from a single cell in the oculomotor nucleus that innervates the inferior rectus muscle. The activity of the neuron is shown along with vertical eye-movement traces. The upper set of records show neuronal activity when spontaneous saccadic eye movements were made with intervening fixations. The lower set of traces show neuronal activity during smooth-pursuit eye movement obtained by moving an object downward in front of the monkey. The rate of maintained activity of the neuron is linearly proportional to the angular displacement of the eye. This is shown for four neurons in (b), the saccadic eye movements in the upper trace of Figure 5.3a are associated with high-frequency bursts, the durations of which are proportional to saccade size. (With kind permission from Springer Science+Business Media: *Experimental Brain Research*, The discharge characteristics of single units in the oculomotor and abducens nuclei of the unanesthetized monkey, 10 (4), 1970, 347–62, Schiller, P. H.)

One more interesting fact about the records shown in Figure 5.2a: Immediately after the execution of a saccadic eye movement brought about by a high-frequency neuronal burst, only a minimal overshoot can be seen. This is not accomplished by some sort of counter activity in neurons innervating the antagonist muscle. If that were the case, one would see in this record a brief burst immediately after the completion of an upward saccade. The remarkable ability of the eye to stop on a dime, so to speak, seems to be simply due to the excellent viscous damping achieved in Tenon's capsule within which the eye resides.

Figure 5.2b shows plots of response rates of five neurons that innervate fibers of the extraocular muscles. There is a linear relationship between the angular deviation of the eye and the discharge rate of the neurons. The slope of each neuron is different, presumably adjusted for the effectiveness with which the fibers can be contracted yielding homogeneous contraction for the entire muscle.

On the basis of these observations, it appears that at the level of the oculomotor complex in the brainstem, where the neurons whose axons innervate the extraocular muscles reside, the saccadic and tracking eye movements are executed by the same set of neurons. The coding operation seen here may be termed a rate/duration code: The higher the maintained rate, the greater the angular deviation of the eye in orbit; the longer the duration of the high frequency burst seen in these neurons, the larger the saccade produced (Robinson 1975; Schiller 1970).

Right above the nuclei innervating the extraocular muscles, there is a complement of neurons in the brain stem in which the various components of the neuronal responses associated with eye movements can be seen separately. Several classes of neurons have been identified (Fuchs, Kaneko, and Scudder 1985). These include the following types: burst neurons that discharge in high frequency bursts during saccadic eye movements but otherwise remain silent; omnipause neurons that fire at a constant rate but pause whenever a saccade is made; and tonic neurons whose discharge rate is proportional to angular deviation of the eye in orbit but do not have bursts or pauses associated with saccadic eye movements. It is assumed that the activity of these and several other classes of neurons drives the cells in the oculomotor, trochlear, and abducens nuclei to produce the desired saccadic and smooth-pursuit eye movements.

5.3 Superior Colliculus and Saccadic Eye Movements

In considering the role of the superior colliculus in eye-movement control, it should first be pointed out that this structure is one that has undergone tremendous changes in the course of evolution. In more primitive animals that have little forebrains, such as toads and fish, this structure, which in these animals is called the optic tectum, is the major site of visual information processing and also participates in converting visual signals into motor outputs. Consequently, ablation of the optic tectum renders these animals virtually blind and incapable of the execution of visually triggered motor commands (Schiller 1984).

In mammals, and particularly in primates that have a greatly expanded neocortex, visual analysis has been relegated largely to the geniculo-striate system and associated higher cortical areas. The superior colliculus, residing on the roof of the midbrain, has taken on a much more modest function that appears to involve predominantly saccadic eye-movement control (Schiller 1984; Sparks 1986; Wurtz and Albano 1980). Figure 5.3a shows a mid-saggital section of the monkey brain showing the location of the superior colliculus.

The superior colliculus has several distinct layers that are revealed in stained tissue. Figure 5.3b shows a coronal section of the cat superior colliculus (Sprague, Berlucchi, and Rizzolatti 1973). Seven distinct layers are shown. The top two, called superficial gray, receives a direct input from the retina. The third layer, called stratum opticum, receives input predominantly from the visual cortex. Subsequent layers receive input from numerous other cortical regions. The lowest layers contain output cells that send signals to the brainstem, in mammals predominantly to regions involved in eye-movement control.

Single cells in layers I–III respond vigorously to visual stimuli, but their receptive field properties, unlike those in the cortex, are not particularly interesting. They prefer small stimuli but are largely insensitive to differences in shape, orientation, and color, and most lack directional selectivity to the movement of stimuli. It is noteworthy, however, that the visual field is laid out in a neat topographic order in the colliculus, with the anterior portion representing the fovea, the posterior portion the periphery, the medial region the upper visual field, and the later region the lower visual field. In each colliculus, the contralateral half of the visual field is represented.

In the deeper layers of the colliculus, there is also an orderly arrangement that has to do with the coding of eye movements. To understand this layout, we shall first consider the effects of electrical stimulation in the superior colliculus in comparison with the effects of electrically stimulating the abducens nucleus that innervates the lateral rectus. In Figure 5.4, the top set of eye-movement traces were obtained when the abducens nucleus was stimulated for various burst durations in the monkey (Schiller and Stryker 1972). The size of the saccade produced increases with increasing durations of the stimulation burst. This fits directly with the single-cell data shown in Figure 5.2. In the center and bottom portions of Figure 5.4a, eye-movement traces are shown that

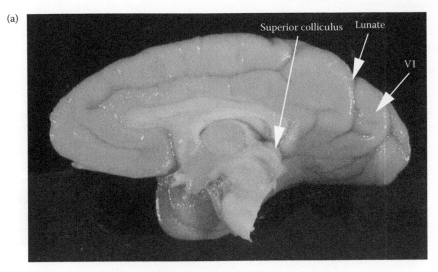

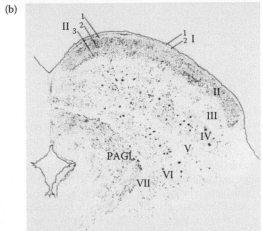

FIGURE 5.3
(See color insert.) (a) Midline saggital section through the monkey brain. The arrows point to the superior colliculus, area V1, and the lunate sulcus. (b) Coronal section through the cat superior colliculus with the layers numbered. Layers I and II are called superficial gray and layer III stratum opticum. (Kanaseki, T. and J. M. Sprague: Anatomical organization of pretectal nuclei and tectal laminae in the cat. *Journal of Comparative Neurology.* 1974. 158 (3): 319–37. Copyright Wiley-VCH Verlag GmbH & Co. KGaA. Reproduced with permission.)

were obtained when the superior colliculus was electrically stimulated. The stimulation produced effects quite different from those obtained by abducens. The amplitude of each saccade in the middle set is unaffected by the duration of the stimulation burst until it becomes 240 and 480 milliseconds. For these longer durations a staircase of identical saccades is elicited. The bottom trace shows a staircase of saccades produced to a long stimulation burst with the electrode placed near the anterior tip of the superior colliculus. Thus, what determines the size and direction of each saccade is where in the colliculus one stimulates (Robinson 1972; Schiller and Stryker 1972). Stimulation of the medial and lateral portions of the colliculus produces upward and downward saccades, respectively.

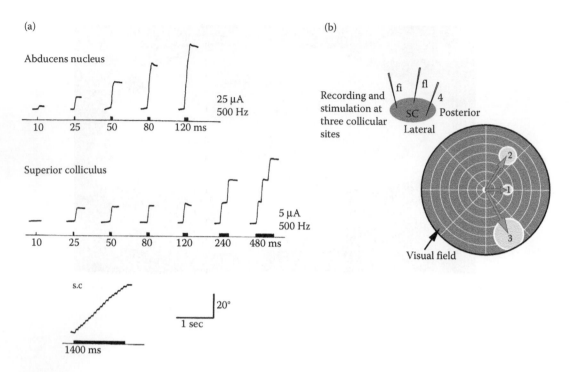

FIGURE 5.4
(See color insert.) (a) The effects of electrically stimulating the abducens nucleus and the superior colliculus. Stimulation frequency was held constant at 500 Hertz while burst duration was systematically varied. Stimulation of the abducens nucleus shows increasing saccade size as a function of increasing burst duration. By contrast, stimulation of the superior colliculus at any given site always produces the same direction and amplitude saccade. For long-duration bursts, staircases of saccades are elicited in the superior colliculus; the size of each saccade remains of the same amplitude and direction. (Adapted from Schiller, P. H. and M. Stryker. 1972. *Journal of Neurophysiology* 35 (6): 915–24.) (b) Schematic representation of saccadic eye movements elicited by stimulation of three sites in the superior colliculus. Electrodes are placed in the anterior, medial, and lateral posterior portions of the colliculus (1–3). The location of the receptive fields recorded from these three recording sites is displayed below (yellow disks) as are the effects of electrically stimulating at these sites (red arrows). The stimulation produces a saccadic eye movement that lands the center of gaze at the location where the receptive field had been prior to the movement of the eyes.

Systematic mapping of the receptive fields and the motor responses in the colliculus reveals a neat correspondence that can best be understood by examining Figure 5.4b. Schematically shown are procedures in which microelectrodes are placed at three sites in the colliculus. First, the location of the receptive field of neurons is plotted and then the same site is electrically stimulated (Schiller and Stryker 1972). The consequence of the stimulation is a saccadic eye movement that shifts the center of gaze, the fovea, to that location of the visual field where the receptive field of the neuron at the tip of the electrode had been located prior to the eye movement. Thus, it appears that we have a targeting system here that can convert a visual signal into a motor output. The calculation seems to be one that computes a retinal error signal, namely the error between the initial gaze position and the location of the target. The consequence of the stimulation is to accurately shift the center of gaze to the intended location, thereby nulling the retinal error. This process has been termed foveation mechanism.

Single cell recordings in the intermediate layers of the colliculus support this inference (Schiller and Koerner 1971; Wurtz and Goldberg 1972). Neuronal activity corresponds with electrical stimulation results. Figure 5.5 provides a demonstration of this. Figure 5.5a–c shows the activity of a superior colliculus neuron in the lower layers of this structure when eye movements of various directions and amplitudes are made. The neuronal responses are limited to small left and up saccades. Figure 5.5d provides a polar plot of eye movements. The center of the display represents the initial fixation spot irrespective of where the center of gaze was directed at in space. The plotted disks represent the size and amplitude of each saccade made. The white disks show saccades not associated with neuronal activity, whereas the red disks show saccades that had been preceded with a burst of neuronal activity. On the basis of such data and on the electrical stimulation effects as depicted in Figure 5.4a and b, collicular neurons have a "motor" or "movement" field that is coded in terms of saccadic vectors (Schiller and Stryker 1972). What this means of course, just to emphasize it, is that the size the direction of a saccade produced by electrical stimulation is independent of the initial position of the eye in orbit; the same is true for single-cell activity. The cell responds in association with the execution of an eye movement of a certain range of sizes and amplitudes and does so irrespective of the initial position of the eye. Many of the cells of this type also have a visual receptive field. For the neuron shown in Figure 5.5d, the receptive field relative to the fovea is located in the same place as the motor field. Thus, the sensory and motor fields are superimposed as indicated also for the stimulation work.

On the basis of these findings it has become evident that the superior colliculus carries a vector code. Different regions of the colliculus code different vectors that are in register with the visual field representation in the superficial layers of the structure (Robinson 1972; Schiller and Sandell 1983; Schiller and Stryker 1972).

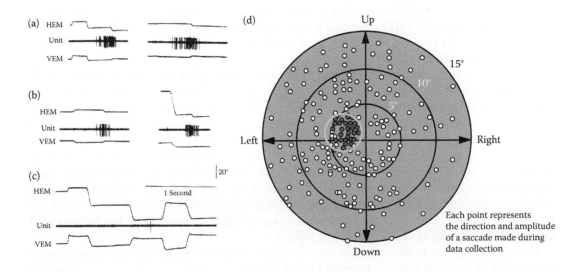

FIGURE 5.5
(See color insert.) (a–c) A montage of horizontal and vertical eye movements and action potentials obtained from a collicular cell. The activity is limited to small left and upward eye movements. (d) A polar plot of the direction and amplitude of saccadic eye movements made. The red disks represent eye movements associated with the activity of a single neuron on the colliculus. The white disks show eye movements that were not associated with neuronal activity.

As an added complication it should be noted that in the deeper layers some cells can be activated not only by visual but also by somatosensory and auditory stimuli (Schiller 1984; Stein, Magahaes-Castro, and Kruger 1976). The somatosensory and auditory representations are arranged topographically. It has been shown, however, that unlike for the visual input, these maps do not conform to the innervation density of the somatosensory and auditory inputs from peripheral receptors. Instead, these maps are in register with the visual map suggesting that the organization in the colliculus is from the point of view of the eye (Drager and Hubel 1975). One might infer, therefore, that when saccadic eye movements are elicited by signals processed by the auditory or somatosensory systems, one pathway by which they reach the brainstem to elicit a saccadic eye movement passes through the superior colliculus (Stein, Magahaes-Castro, and Kruger 1976).

5.4 Cortical Control of Saccadic Eye Movements

It is a well-known fact that quite a few structures in the cortex play significant roles in eye-movement control. These include regions of the occipital, parietal, temporal, and frontal cortices. Some of the structures in the monkey cortex are depicted in Figure 5.6a. Electrical stimulation of most of these areas can elicit saccadic eye movements. This is depicted in Figure 5.6b in more detail where the superior colliculus stimulation effects are also included. Stimulation of the superior colliculus, the visual cortex, regions of the parietal cortex, and the frontal eye fields (FEFs) elicit constant vector saccades. The direction and amplitude of the saccade depends on the site of stimulation. In the visual cortex, as in the superior colliculus, the saccade elicited by electrical stimulation shifts the center of gaze into the receptive field of the stimulated neurons. In contrast with these areas, stimulation of the medial eye fields (MEFs) reveals a different coding operation: in this area electrical stimulation moves the eye to a certain orbital location. Different sites within the MEFs code different orbital positions.

Given all these cortical areas involved in the generation of saccadic eye movements, the next central question one needs to pose is: how do the signals from these areas reach the brainstem oculomotor centers? Anatomical studies have shown extensive connections from these cortical regions to the superior colliculus but have also shown connections to the brainstem oculomotor centers directly from the FEFs and MEFs.

One procedure to address this question is to electrically stimulate various cortical areas before and after removal of the superior colliculus. The results of such experiments yield straightforward answers and are depicted schematically in Figure 5.6c. Following ablation of the superior colliculus, eye movements can no longer be elicited from the occipital and parietal cortices, even at very high currents, but can still be produced by frontal and MEF stimulation (Keating et al. 1983; Schiller 1977).

These findings, therefore, suggest that there are at least two parallel pathways for the generation of saccadic eye movements. One of these involves the posterior cortex and the superior colliculi. The other involves the frontal cortex that, in addition to projections to the superior colliculus, has direct access to the brainstem. These findings have led to the idea that there are two major parallel systems of visually guided eye movements, the anterior and the posterior, which will be discussed in more detail below.

In what follows, several different experimental procedures are described that have contributed to our understanding of how the brain controls eye movements.

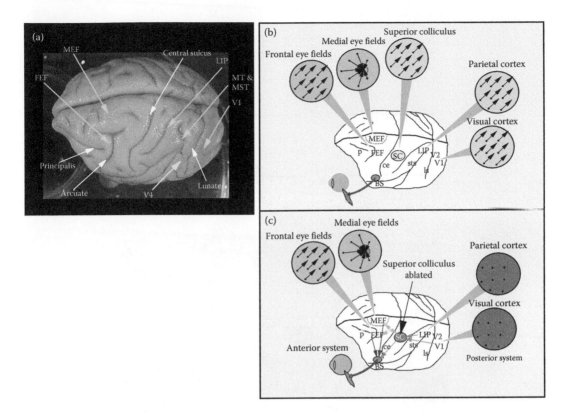

FIGURE 5.6
(See color insert.) (a) Top view of a monkey brain. Indicated in blue are some of the areas believed to be involved in eye-movement generation; shown in white are a few of the relevant sulci. (b) Schematic of the saccadic eye movements elicited by electrical stimulation of five areas of the rhesus monkey: area V1, the lateral intraparietal sulcus, the superior colliculus, the frontal eye fields (FEFs), and the medial eye fields (MEFs). Electrical stimulation in all of these areas, except for the MEFs, elicits constant vector saccades whose direction and amplitude depend on the site stimulated within each of these structures. Stimulation of the MEFs produces saccades to a particular orbital location; different regions within this structure code different orbital locations. (c) The effect of superior colliculus ablation on electrical stimulation in the cortex. After superior colliculus removal, even many months later, electrical stimulation of the posterior cortex no longer generates saccadic eye movements. However, stimulation of the FEFs and MEFs continue to be effective.

5.4.1 Effects of Inactivating Area V1 on the Superior Colliculus

Several investigators have examined the consequences of inactivating the visual cortex on the responses of single cells in the superior colliculus. One procedure that allows for reversible inactivation is to cool the visual cortex while recording from individual neurons in the superior colliculus. This kind of work has been carried out in both cats and monkeys (Schiller et al. 1974; Wickelgren and Sterling 1969). Figure 5.7a shows examples of recordings made in the superficial gray and in the intermediate layers of the monkey superior colliculus before, during, and after area V1 has been inactivated by cooling. The cells were driven by visual stimuli that either were flashed stationary spots or were moved across the receptive fields of the neurons. The data show that the cooling had no effect on cells in the superficial layers but that cells in the intermediate layers became unresponsive. This was the case for all the cells studied in the intermediate layers.

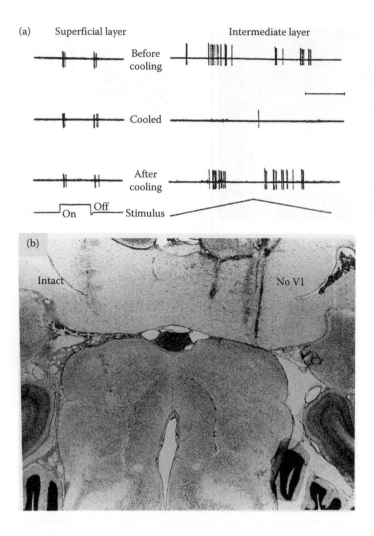

FIGURE 5.7

(See color insert.) (a) The effect of inactivating area V1 in the monkey on the responses of neurons in the superficial and the intermediate layers of the superior colliculus to visual stimuli presented in their receptive fields. In the superficial layers, which receive input directly from the retina, V1 cooling has no effect. In the intermediate layers, which receive input from area V1, cooling of V1 eliminates neuronal responses. (b) Coronal section of a monkey superior colliculus. The left hemifield is intact. In the right hemifield, area V1 has been removed. Recordings made several months later show no responses to visual stimuli in the right superior colliculus below the superficial layers. The marker lesions depicted in red were made at the tip of the recording electrode at the sites where visual responses could no longer be elicited.

To determine whether this effect is temporary or long-lasting, experiments had been carried out in which recordings were made in the monkey superior colliculus many months after area V1 had been removed unilaterally. Marker spots were then placed in the superior colliculus at the point where visual responses could no longer be elicited on the intact side and on the side where the V1 had been blocked. Figure 5.7b shows a coronal section from such an animal. The data show that neuronal responses could not be elicited below the superficial gray on the side that did not have an area V1.

These findings indicate that in the monkey, as is most likely in all primates, the intermediate and lower layers of the colliculus are controlled by cortical downflow.

Furthermore, the data indicate that in the adult animal there is no discernible change in this state of affairs. Even after many months, the deeper layers do not become responsive to visual stimuli. This suggests that the saccadic eye movements generated in such animals are under the control of input to the brainstem oculomotor centers from brain areas other than the superior colliculus. This issue will be considered in more detail below.

5.4.2 Effects of Cortical Electrical Stimulation on Target Selection

One of the central tasks in generating saccadic eye movements to visual stimuli is to select one visual stimulus in the plethora of stimuli in the visual scene. Typically, with each shift in gaze, the image of numerous objects impinges on the retina. To be able to make an accurate saccadic eye movement to one of these targets, a selection process has to take place. Primates are very good at this task and can generate an accurate saccade to the desired target with 90% accuracy. A variety of experiments have been carried out examining this process.

Figure 5.8a shows a simple paradigm used with monkeys in which following fixation two targets appear which are presented either simultaneously or with various temporal asynchronies. Below are shown three sets of eye movement traces under three conditions, in which either the left or the right target appeared 34 milliseconds prior to the other target or both appeared simultaneously. Two points should be noted here: (a) When the targets were simultaneous the monkeys made saccades either to the left or to the right target; and (b) the monkey selects either of the two targets with equal probability. However, when the targets were presented with a temporal offset, the monkey showed a strong preference for the one that had appeared first.

Figure 5.8b shows eye movements made by a monkey to single or paired targets presented simultaneously with various angular separations. Single target performance is shown on the left. Corresponding eye-movement traces for the paired targets appear on the right for two angular separations, 90 and 20 degrees. The inset shows the percent of vector-averaged saccades, which are eye movements that land within ±4.5 degrees of the midpoint. With an angular separation of 90 degrees most saccades are made quite accurately to one or the other of the targets. However, when the angular separation is 20 degrees, most of the saccades land in-between the two targets (73.1%). The relationship between angular separation and vector averaging is depicted in the inset.

Figure 5.9 shows, schematically, the effects of electrically stimulating two sites simultaneously in the superior colliculus, the FEFs, and with one electrode in each structure. Simultaneous electrical stimulation at two sites with currents adjusted for equality always produces vector-averaged saccades (Robinson 1972; Robinson and Fuchs 1969; Schiller and Stryker 1972). This is so dramatic that when sites are stimulated which elicit equal magnitude straight left and right saccades, the paired stimulation vector averages perfectly and creates no discernible eye movement.

The dramatic differences seen between saccades made to visual targets and in response to electrical stimulation highlight the fact that under the former condition a decision is made as to which target to select, which is not the case with electrical stimulation.

5.4.3 Effects of Blocking Various Brain Regions on Saccadic Eye Movements

Several experiments are described here in four subsections that examine the effects of selected brain lesions on the generation of saccadic eye movements.

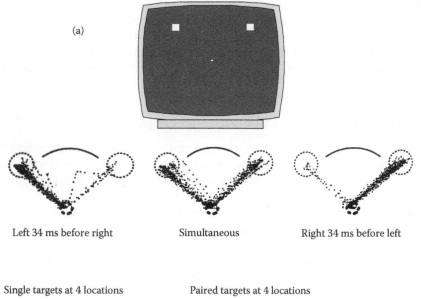

(a)

| Left 34 ms before right | Simultaneous | Right 34 ms before left |

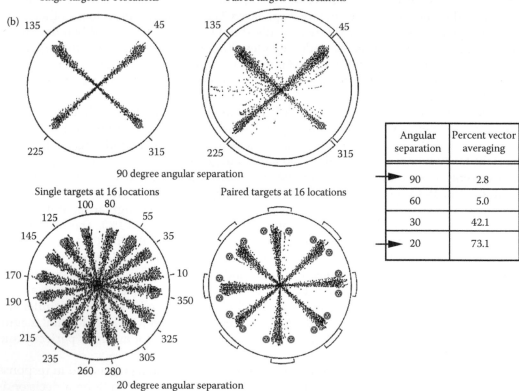

(b)

Single targets at 4 locations

Paired targets at 4 locations

90 degree angular separation

Single targets at 16 locations

Paired targets at 16 locations

20 degree angular separation

Angular separation	Percent vector averaging
90	2.8
60	5.0
30	42.1
20	73.1

FIGURE 5.8

(See color insert.) (a) Traces of eye movements made to two targets that appear either simultaneously (center) or with a temporal offset of 34 milliseconds (left target first on left, right first on right). (b) Traces of eye movements made to single or paired simultaneous targets shown respectively on the left and right. The inset shows the percent of vector-averaged saccades under four angular separation conditions (±4.5° from midpoint between the two targets).

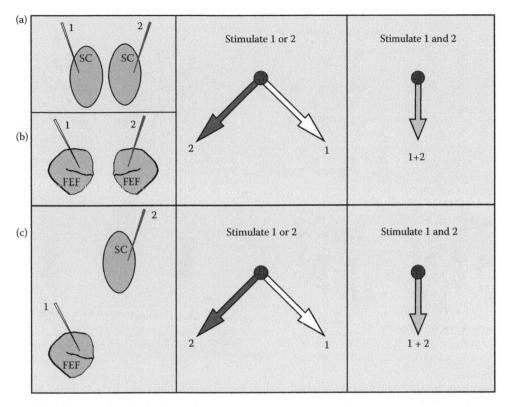

FIGURE 5.9
(**See color insert.**) Shown schematically are the effects of electrically stimulating two sites in the superior colliculus (a), the frontal eye fields (b), and in each of the two structures (c). Shown are the effects of stimulating each site singly and stimulating them simultaneously. Simultaneous stimulation produces vector-averaged saccades.

5.4.3.1 Hand–Eye Coordination Task

In this set of experiments, monkeys were trained to pick apple pieces out of a board, which necessitated them to properly adjust their hands and fingers to succeed in retrieving each apple piece from the nine slots. The layout of the board is shown in Figure 5.10a. While performing this task the monkey's eye movements were recorded, and from the data collected each fixation point was marked by a square as shown in the rest of the figure. Each set is based on 10 repeated trials. Data are shown from two monkeys before and after the superior colliculus and the FEFs were removed. For monkey 1, preoperative performance is shown in Figure 5.10b. In Figure 5.10c and d, data are shown for performance 4 days and 20 days after bilateral ablation of the FEFs, respectively. Below are shown quantitative data for the length of time it took to complete a trial (T), the mean number of saccades per seconds (S), the mean saccadic amplitude (A), the mean saccadic velocity (V), and the mean number of errors in retrieval (E). The preoperative data for monkey 2 are shown in Figure 5.10e. In Figure 5.10f, the data shown were obtained 4 days after bilateral superior colliculus removal. In Figure 5.10g, the data shown were collected 57 days subsequent to removing the FEFs in addition to the superior colliculus. In Figure 5.10h, similar data were collected 134 days later.

These data establish the following: The bilateral FEF and the bilateral superior colliculus lesions produced relatively mild deficits in eye movements. Notable are the somewhat

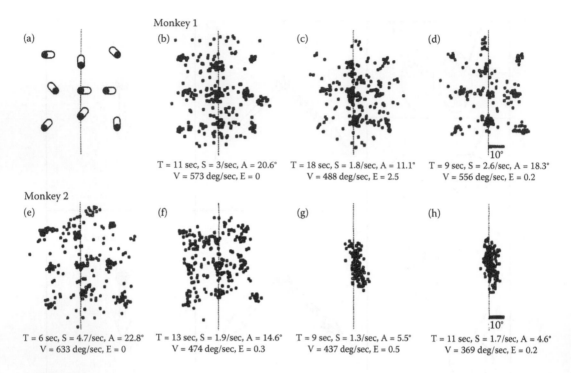

FIGURE 5.10

Eye fixation patterns of two monkeys at various stages in an experiment in which the task was to pick out apple pieces in an apple board shown in (a). (b) Fixation patterns of monkey 1 produced in the course of 10 repeated preoperative trials. (c) Data collected 4 days after bilateral ablation of the frontal eye fields (FEFs). (d) Data collected 20 days later. (e) Preoperative fixation patterns for monkey 2. (f) Data collected 4 days after bilateral superior colliculus ablations. (g) Performance of the second monkey 57 days after adding bilateral FEF lesions to the bilateral superior colliculus lesions. (h) Re-test of the second monkey after 134 days. Quantitative data below each display show mean number of seconds to complete a trial (T), mean number of saccades per second (S), mean saccade amplitude (A), mean saccade velocity (V), and mean number of errors (E). FEF lesions alone produce no lasting deficits. Superior colliculus lesions show mild deficits on all quantitative measures. Paired FEF and superior colliculus lesions devastate performance to the extent that the animal is virtually incapable of directing his eyes to visual targets. At this stage, however, the animal can still pick the apple board clean. (Adapted from Schiller, P. H., S. D. True, and J. L. Conway. 1980. *Journal of Neurophysiology* 44 (6): 1175–89.)

reduced amplitudes of saccades after the collicular lesion and the decrease in the number of saccades made per second. However, after both structures have been removed there is a dramatic deficit, with the monkeys having very limited eye movements, most of which are along the vertical which is probably attributable to some sparing of tissue representing the vertical meridian. There is virtually no recovery over time even more than a year later. Films made of such monkeys show virtually no visible eye movements.

These findings, taken along with the stimulation data shown in Figure 5.6b and c, suggest that two major systems are involved in the control of saccadic eye movements: the anterior system from the FEFs and MEFs that have direct connections to the brainstem oculomotor centers in addition to the connections made to the superior colliculus; and the posterior system that reaches the brainstem predominantly through the superior colliculus.

In addition to these inferences, it is also noteworthy that the bilateral superior colliculus lesions produced relatively limited deficits even when tested just 4 days after their removal.

This stands in contrast with what happens when unilateral lesions are made which produce much more dramatic effects. After unilateral lesions, monkeys tend to rotate toward the side of the lesions and they have their eyes strongly deviated to that side. It takes months to recover. Similar rotations have been found also in cats and in many rodents.

It has been suggested that in intact monkeys the information from the frontal areas does not effectively reach the brainstem areas directly but instead passes through the superior colliculus (Hanes and Wurtz 2001). Eye movements become effective again after collicular lesions by virtue of plasticity. While this hypothesis is in need of testing, strong arguments exist favoring an effective functional projection from the frontal lobe to the brainstem. Notable among these is that just 4 days after bilateral removal of the superior colliculus eye-movement performance is quite strong. Plasticity is unlikely to become effective so rapidly.

5.4.3.2 Generation of Express Saccades

One of the fascinating discoveries that has been made about saccadic eye movements is that under certain conditions a bimodal distribution of saccadic latencies can be obtained

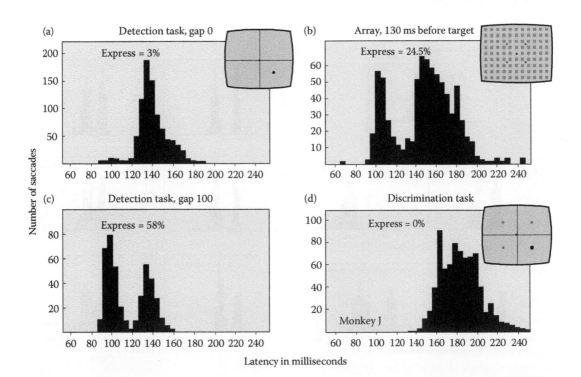

FIGURE 5.11
(See color insert.) The distribution of saccadic latencies to visual targets. (a) Following fixation a single target appears in one of two locations; the target appears upon the termination of the central fixation spot. (b) The single target appears in one of two locations 100 milliseconds after the termination of the fixation spot. As a result, a distinct bimodal distribution of saccadic latencies is obtained, the first mode of which is called express saccades. (c) An array of stimuli appears 130 milliseconds prior to the target. The fixation spot terminates upon the appearance of the target. This condition also produces a bimodal distribution of saccadic latencies. (d) A discrimination task is used in which one of the four targets is different from the other three identical stimuli. This condition yields no express saccades and the overall latency is longer than the second mode in the detection task.

as discovered by Fischer and Boch (1983). They named the first mode of this distribution, which peaks near a latency of 100 milliseconds, "express saccades," and the second mode as "regular saccades." This interesting finding has triggered numerous experiments. Figure 5.11 describes some of the basic conditions that do and do not generate express saccades. In these experiments, monkeys were trained to make a saccadic eye movement to a target that appeared subsequent to the central fixation spot. Figure 5.11a shows the distribution of saccadic latencies when a single target appeared on a homogeneous background immediately after the fixation spot has been turned off, whereas Figure 5.11b shows the distribution when the fixation spot is terminated 100 milliseconds prior to the target. The intervening period is called the "gap." The percent of express saccades (those between 85 and 120 milliseconds) is indicated in each section. More than half the saccades under the 100-millisecond gap condition are in the express range. As shown in Figure 5.11c, express saccades are also readily produced when an array of stimuli precedes the target even when the fixation spot is terminated on the appearance of the target. By contrast, express saccades are practically never produced when an oddities discrimination task is used, as depicted in Figure 5.11d; for this task four stimuli appear one of which, the target, is different from the others. To be rewarded, the monkey had to make a saccadic eye movement directly to the target.

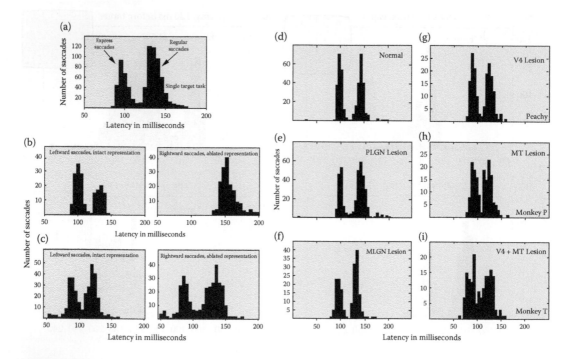

FIGURE 5.12
The effects various lesions on the temporal distribution of saccadic latencies. (a) Distribution of saccadic latencies in an intact monkey yielding a bimodal distribution. (b) Subsequent to a left superior colliculus removal express saccades are no longer produced, even many months later, to the right. The bimodal distribution to the left, governed by the intact superior colliculus, persists. (c) After frontal eye field removal, the bimodal distribution of saccadic latencies persists. (d) The bimodal distribution of saccadic latencies in another intact monkey. (e) Saccadic latency distributions after inactivation of the parvocellular lateral geniculated nucleus that blocks the midget system. (f) Saccadic latency distributions after inactivation of the magnocellular lateral geniculate nucleus that blocks the parasol system. (g) Saccadic latency distributions after V4 removal. (h) Saccadic latency distributions after removal of area MT. (i) Saccadic latency distributions after removal of both V4 and MT.

Responding quickly to events in the world is an essential requirement for survival in most species. The generation of quick, short-latency eye movements plays a significant role in this process. How this is accomplished has been examined in numerous experiments by selective removal of brain areas involved in eye-movement control. Figure 5.12a–c shows the effects of collicular and FEF blocks on the generation of express saccades. Figure 5.12a shows the intact monkey's performance on a task similar to that described for Figure 5.11. Subsequent to the unilateral collicular lesions, as shown in Figure 5.11b, express saccades are no longer made toward the side that had been represented by the now missing colliculus. This effect is powerful, and even after many months express saccades are never made again. By contrast, as shown in Figure 5.12c, after FEF lesions express saccades continue to be made. These findings suggest that the posterior system through the superior colliculus plays an essential role in saccade production.

To examine other pathways and structures that may play a role in express saccade generation several other areas had been blocked. Figure 5.12d–i shows some of these. One hypothesis was that of the two major pathways originating in the retina, the midget and parasol, one of them may selectively contribute to express saccade generation. These two systems pass through the lateral geniculate nucleus, with the midget system projecting to V1 through the parvocellular layers (PLGN) and the parasol system through the magnocellular layers (MLGN). Blocking either of these channels, as shown in Figure 5.12e and f, failed to selectively alter express saccade generation, suggesting that both systems play a role in the generation of such rapid eye movements. Also ineffective were lesions of areas V4 and MT made singly and in combination (Figure 5.12g–i).

5.5 Role of Frontal Cortical Areas in the Generation of Saccadic Eye Movements

As has already been noted with reference to Figure 5.6b and c, in the frontal cortex two major areas have been shown to play a significant role in saccadic eye-movement generation (Bizzi 1967; Bruce and Goldberg 1984; Chen and Wise 1995a,b; Mann, Thau, and Schiller 1988; Schall 1991a,b; Schlag, Schlag-Rey, and Pigarev 1992; Tanji and Kurata 1982; Tanji and Shima 1994; Tehovnik 1995; Tehovnik and Lee 1993). These two areas are the FEFs and the MEFs. For the most part, the FEFs carry a vector code and the MEFs and orbital position code. Electrical stimulation of different regions of the FEFs yields different constant vector saccades. In the MEFs, different subregions code different orbital positions. These findings have been established both with single-cell recordings and with microstimulation (Bizzi 1967; Bruce and Goldberg 1984; Robinson and Fuchs 1969; Schiller and Sandell 1983).

That the operational principles of the FEFs and the dorsomedial frontal cortical area (MEFs) are different is also supported by two other lines of evidence. The neuronal properties of single cells in these two areas are notably different: in the MEFs, it has been shown that many cells respond to both eye and limb movements, suggesting that they have multifunctional characteristics (Mann, Thau, and Schiller 1988; Tanji and Kurata 1982; Tanji and Shima 1994). This is not seen in the FEFs. Selective inactivation of these two areas also yields quite different effects. Acute inactivation of the FEFs has rather pronounced effects: animals have difficulties in making saccadic eye movements to briefly flashed visual targets that appear in the visual field contralateral to the inactivation; however, less of a deficit is evident when the targets are bright and are not extinguished prior to the initiation of a saccadic eye movement (Dias, Kiesau, and Segraves 1995; Sommer and Tehovnik 1999). By contrast, inactivation of the dorsomedial frontal cortex produces practically no deficits to briefly presented targets. Inactivation in these kinds of experiments is accomplished by injecting various chemical agents, such as lidocaine or neurotransmitter analogs and antagonists, through a fine tube inserted into the region. Current ablation studies of MEFs have also failed in revealing any clear-cut deficits in eye-movement control (Schiller and Chou 1998).

The aspects of saccadic eye-movement generation in which the FEFs and MEFs are involved have been addressed in several ways. One approach is to examine the consequences of inactivating or removing these areas on a variety of eye-movement tasks. As already shown in Figure 5.12c, the FEFs do not seem to play a role in the generation of express saccades. This is also the case for the MEFs as their removal does not alter express saccade generation either (Schiller and Chou 1998).

Two other aspects of eye-movement generation examined in lesion studies have been target selection and the execution of sequences of saccadic eye movements. Target selection is a process that occurs during each fixation. In natural settings, every time a saccadic eye movement is made to a visual stimulus, numerous stimuli impinge on the retina; one has to be selected for the next eye movement. This is not a trivial task as it requires a selection process and the subsequent generation of an accurate saccade to the desired location. Studies suggest that the FEFs play a significant role in this process.

Figure 5.13 shows examples of such an experiment. The procedure was similar to that shown in Figure 5.8a: Following fixation, two targets were presented with varied temporal asynchronies. The monkey chose one of these targets with a saccadic eye movement and was rewarded irrespective of which target ended up being the choice. The temporal asynchrony between the appearances of the two targets was randomly varied. After extensive training on this task, either the FEFs or the MEFs were removed and the animal was tested repeatedly over time. The angular separation for the data shown in Figure 5.13a was 90 degrees.

The data in Figure 5.13a shows that in the intact monkey the equal probability point of target selection occurred when the two targets were presented simultaneously (pre-op condition). The subsequent unilateral FEF lesion produced a sizable deficit; the equal probability point of choosing one or the other of the targets 2 weeks after the lesion shifted dramatically; the target presented in the right contralateral hemifield relative to the lesion had to appear 116 milliseconds prior to the other target to obtain equal probability choice. This effect declined moderately, but even 4 years later a sizable deficit remained. Thus, target choice shifted dramatically toward the side of the visual field represented by the intact FEF.

In contrast with the data obtained after an FEF lesion, removal of the right MEF in another monkey produced only a mild deficit that recovered quite rapidly. Sixteen weeks after the lesion performance was back to normal.

In Figure 5.13b, eye-movement traces are shown to visual targets presented with angular separations of 40 degrees. Various temporal asynchronies were used as marked in the figure. Under conditions like these, as has been shown in Figure 5.8b, vector-averaged saccades become common in intact monkeys when the two targets are presented simultaneously. The upper section of Figure 5.13b shows such eye-movement traces in a normal monkey using four different temporal asynchronies. The maximum number of vector-averaged saccades occurred when the two targets were presented simultaneously (asynchrony of 0 milliseconds). After the left FEF lesion, the maximum number of vector-averaged saccades was obtained not when the targets were presented simultaneously, but

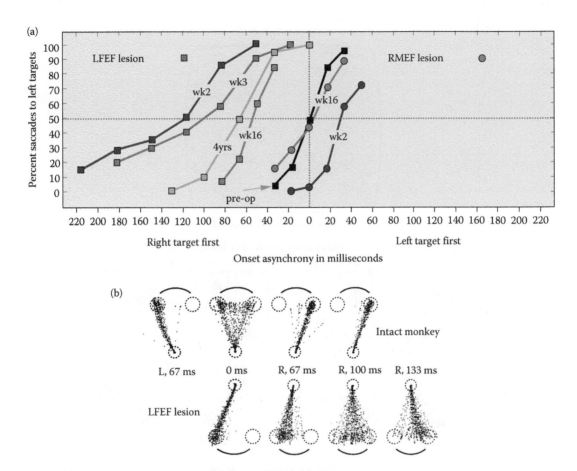

FIGURE 5.13

(a) The percent of saccades made to the left of two targets presented with various temporal asynchronies as indicated on the x-axis using procedures similar to those shown in Figure 5.8a, with the targets separated by 90 angular degrees. Data are shown before and various times after frontal eye field (FEF) and medial eye field (MEF) lesions. After the FEF lesion, deficits are evident even 4 years later. After the MEF lesion, there is full recovery after 16 weeks. (b) Eye-movement records are shown to paired targets separated by 40 angular degrees. Under such conditions, as had been shown in Figure 5.8b, vector-averaged saccades become common. The upper traces show performance in the intact monkey; vector-averaged saccades occur most frequently when the two targets appear simultaneously. After left FEF lesion, as shown in the lower set of traces, vector-averaged saccades occur most frequently when the target in the representation of the ablated FEF appears 100 milliseconds prior to the target in the intact representation.

when the target in the hemifield contralateral to the lesion was present 100 milliseconds prior to the target in the intact field. These findings show a selection bias that is similar to that shown in Figure 5.13a.

These findings indicate, then, that the FEFs play a significant role in the target selection process whereas the MEFs do not appear to do so. The effect of FEF removal is long lasting, suggesting that in the adult monkey there is limited plasticity for recovery of this process.

Another important aspect of eye-movement control involves the execution of planned sequences of eye movements. Figure 5.14 describes an experimental procedure that has examined the effects of FEF removal on the generation of sequences of eye movements. Following fixation, as shown in the inset on the top of the figure, two targets were presented

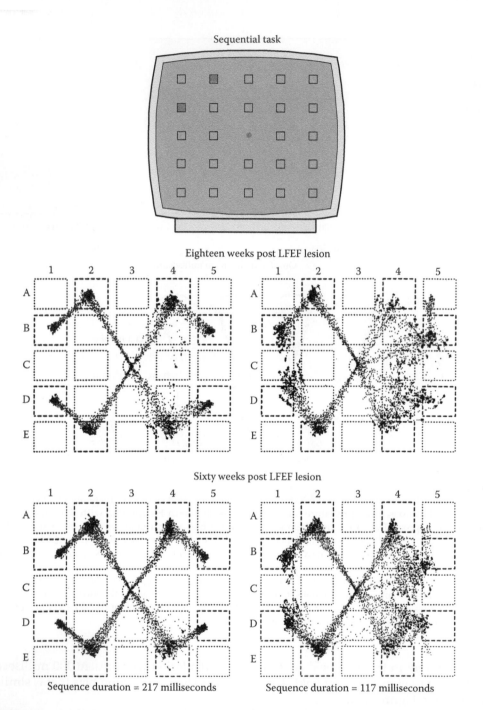

FIGURE 5.14

(See color insert.) Eye-movement traces collected when two targets are presented in succession as shown in the top of the figure. Following fixation, two targets were presented successively at four sets of locations with sequence durations of either 217 or 117 milliseconds. Performance is shown 18 and 60 weeks following a left frontal eye field removal. Performance for the shorter sequence is quite poor for rightward saccadic sequences even 60 weeks after the lesion.

with varied temporal sequences. The sequences were brief and were terminated before the initiation of the eye movements, so the monkey had to plan the saccadic sequence. Reward was given only when both target locations were correctly targeted in succession. Four pairs of sequences were used for the figure shown, two to the left and two to the right. The inset shows one such sequence to the top left of the display indicated by red squares. The data were obtained from a monkey with a left FEF lesion that affected rightward saccades. Thus, the saccadic eye movements made to the left represent normal performance and saccades made to the right performance carried out in the absence of the FEF. Data are presented for two sequence durations, 217 and 117 milliseconds. With the longer sequence there is little deficit. However, with the shorter sequence performance for rightward saccades is quite poor. This deficit also showed little recovery over time.

These findings suggest that the FEFs play a significant role both in the process of target selection and in the execution of sequences of saccadic eye movements.

5.6 Role of Excitatory and Inhibitory Circuits in the Generation of Saccadic Eye Movements

Two types of experiments will be described here. The first examines how low levels of electrical stimulation can influence the target selection process. The second examines the consequences of infusing pharmacological agents into various brain areas that affect inhibitory circuits.

The experimental procedures used in these studies are described in Figure 5.15. The top left panel shows the brain structures into which microelectrodes had been placed, allowing for recording of neurons, electrical microstimulation, and the infusion of pharmacological agents. The monkeys were trained to perform on five tasks. In the first, monkeys had to maintain fixation briefly that made it possible to map the location of the receptive fields of the neurons at the tip of the electrode. In the second, the monkeys simply fixated a central fixation spot which, upon termination, was followed by electrical stimulation that elicited a saccadic eye movement. In the third, the monkeys had to make saccadic eye movements to singly appearing targets. In the fourth, paired targets were presented with various temporal asynchronies as already described in Figure 5.13. In the fifth, the monkeys were trained on an oddities discrimination task in which four stimuli were presented, one of which was different from the other three identical stimuli. The task was to make a saccadic eye movement to the target that was different from the others.

Figure 5.16 shows data obtained with low-level electrical stimulation of areas V1, the lateral intraparietal (LIP) area, the MEF, and the FEF. Following mapping of the receptive or motor fields, the threshold for eliciting eye movements was determined using procedure number 2 shown in Figure 5.15. This was followed by the presentation of single targets, one of which was placed into the receptive or motor field area of the neurons at the tip of the electrode, as depicted in Figure 5.15, number 3. Correct alignment was confirmed by the generation of identical saccades for conditions 2 and 3. The next step involved the presentation of two visual targets, with one in the receptive or motor field of the neurons to be stimulated. The second target was either in the contralateral visual field or in the upper visual field, as depicted in each inset of Figure 5.15. Electrical stimulation then was administered at a variety of current levels on selected trials in conjunction with the appearance of the two visual targets. The temporal asynchrony of the two targets was systematically varied.

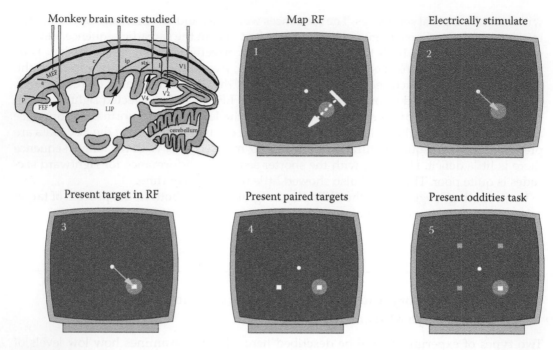

FIGURE 5.15
(See color insert.) Experimental procedures for recording, electrically stimulating, and infusing pharmacological agents into various brain areas. The top left figure shows monkey brain and the six areas studied: areas V1, V2, V4, the lateral intraparietal sulcus (LIP), the frontal eye fields (FEFs), and the medial eye fields (MEFs). ce, central sulcus; p, principal sulcus; ip, intraparietal sulcus; sts, superior temporal sulcus; ls, lunate sulcus. The following steps were taken in experimental sessions: (1) The receptive field (RF) of the neurons recorded from was mapped. (2) The motor field (MF) was established by eliciting saccadic eye movements with electrical stimulation. (3) One target was then placed into the RF/MF that elicited saccades with the same vector. (4) Two targets were presented with varied temporal asynchronies with one of them placed into the RF/MF. (5) Four targets were presented, one of which was different from the others in luminance. The luminance, size, wavelength, and shape of the three identical distracters could be systematically varied. Data were collected pairing electrical stimulation with target presentation and examining the effects of infusing pharmacological agents.

The effects of the electrical stimulation at various current levels were examined in areas V1, LIP, the MEF, and the FEF (Schiller and Tehovnik 2001). For each curve shown, the current levels used are noted as is the percent of saccades elicited by the electrical stimulation when no visual target accompanied the stimulation (Figure 5.15, condition 2).

Examination of other structures using these procedures has revealed that electrical stimulation in the upper layers of V1 produces interference, and stimulation of the lower layers produces facilitation. Similar results have been obtained in area V2. Electrical stimulation of area V4 is largely ineffective in influencing target choice at current levels up to 150 µA.

In the LIP area, in addition to regions in which electrical stimulation elicits saccadic eye movements, neurons have been found that discharge vigorously while the animal maintains fixation. Such activity is largely independent of the orbital position of the eyes. Such neurons, which are found in batches in the LIP, were reported several years ago by Motter and Mountcastle (1981). They discharge during fixation irrespective of gaze angle. A saccadic eye movement arises when such cells stop discharging. Electrical stimulation in the LIP at these sites prolongs fixation time as made evident by the increased latencies with

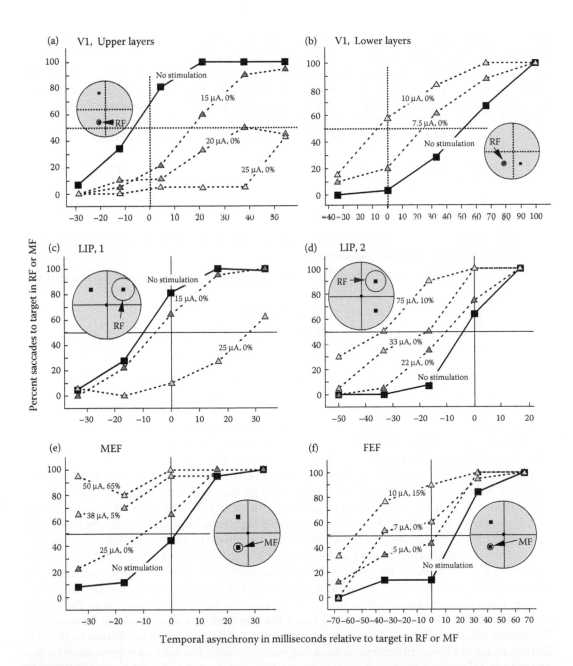

FIGURE 5.16
(See color insert.) The effects of electrical stimulation of area V1, the lateral intraparietal sulcus (LIP), the medial eye fields (MEFs), and the frontal eye fields (FEFs) on target selection using the two-target task. Plotted are curves showing the probability with which targets presented in the receptive field are chosen as a function of the temporal asynchrony of the two targets and the current of electrical stimulation used. The current levels used are indicated for each curve. The percent values that follow indicate the percent of saccades generated to electrical stimulation when it was administered in the absence of any target. The insets show the location of the receptive fields and the layout of the targets. RF, receptive field; MF, motor field. (a) Stimulation of the upper layers of V1 produces interference. (b) Stimulation of the lower layers of V1 produces interference. (c) In some regions of the LIP, stimulation produces interference. (d) In other regions of the LIP, facilitation is produced by electrical stimulation. (e) In the MEF, stimulation produces facilitation. (f) In the FEF, stimulation produces facilitation.

which saccades are initiated. This indicates that the LIP area plays a significant role in determining how long each fixation should be maintained.

Another interesting aspect of MEF stimulation is that when the eye is placed at the orbital position represented by the neurons to be stimulated by placing the fixation spot so as to create this orbital position, electrical stimulation keeps the eye at that position. The animal has difficulty initiating any eye movement under such conditions.

The results of the microstimulation studies may be summarized as follows:

1. Stimulation of the upper layers of V1 and V2 produces interference and of the lower layers produces facilitation.

2. Area V4 does not seem to play a direct role in saccade initiation or in target selection with saccadic eye movements.

3. Stimulation of some regions of the LIP produces facilitation whereas stimulation of other regions produces interference.

4. Stimulation of those regions of the LIP that contain fixation cells prolongs fixation time.

5. Stimulation of the FEF always produces facilitation.

6. Stimulation of the MEF produces facilitation when the target is in the terminal zone and produces increased fixation time when fixation spot is in the terminal zone.

These results suggest that the generation of saccadic eye movements involves several steps that include: (a) analysis of the visual scene, (b) selection of the target to be looked at next, (c) rejection of other targets, (d) decision as to when to initiate a saccade, and (e) computing the trajectory (size and direction) of an accurate saccadic vector.

The fact that electrical stimulation can produce not only facilitation but also interference in some brain regions suggests saccade generation involves interplay between excitatory and inhibitory neural circuits. This has already been shown to be the case in an elegant study by Hikosaka and Wurtz (1985). They showed that when inhibition is increased in the superior colliculus by infusion of gamma-aminobutyric acid (GABA) agonist muscimol, monkeys have great difficulties in generating saccades. Conversely, they showed that when the GABA antagonist bicuculline is infused into the superior colliculus, saccade production is increased; monkeys make irrepressible saccades with vectors that are represented by the disinhibited neurons in the superior colliculus. These findings are depicted schematically in Figure 5.17. Infusion is made into the superior colliculus, as shown on the top through a microelectrode. Electrical stimulation at that site establishes the saccadic vector coded by the neurons at the tip of the electrode, as shown on the bottom left. Following infusion of the GABA agonist muscimol, which increases inhibition in the colliculus, monkeys have difficulties generating saccades with the vectors represented by the neurons in this area. Conversely, when bicuculline is injected, which blocks GABAergic inhibition, many spontaneous saccades are produced with the vectors represented at the disinhibited site.

The role of cortical inhibitory circuits in vision and saccadic eye-movement generation has also been examined (Schiller and Tehovnik 2003). Figures 5.18 and 5.19 show the results of such experiments using the procedures described in Figure 5.15. Performance was assessed using the two-target task and the discrimination task as depicted in Figure 5.15, numbers 4 and 5.

Figure 5.18 shows performance on these two tasks when muscimol was infused into V1, the FEF, and the LIP. The dosages we used were 0.8 μL for V1, 0.5 μL for the FEF, and

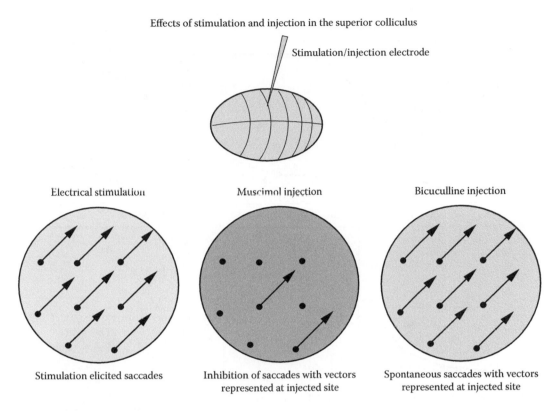

FIGURE 5.17
(See color insert.) Schematic of the effects of infusing muscimol or bicuculline into the superior colliculus on eye movements as reported by Hikosaka and Wurtz (1985). At the site of the electrode in the superior colliculus, saccades of a specific vector are elicited at low currents as shown on the left. After muscimol injection, few spontaneous saccades are made with that vector as shown in the center. After bicuculline injection, numerous spontaneous saccades are generated with the vector represented at that site.

1.5 μL for the LIP of a 0.5 μg/μL solution. Examination of the data for the two-target task shows that in both V1 and the FEF muscimol infusion produced a major interference effect (panels a and c): the target in the receptive fields of the infused neurons was chosen much less frequently after the infusion. In the LIP, however, only a mild effect was obtained even though a higher volume of muscimol was infused (panel e). With infusion levels similar to those at which major effects were obtained in V1 and the FEF, no effect was obtained in the LIP.

Performance on the discrimination task was devastated when muscimol was infused into V1 (panel b), but had only a small effect with FEF infusion (panel d) and no significant effect in the LIP (panel f).

Figure 5.19 shows what happens when these same areas are infused with the GABA antagonist bicuculline. In V1 this agent, just like muscimol, produced major interference in target selection and disrupted visual discrimination (panels a and b). By contrast, infusion of bicuculline into the FEF had a major facilitatory effect on the two-target task (panel c). The inset showing the eye movements demonstrates that the monkey after the infusion made many irrepressible saccades. On the discrimination task performance was unaffected, indicating that the monkey's ability to process visual information was not affected

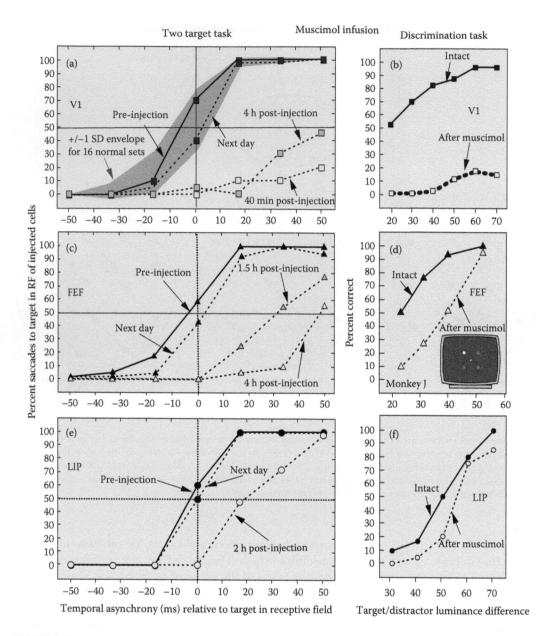

FIGURE 5.18

The effects of infusing muscimol into areas V1, lateral intraperietal sulcus (LIP), and frontal eye field (FEF) on the two-target task and the discrimination task. Plotted on the left (two-target task: a, c, and e) is the percent of time the target presented in the receptive and motor fields of the neurons was chosen as a function of the temporal asynchrony between the two targets. Muscimol injections in V1 were 0.8 μL, in the FEF 0.5 μL, and in the LIP 1.5 μL of 0.5 μg/μL solution. Each data point shown in the graphs (here and in all other figures) is based on a minimum of 20 and a maximum of 100 trials. Each block had 15 conditions consisting of 8 single targets presented at 4 target locations and 7 paired targets presented with various temporal asynchronies. On the right (discrimination task: b, d, and f) the effects of muscimol infusion on the concurrently collected brightness discrimination task are shown. Inset in the center panel shows the brightness discrimination task. The percent contrast difference between the target (bright stimulus) and the distracters was presented in a randomized order. The luminance of the background and the target was kept constant. In area V1, the muscimol infusion produced a significant loss in the ability to discriminate brightness differences. In the FEF and LIP, the infusion produced only a mild deficit.

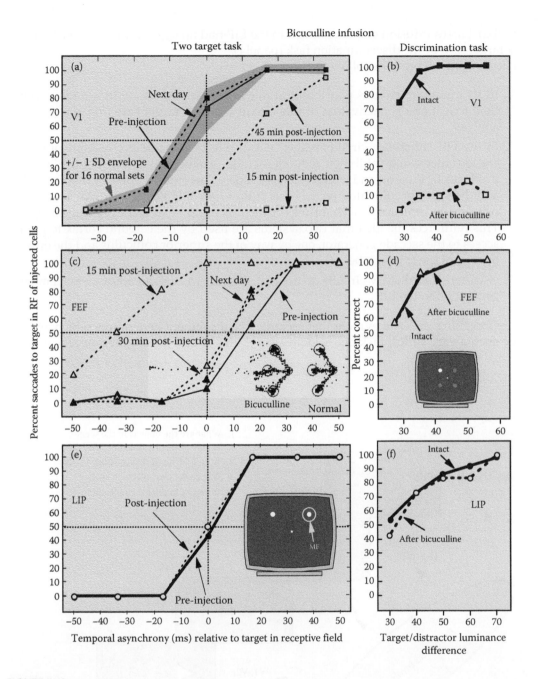

FIGURE 5.19

The effects of infusing bicuculline into areas V1, lateral intraprietal sulcus (LIP), and frontal eye field (FEF) on the two-target task and the discrimination task. On the left (two-target task: a, c, and e) plotted is the percent of time the target presented in the receptive and motor fields of the neurons is chosen as a function of the temporal asynchrony between the two targets. Bicuculline injections in V1 were 0.5 μL, in the FEF 0.3 μL, and in the LIP 0.4 μL of 1 μg/μL solution. In V1, the bicuculline infusion produced a major deficit. In the FEF, the infusion produced facilitation and irrepressible saccades. In the LIP, the infusion was ineffective. On the right (discrimination task: b, d, and f) the effects of bicuculline infusion on the concurrently collected brightness discrimination task are shown. In V1 the infusion caused a major deficit in visual discrimination whereas in the FEF and LIP the infusion had no effect on this task. Each data point is based on 20 to 100 trials.

(panel d). Lastly, infusion of bicuculline into the LIP had no significant effect on either the two-target task or the discrimination task (panel f).

These results suggest the following:

1. In V1 inhibitory circuits play a central role in processing visual information such that activation or inactivation of this circuit disrupts target selection and visual analysis.

2. In the FEF inhibitory circuits play a central role in saccadic eye-movement generation. Increasing inhibition reduces saccade production; decreasing inhibition produces facilitation and irrepressible saccades. Therefore, it appears that the FEF and the superior colliculus, on the basis of the work of Hikosaka and Wurtz (1985), use similar inhibitory mechanisms for the execution of saccadic eye movements. This reinforces the idea that two systems are used by the cerebral cortex to gain access to the saccade generator, one by way of the superior colliculus and the other by way of the frontal lobe.

3. GABAergic inhibitory circuits do not play a direct role in saccadic eye-movement generation in the LIP.

The foregoing makes it evident that saccadic eye-movement generation, which appears to be such a very simple task one seldom even thinks about, is a highly complex process.

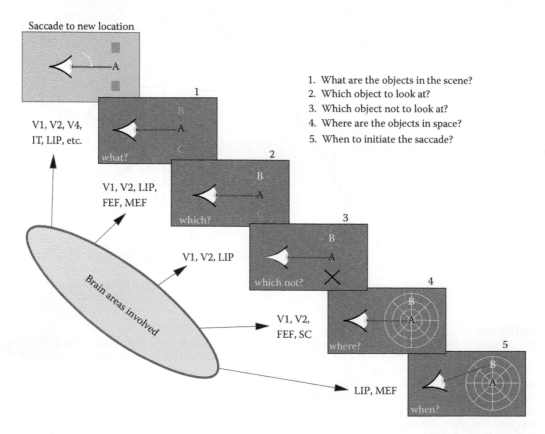

FIGURE 5.20
(See color insert.) Schematic representation of the tasks involved in generating a saccadic eye movement.

It involves numerous brain areas that interact utilizing both excitatory and inhibitory circuits to yield the decisions involved in the generation of accurate eye movements to desired target locations that then allows detailed, fine-grain analysis of the visual percept at that site.

The basic tasks and neural structures involved in the execution of saccadic eye movements are depicted in Figure 5.20. Beginning with a fixation at a specific location in space (A) the visual scene is rapidly analyzed to determine, at a coarse level, what the essential objects are and where they are located. The second step involves a decision to be made as to which object the center of gaze should be shifted with the next saccadic eye movement. This decision process also necessitates a decision as to which objects not to look at. This is necessary for the activation of inhibitory circuits that make it possible to assure accurate saccade generation. The processing of the location of the objects in space coded in topographic sensory and motor maps is another important step as depicted in number 4. The last step involves a decision as to when to initiate the eye movement, which presumably will take place after the objects in the center of gaze have been satisfactorily processed.

The numerous brain areas involved are listed in red. Actually several additional areas contribute to these processes, which have not been dealt with in this chapter. Such areas include V4, MT, MST, the inferotemporal cortex, and several frontal cortical areas in addition to the FEF and MEF.

A schematic diagram of the brain areas involved and their interconnections is shown in Figure 5.21. Depicted here are the several parallel pathways that originate in the retina that project to the visual cortex through the lateral geniculate nucleus and to the superior

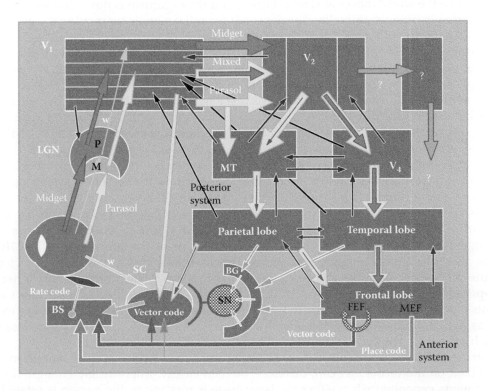

FIGURE 5.21
(See color insert.) The neural structures and circuitry involved in the generation of visually guided saccadic eye movements.

colliculus. The visual information then passes through several parallel channels to V2, V4, and MT and from there proceed to the parietal, temporal, and frontal lobes. From these regions information is sent to the superior colliculus and, also, directly to the brainstem oculomotor centers from the frontal lobe. Feedback circuits as well as inhibitory circuits are prominent throughout.

5.7 Tracking Eye Movements for Image Stabilization

The next three sections will deal with three aspects of tracking eye movements. In this section, eye movements to stabilize the images on the retina will be considered.

The movement by living organisms in the world is pervasive. Two major systems combat the blurring of visual images on the retina that would occur under such conditions without them: the vestibular system and the accessory optic system.

Neurons from the semicircular canals of the vestibular system make connections with the extraocular muscles through the brainstem oculomotor complex with just a few synaptic connections. The neural signals generated produce extremely rapid eye-movement responses that result in counter rotating the eye with respect to the motion of the head, resulting in the stabilization of the eye with respect to the world.

The accessory optic system produces the visual signals that contribute to this stabilization. When the world moves at slow velocities and the organism is not in motion, it is this system that in many mammalian species sends essential signals for moving the eyes so as to stabilize them with respect to the visual scene.

These two systems are interlinked, as will be described next. An example of this interlinking can readily be experienced when one goes to a 360-degree cinema as seen, for example, in Disney parks. At such panoramic cinemas, there are typically rails to which one is admonished to hang on. The reason is that when the world begins to move and seems to tilt by virtue of the film shown projected all the way around the 360-degree screen, there is a strong tendency to lose one's balance. This is because the brain under these conditions receives conflicting signals from the vestibular and accessory optic systems.

To better understand the eye movements that arise when either the organism or a large portion of the visual scene is in motion, experiments can be carried out in which a person is placed into a round enclosure that allows one to rotate either the person or the walls of this enclosure. This can be done quite simply actually by just about anyone by using a rotating chair and a large lampshade with displays on it such as vertical stripes. This arrangement makes it possible to rotate either the chair or the lampshade. When this is done, the horizontal eye-movement signals obtained look much like those depicted in Figure 5.22a. Schematically shown in this figure is how the eyes move when either the lampshade or the subject is moved at three different velocities. Two kinds of eye movements can be seen: the slow phase of tracking movements, often called pursuit eye movements, which follow the moving edges, and the fast phase of saccadic eye movements, which arise once the eye has deviated in orbit and needs to be reset.

During the slow phase of pursuit eye movements the stripes on the lampshade are stabilized on the retina and can, therefore, be seen clearly. Interestingly enough, the eye movements generated when either the lampshade is rotating or the person is rotated are quite similar. But they do have different names as they are initiated by different receptor organs. The eye movement generated when the lampshade is moving and the person is

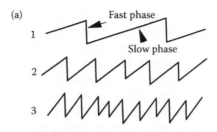

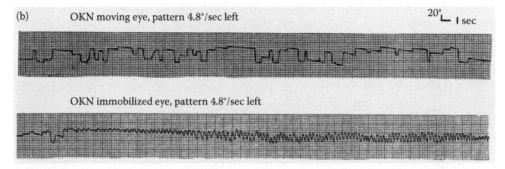

FIGURE 5.22

(a) Schematic representation of nystagmic eye movements produced by a set of moving vertical bars either while a subject is stationary or while the subject is rotated and the bars are stationary using three different velocities. The slow phase on the nystagmus occurs during tracking. The fast phase resets the eye with saccadic eye movements. (b) Horizontal eye movements shown for a monkey with one eye immobilized. The top trace shows the eye movements of the normal eye to a set of vertical stripes presented to that eye moving 4.8 degrees per second. The bottom trace shows the eye movements of the same eye when the moving stripes are presented only to the immobilized eye. The velocity of tracking is constant and accurate when the stripes are seen by the normal eye and rapidly increases when presented to the immobilized eye.

stable is called optokinetic nystagmus; it is initiated by the visual input. The eye movement generated when the person is rotating and the lampshade is stationary is referred to as vestibulo-ocular nystagmus; it is initiated in a reflex-like manner by the semicircular canals. This, as already noted, is a very rapidly conducting pathway that can start the eyes moving in less than 10 milliseconds after the head begins to rotate.

The manner in which the vestibulo-ocular reflex operates to produce vestibular nystagmus has been extensively studied. One of the interesting questions investigators had asked is: how can this system accurately stabilize the eyes with respect to the world for one's entire lifetime? To do so, the vestibulo-ocular reflex must have a gain of 1; thus when the head moves, the eye is counter-rotated so as to keep the center of gaze stationary with respect to the visual scene. It turns out that the gain of the reflex can be changed by exposing the organism to different situations (Miles 1983). It has been shown, for example, that if one wears lenses that magnify or minify the image, the gain of the reflex changes accordingly so that, once again, the eyes become stabilized with respect to the world when the head is rotated while one is wearing the lenses; apparently, the gain can be doubled or halved within a few days by continuously wearing a set of lenses. This suggests that under normal circumstances inputs from the visual system can adjust the vestibulo-ocular reflex so as to have a gain of 1. The cerebellum plays an important role in this process. It has been shown that selected lesions of the cerebellum reduce or eliminate the ability to adjust, or modify the grain of the vestibulo-ocular reflex (Robinson 1976).

In contrast to eye movements triggered by the vestibular system, visually triggered pursuit movements have a much longer onset latency. However, this latency, as shown in Figure 5.1, is still quite a bit shorter than the latency with which saccadic eye movements are generated. The difference in latency between smooth-pursuit eye movements elicited by the vestibular and the visual systems can be readily experienced. If one takes a lined pad placed sideways so that the lines run vertically, rocking the head back and forth sideways keeps the vertical lines in sharp focus up to relatively high velocities owing to the input from the vestibular system that counter-rotates the eye. When instead the head is kept stable and the pad is moved back and forth horizontally, the image will start to blur at much lower velocities. In this case, stabilization is accomplished by the accessory optic system; blurring arises because of the slower velocities with which the visual information can be transferred into motor signals to move the eyes.

For the most part, the generation of tracking eye movements, even as seen under conditions of nystagmus as just described, can occur effectively only when visual or vestibular information is continuously supplied. It is next to impossible to will smooth pursuit in the absence of visual or vestibular input. When pursuit is initiated to a moving target, after a very brief period, the velocity of the eye movement matches the velocity of the target so that its image remains accurately within the fovea. This condition is referred to as pursuit maintenance or closed-loop operation (Keller and Heinen 1991; Koerner and Schiller 1972). One can artificially open the loop by decoupling the eye movements from the movement of the visual scene. What happens under such conditions is quite curious. In one set of experiments investigators immobilized one eye to which moving targets were presented while measuring the movement of the other eye, which is occluded. TerBraak (1936) was the first person to do this clever manipulation in the rabbit. Subsequently, this has also been done in the monkey by immobilizing one eye by transecting the third, fourth, and sixth cranial nerves (Koerner and Schiller 1972). Eye movements for the occluded intact eye were then generated by presenting evenly spaced black and white vertical stripes to the immobilized eye at a slow, steady velocity. Such stripes are excellent for producing optokinetic nystagmus. When this is done, the movement of the intact eye gradually increases in velocity until it exceeds the rate of target movement several-fold. This is demonstrated in Figure 5.22b. Eye tracking is shown for the moving eye when the moving visual stripes are presented to that eye, as shown in the upper trace, and when they are shown to the immobilized eye. The velocity of the tracking eye movements (the slow phase) is constant and keeps the stripes accurately positioned on the retinal surface. When the display is presented to the immobilized eye, there is a gradual increase in the tracking velocity. The question is: why does the intact eye "run away" under this condition generally called the open-loop condition? Without going into technical details, it can be said that the position of the target, in this case a vertical edge, is continuously monitored by the visual system relative to the position of the fovea. The disposition is to minimize the error between the two. This error keeps increasing as the eye is immobilized; therefore, a central processor sends a command to the motor plant to increase the rate of tracking. Continued lack of success in catching the moving target results in further signals to increase the speed of the pursuit. From this it is clear that the tracking system at large has several components, some of which deal with the velocity and direction of the moving visual scene, some of which generate the motor commands to move the eyes, and some of which assess the accuracy of the tracking process.

The visual signals involved in the generation of optokinetic nystagmus and pursuit tracking of objects come predominantly from direction and velocity-selective neurons found in the retina and in many other parts of the visual system. The accessory optic system makes a central contribution to this process; it is involved in the stabilization of the eye with respect to the visual scene at slow velocities of movement. The accessory optic system has been studied most extensively in the rabbit, but has also been explored in birds and cats (Collewijn 1975; Karten, Fite, and Brecha 1983; Simpson 1984). In the rabbit there are approximately 350,000 ganglion cells in each eye. A small subgroup of these, some 6000 to 7000 cells, are the displaced cells of Dogiel. These cells are called "displaced" because their cell bodies, instead of being in the ganglion-cell layer, are closer to the cell bodies of the amacrine cells in the inner plexiform layer of the retina, and "Dogiel" after the person who discovered them.

Physiological studies of the cells of Dogiel of the rabbit have established that these cells respond in a directionally selective manner and do so to slow velocities ranging between 0.1 and 1.0 degree per second. Furthermore, examination of the distribution of direction selectivities reveals that the prime axes form three lobes, as shown on the top left of Figure 5.23. What is remarkable about this layout is that these three lobes correspond to the direction of action of the semicircular canals indicated on the bottom right of the figure. The cells of Dogiel project to the three terminal nuclei in the anterior portion of the midbrain—the dorsal, medial, and the lateral. From here cells project to the dorsal cap of Kooy in the inferior olive which in turn has cells whose axons form one set of climbing fibers that project to the cerebellum. Another group of direction-selective cells in the retina projects to the nucleus of the optic tract and is part of the same circuit although the cells here are selective for more rapid velocities of movement. The relevant portions of the circuit then project from the cerebellum to the vestibular nuclei which, of course, as the name implies, receive a major input from the semicircular canals. The circuit is completed by the projections from the vestibular nucleus to the brainstem where connections are made with the brainstem oculomotor centers to generate the appropriate eye movements.

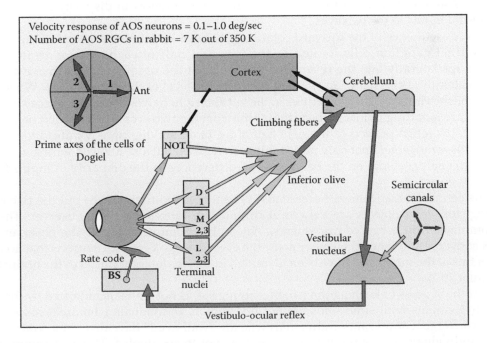

FIGURE 5.23

(See color insert.) Diagram of the structures and connections involved in eye stabilization by the accessory optic system. NOT, nucleus of the optic tract; BS, brain stem; D, dorsal; M, medial; L, lateral terminal nuclei.

Simpson (1984) conjectured that these two systems, the vestibular and the accessory optic, enable the organism to stabilize the eyes over the great range of velocities encountered in real life. At very low velocities the vestibular system works poorly; hence the accessory optic system, beginning with the retinal direction selective cells, provides the crucial information for eye stabilization. At higher velocities, the vestibular system kicks in and stabilizes the eyes with respect to the visual scene by virtue of the signals generated in the semicircular canals. The vestibular system, however, can stabilize the eyes only when the organism is in motion. To stabilize the objects in the visual scene when they move at higher velocities, yet another system is needed.

5.8 Eye Movements That Keep the Two Eyes in Register

In most vertebrate animals at lower levels of the phylogenetic scale, the two eyes perceive different portions of the world; the left eye perceives the visual scene to the left of the animal and the right eye the visual scene to the right. There is relatively little binocular overlap. In such animals, the retinal ganglion cells of each eye cross over almost entirely at the level of the optic chiasm, thereby sending the signals from the left eye to the right half of the brain and the signals from the right eye to the left half of the brain. In some animals, such as the chameleon, the two eyes move about independently. A major evolutionary change occurred in higher mammals. The eyes moved to the front. Sacrificed in this process was the ability to perceive the visual scene behind the head. But what was gained was obviously of great benefit: one of these is the ability to process depth information well by virtue of stereopsis which hinges on analyzing the differences in disparity produced by the visual inputs to the two eyes.

As a consequence of the forward rotation of the eye, a major change in wiring arose: The retinal ganglion cells located in the temporal half of each eye are arranged to project ipsilaterally and the retinal ganglion cells of the nasal half of each eye project contralaterally. This change in crossing occurs at the level of the optic chiasm. What this accomplishes is that visual structures in the left and right halves of the brain receive input from corresponding points in the visual scene from the two eyes. Thus, the left hemifield through the retina projects to the right half of the brain and the right hemifield to the left half. This arrangement not only placed things in register, but also allowed wiring arrangements to analyze depth on the basis of small differences in the disparity of inputs from the two eyes.

This complex arrangement necessitated yet another requirement: to put the two eyes in register when objects are viewed at different distances from the observer. This is accomplished by vergence movements. When objects move closer to the observer the eyes converge and when they move away the eyes diverge. Vergence neurons that accomplish this at the motor end have been identified in the oculomotor nuclei of the brainstem (Schiller 1970).

That the process of keeping the two eyes in register is not trivial is indicated by the fact that individuals with strabismus are not uncommon. Individuals who are "cross-eyed" have convergent strabismus; individuals who are "wall-eyed" have divergent strabismus. Such individuals have a problem to solve: how not to see double. This is accomplished either by suppressing the input from one of the eyes or by alternating between the two eyes in analyzing the visual scene. Such individuals typically are stereoblind.

5.9 Smooth-Pursuit Tracking of Moving Visual Objects

The tracking of moving visual objects by smooth-pursuit eye movements is an essential part of eye-movement control. To be able to analyze fine detail in objects that move, for example, the center of gaze needs to be maintained on that object. For example, when we wish to identify the species of the bird that flies in the sky, we need to track it. Several neural mechanisms in addition to the ones we have so far discussed are involved in this process. Single-cell recordings, microstimulation, and lesion studies have made significant contributions toward the understanding of eye-movement tracking.

Two of the cortical regions involved in this process are the areas MT and MST. Studies have shown that electrical stimulation in these areas during active pursuit accelerates the pursuit speed when the eye moves toward the side of the brain that is being stimulated. Conversely, when the eye pursues a target that is moving away from that side, the pursuit movement of the eye is slowed down (Komatsu and Wurtz 1989). Both of these conditions lead to retinal slip; the retinal error so produced is often reduced by initiation of a saccadic eye movement. Stimulation of these brain sites during fixation has little effect. Similar results have also been obtained with stimulation of various pontine nuclei implicated in the generation of smooth-pursuit eye movements (May, Keller, and Crandall 1985; Suzuki et al. 1990).

As one might expect on the basis of these considerations, inactivation of areas MT and MST should produce deficits in the execution of accurate smooth-pursuit eye movements. This is indeed the case. After such inactivation, monkeys tend to compensate by making repeated saccadic eye movements to catch up to targets that are in motion (Newsome and Wurtz 1988). Interestingly enough, though, the deficits seen after MT and MST lesions are transitory. Even with relatively large lesions there is striking recovery after 3 months (Yamasaki and Wurtz 1991). Similar deficits and recovery have been reported for lesions made in the pontine nuclei (May and Keller 1988; May, Keller, and Suzuki 1988).

The relatively rapid recovery after these lesions suggests that several pathways and neural structures must be involved in smooth-pursuit tracking of moving objects in the visual scene. Indeed, single-cell recording work has shown that cells responding during pursuit can be seen in area 7a of the parietal lobe, in the FEFs and in the dorsomedial frontal cortex (Hyvarinen and Poranen 1974; MacAvoy, Gottlieb, and Bruce 1991; Mountcastle et al. 1975). Lesion work has shown pursuit deficits after FEF lesions (Lynch 1987). Anatomical work supports the possibility that the signals necessary for pursuit can bypass area MT and MST. For example, areas V2 and V3, where direction-selective cells are common, could supply the visual signals necessary and send them to the FEFs or to the dorsomedial frontal cortex. From there the information could be channeled down to the pons and then of course to the brainstem. These considerations highlight the fact that the execution of most tasks involves several pathways. Such an arrangement often makes it possible to survive unscathed when various portions of the brain are damaged or at least to effectuate considerable recovery over time.

5.10 Summary

In this chapter, the neural mechanisms underlying visually guided saccadic eye movements and tracking eye movements have been delineated. While the neurons in the oculomotor, trochlear, and abducens nuclei control both saccadic and tracking eye movements conjointly, in higher brain areas for the most part these two types of eye movements are controlled by different neural systems.

The networks controlling visually guided saccadic eye movements appear to form two major systems: the anterior and the posterior. The posterior system consists of the visual pathways originating in the retina that pass through the lateral geniculate nucleus on the way to the visual cortex from where outputs stream to the superior colliculus and then to the brainstem oculomotor complex. This posterior system utilizes a vector code that computes predominantly a retinal error signal. The anterior system of visually guided saccadic eye movements receives input from the occipital, parietal, and temporal cortices and consists of two subdivisions, one of which passes through the FEFs and the other through the dorsomedial frontal cortex (MEFs). The subdivision of which the FEFs are a part also carries a vector code. In contrast, the subdivision that passes through the dorsomedial frontal cortex carries a place code. The posterior system appears to play an important role in the generation of rapid, reflex-like eye movements called express saccades that enable the organism to respond quickly to suddenly appearing visual stimuli. In line with this view is the fact that express saccades are eliminated by lesions of the superior colliculus. The portion of the anterior subsystem that involves the FEFs is believed to contribute to higher-level eye-movement generation important for object selection and for planning sequences of eye movements. The portion of the anterior subsystem that includes the dorsomedial frontal cortex is believed to integrate information about the location of objects in space and also plays a role in hand–eye coordination as well as visuo-motor learning.

Tracking eye movements perform several tasks, three of which had been noted. The first task is image stabilization that involves the vestibular system and the accessory optic system. The vestibulo-ocular reflex assures rapid, short-latency stabilization whereas the accessory optic system, which receives its prime visual input from the retinal ganglion cells of Dogiel, stabilizes the eye at low velocities of motion. The vestibular and accessory optic systems are interlinked. The visual input sets the gain of the vestibulo-ocular reflex to assure accurate stabilization over time. The second task is to keep the two eyes in register to allow for integrated vision in the two eyes. The third system involves the smooth-pursuit tracking of objects when there is motion. This system can analyze several different kinds of motion including those that necessitate interpretation of the scene in depth. Several cortical areas are involved, as a result of which lesions to any one of them produce neither unique nor long-term deficits in smooth pursuit.

Inhibitory circuits play a central role in eye-movement generation. Such circuits for saccadic eye movement generation allow for target selection and the execution of accurate saccadic eye movements to the target chosen to which the center of gaze is to be shifted at the end of each fixation. Many of these circuits involve GABAergic neurons.

References

Bizzi, E. 1967. Discharge of frontal eye field neurons during eye movements in unanesthetized monkeys. *Science* 157 (796): 1588–90.

Bruce, C. J. and M. E. Goldberg. 1984. Physiology of the frontal eye fields. *Trends in Neurosciences* 7 (11): 436–41.

Chen, L. L. and S. P. Wise. 1995a. Neuronal activity in the supplementary eye field during acquisition of conditional oculomotor associations. *Journal of Neurophysiology* 73 (3): 1101–21.

Chen, L. L. and S. P. Wise. 1995b. Supplementary eye field contrasted with the frontal eye field during acquisition of conditional oculomotor associations. *Journal of Neurophysiology* 73 (3): 1122–34.

Collewijn, H. 1975. Oculomotor areas in the rabbits midbrain and pretectum. *Journal of Neurobiology* 6 (1): 3–22.

Dias, E. C., M. Kiesau, and M. A. Segraves. 1995. Acute activation and inactivation of macaque frontal eye field with GABA-related drugs. *Journal of Neurophysiology* 74 (6): 2744–8.

Drager, U. C. and D. H. Hubel. 1975. Responses to visual stimulation and relationship between visual, auditory, and somatosensory inputs in mouse superior colliculus. *Journal of Neurophysiology* 38 (3): 690–713.

Fischer, B. and R. Boch. 1983. Saccadic eye movements after extremely short reaction times in the monkey. *Brain Research* 260 (1): 21–6.

Fuchs, A. F., C. R. Kaneko, and C. A. Scudder. 1985. Brainstem control of saccadic eye movements. *Annual Review of Neuroscience* 8: 307–37.

Hanes, D. P. and R. H. Wurtz. 2001. Interaction of the frontal eye field and superior colliculus for saccade generation. *Journal of Neurophysiology* 85 (2): 804–15.

Hikosaka, O. and R. H. Wurtz. 1985. Modification of saccadic eye movements by GABA-related substances. I. Effect of muscimol and bicuculline in monkey superior colliculus. *Journal of Neurophysiology* 53 (1): 266–91.

Hyvarinen, J. and A. Poranen. 1974. Function of the parietal associative area 7 as revealed from cellular discharges in alert monkeys. *Brain* 97 (4): 673–92.

Kanaseki, T. and J. M. Sprague. 1974. Anatomical organization of pretectal nuclei and tectal laminae in the cat. *Journal of Comparative Neurology* 158 (3): 319–37.

Karten, H. J., K. V. Fite, and N. Brecha. 1983. Specific projection of displaced retinal ganglion cells upon the accessory optic system in the pigeon (*Columbia livia*). *Proceedings of the National Academy of Sciences of the United States of America* 74: 1753–6.

Keating, E. G., S. G. Gooley, S. E. Pratt, and J. E. Kelsey. 1983. Removing the superior colliculus silences eye movements normally evoked from stimulation of the parietal and occipital eye fields. *Brain Research* 269 (1): 145–8.

Keller, E. L. and S. J. Heinen. 1991. Generation of smooth-pursuit eye movements: Neuronal mechanisms and pathways. *Neuroscience Research* 11 (2): 79–107.

Koerner, F. and P. H. Schiller. 1972. The optokinetic response under open and closed loop conditions in the monkey. *Experimental Brain Research* 14 (3): 318–30.

Komatsu, H. and R. H. Wurtz. 1989. Modulation of pursuit eye movements by stimulation of cortical areas MT and MST. *Journal of Neurophysiology* 62 (1): 31–47.

Lynch, J. C. 1987. Frontal eye field lesions in monkeys disrupt visual pursuit. *Experimental Brain Research* 68 (2): 437–41.

MacAvoy, M. G., J. P. Gottlieb, and C. J. Bruce. 1991. Smooth-pursuit eye movement representation in the primate frontal eye field. *Cerebral Cortex* 1 (1): 95–102.

Mann, S. E., R. Thau, and P. H. Schiller. 1988. Conditional task-related responses in monkey dorsomedial frontal cortex. *Experimental Brain Research* 69 (3): 460–8.

May, J. G. and E. L. Keller. 1988. Recovery from smooth pursuit impairments after successive unilateral and bilateral chemical lesions in the dorsolateral pontine nucleus of the monkey. In *Post-Lesion Neural Plasticity*, edited by H. Flohr, 413–20. Berlin: Springer-Verlag.

May, J. G., E. L. Keller, and W. F. Crandall. 1985. Changes in eye velocity during smooth pursuit tracking induced by microstimulation in the dorsolateral pontine nucleus of the macaque. *Society for Neuroscience Abstracts* 11: 79.

May, J. G., E. L. Keller, and D. A. Suzuki. 1988. Smooth-pursuit eye movement deficits with chemical lesions in the dorsolateral pontine nucleus of the monkey. *Journal of Neurophysiology* 59 (3): 952–77.

Miles, F. A. 1983. Plasticity in the transfer of gaze. *Trends in Neuroscience Research* 6: 57–60.

Miles, F. A., K. Kawano, and L. M. Optican. 1986. Short-latency ocular following responses of monkey. I. Dependence on temporospatial properties of visual input. *Journal of Neurophysiology* 56 (5): 1321–54.

Motter, B. C. and V. B. Mountcastle. 1981. The functional properties of the light-sensitive neurons of the posterior parietal cortex studied in waking monkeys: Foveal sparing and opponent vector organization. *Journal of Neuroscience* 1 (1): 3–26.

Mountcastle, V. B., J. C. Lynch, A. Georgopoulos, H. Sakata, and C. Acuna. 1975. Posterior parietal association cortex of the monkey: Command functions for operations within extrapersonal space. *Journal of Neurophysiology* 38 (4): 871–908.

Newsome, W. T. and R. H. Wurtz. 1988. Probing visual cortical function with discrete chemical lesions. *Trends in Neuroscience* 11 (9): 394–400.

Rashbass, C. 1961. The relationship between saccadic and smooth tracking eye movements. *Journal of Physiology (London)* 159: 326–38.

Robinson, D. A. 1972. Eye movements evoked by collicular stimulation in the alert monkey. *Vision Research* 12 (11): 1795–808.

Robinson, D. A. 1975. Oculomotor control signals. In *Basic Mechanisms of Ocular Motility and their Clinical Implications*, edited by G. Lennerstrand and P. Bach-y-Rita, 337–374. Oxford: Pergamon.

Robinson, D. A. 1976. Adaptive gain control of vestibulocular reflex by the cerebellum. *Journal of Neurophysiology* 39 (5): 954–69.

Robinson, D. A. and A. F. Fuchs. 1969. Eye movements evoked by stimulation of frontal eye fields. *Journal of Neurophysiology* 32 (5): 637–48.

Schall, J. D. 1991a. Neuronal activity related to visually guided saccadic eye movements in the supplementary motor area of rhesus monkeys. *Journal of Neurophysiology* 66 (2): 530–8.

Schall, J. D. 1991b. Neuronal activity related to visually guided saccades in the frontal eye fields of rhesus monkeys: Comparison with supplementary eye fields. *Journal of Neurophysiology* 66 (2): 559–79.

Schiller, P. H. 1970. The discharge characteristics of single units in the oculomotor and abducens nuclei of the unanesthetized monkey. *Experimental Brain Research* 10 (4): 347–62.

Schiller, P. H. 1977. The effect of superior colliculus ablation on saccades elicted by cortical stimulation. *Brain Research* 122 (1): 154–6.

Schiller, P. H. 1984. The superior colliculus and visual function. In *Handbook of Physiology, Section 1, The Nervous System*, edited by I. Darian-Smith, 457–505. New York: Oxford University Press.

Schiller, P. H. and I. H. Chou. 1998. The effects of frontal eye field and dorsomedial frontal cortex lesions on visually guided eye movements. *Nature Neuroscience* 1 (3): 248–53.

Schiller, P. H. and F. Koerner. 1971. Discharge characteristics of single units in superior colliculus of the alert rhesus monkey. *Journal of Neurophysiology* 34 (5): 920–36.

Schiller, P. H. and N. K. Logothetis. 1987. The effect of frontal eye field and superior colliculus lesions on saccadic and pursuit eye-movement initiation. *Association for Research in Vision and Ophthalmology* 303: 11.

Schiller, P. H. and J. H. Sandell. 1983. Interactions between visually and electrically elicited saccades before and after superior colliculus and frontal eye field ablations in the rhesus monkey. *Experimental Brain Research* 49 (3): 381–92.

Schiller, P. H. and M. Stryker. 1972. Single-unit recording and stimulation in superior colliculus of the alert rhesus monkey. *Journal of Neurophysiology* 35 (6): 915–24.

Schiller, P. H., M. Stryker. M. Cynader, and N. Berman. 1974. Response characteristics of single cells in the monkey superior colliculus following ablation or cooling of visual cortex. *Journal of Neurophysiology* 37: 181–84.

Schiller, P. H. and E. J. Tehovnik. 2001. Look and see: How the brain moves your eyes about: Chapter 9. In *Vision: From Neurons to Cognition. Progress in Brain Research*, Volume 134, edited by C. Casanova and M. Ptito. 127–42. Amsterdam: Elsevier.

Schiller, P. H. and E. J. Tehovnik. 2003. Cortical inhibitory circuits in eye-movement generation. *European Journal of Neuroscience* 18 (11): 3127–33.

Schiller, P. H., S. D. True, and J. L. Conway. 1980. Deficits in eye movements following frontal eye-field and superior colliculus ablations. *Journal of Neurophysiology* 44 (6): 1175–89.

Schlag, J., M. Schlag-Rey, and I. Pigarev. 1992. Supplementary eye field: Influence of eye position on neural signals of fixation. *Experimental Brain Research* 90 (2): 302–6.

Sekuler, R. and R. Blake. 1990. The Human Eye. In *Perception*, 2nd ed., edited by B. R. Fetterolf and T. Holton, 23–60. New York: McGraw-Hill Publishing.

Simpson, J. I. 1984. The accessory optic system. *Annual Review of Neuroscience* 7: 13–41.

Sommer, M. A. and E. J. Tehovnik. 1999. Reversible inactivation of macaque dorsomedial frontal cortex: Effects on saccades and fixations. *Experimental Brain Research* 124 (4): 429–46.

Sparks, D. L. 1986. Translation of sensory signals into commands for control of saccadic eye movements: Role of primate superior colliculus. *Physiological Review* 66 (1): 118–71.

Sprague, J. M., G. Berlucchi, and G. Rizzolatti. 1973. The role of the superior colliculus and pretectum in vision and visually guided behavior. In *Handbook of Sensory Physiology*, Volume VII/3B edited by R. Jung, 27–101. Berlin: Springer-Verlag.

Stein, B. E., B. Magalhaes-Castro, and L. Kruger. 1976. Relationship between visual and tactile representations in cat superior colliculus. *Journal of Neurophysiology* 39 (2): 401–19.

Suzuki, D. A., J. G. May, E. L. Keller, and R. D. Yee. 1990. Visual motion response properties of neurons in dorsolateral pontine nucleus of alert monkey. *Journal of Neurophysiology* 63 (1): 37–59.

Tanji, J. and K. Kurata. 1982. Comparison of movement-related activity in two cortical motor areas of primates. *Journal of Neurophysiology* 48 (3): 633–53.

Tanji, J. and K. Shima. 1994. Role for supplementary motor area cells in planning several movements ahead. *Nature* 371 (6496): 413–6.

Tehovnik, E. J. 1995. The dorsomedial frontal cortex: Eye and forelimb fields. *Behavioral Brain Research* 67 (2): 147–63.

Tehovnik, E. J. and K. Lee. 1993. The dorsomedial frontal cortex of the rhesus monkey: Topographic representation of saccades evoked by electrical stimulation. *Experimental Brain Research* 96 (3): 430–42.

TerBraak, J. W. G. 1936. Untersuchungen uber optokinetischen nystagmus. *Archives Neerlandaises de Physiologie* 21: 308–76.

Wickelgren, B. G. and P. Sterling. 1969. Influence of visual cortex on receptive fields in the superior colliculus of the cat. *Journal of Neurophysiology* 32 (1): 16–23.

Wurtz, R. H. and J. E. Albano. 1980. Visual-motor function of the primate superior colliculus. *Annual Review of Neuroscience* 3: 189–226.

Wurtz, R. H. and M. E. Goldberg. 1972. Activity of superior colliculus in behaving monkey. 3. Cells discharging before eye movements. *Journal of Neurophysiology* 35 (4): 575–86.

Yamasaki, D. S. and R. H. Wurtz. 1991. Recovery of function after lesions in the superior temporal sulcus in the monkey. *Journal of Neurophysiology* 66 (3): 651–73.

6

Sleep Deprivation and Error Negativity: A Review and Reappraisal

Shulan Hsieh

CONTENTS

6.1 Introduction

Performance monitoring is an aspect of cognitive control that is crucial to optimal task performance. Error monitoring is a major domain of performance monitoring. In everyday life, people commit action slips that indicate losses of intentional control. Reason (1979) argues that "central to the notion of error is the failure of 'planned actions' to achieve a desired outcome" (p. 69). The key factor mediating action slips is the lack of close monitoring of ongoing activity by attentional control, even in a well-learned and familiar situation. In addition, these lapses also occur when exercising any well-learned behavior in daily life, particularly in states of reduced arousal and attention, such as during periods of extended wakefulness or sleep deprivation. Learning from errors is also critical to almost every newly learned psychomotor and cognitive behavior. When errors are detected during or after their commission, based on self-generated feed-forward and feedback information and/or externally provided feedback information, post-error remedies and adjustments become critical to achieving the intended goal.

In modern society, there are not only increasing risk factors for developing sleep disorders, but many healthy young adults suffer from partial sleep loss without even being aware of it. Therefore, it is timely and important to evaluate the possible adverse effects of sleep loss on error monitoring, including error detection and error correction. This chapter focuses on studies examining the impact of one night of total sleep deprivation on error monitoring by using event-related potentials (ERPs) to complement the usual behavioral measures (e.g., reaction time, accuracy, error rate, and omission rate). Some possible functions of sleep and possible impacts of sleep loss on various psychological performance tests, including simple tasks and higher-level control (or frontal-sensitive) tasks, are first introduced. The chapter then introduces two error-related ERP components, the error-related negativity (ERN or Ne) and the error positivity (Pe), focusing on their neural correlates and functional significance. The chapter then describes why and how sleep deprivation may impair error-monitoring functions and how these impairments may be reflected in the ERN and/or Pe. How the impact of sleep deprivation on error monitoring may be further modulated by other factors, such as task difficulty, explicit instruction to immediately correct errors, and motivational incentives, is then discussed. Finally, the chapter focuses on how sleep deprivation and other factors affect post-error remedial actions, how the impairment of remedial actions may be related to Pe modulations, and the implications of these findings for the linkage between Pe and post-error adjustments. Future directions for research on the prevention and mitigation of human errors are also discussed.

6.2 Sleep and Sleep Deprivation

6.2.1 Functions of Sleep

Almost every animal species needs sleep; at least, there is no clear evidence of any animal species that does not need sleep. Even the dolphin, which does not appear to sleep because it moves continuously, has now been shown to engage in "unihemispheric sleep." But why is it that all species need sleep? What kind of core function does sleep perform? Is sleep essential for all animals? Some researchers argue that, despite the fact that all animal species need sleep, sleep may not be essential but rather reflects a convenient choice that is less dangerous than roaming around, wasting energy, and risking exposure to predators (Rail et al. 2007). Nevertheless, Cirelli and Tononi (2008) have raised doubts about this hypothesis. In addition to the evidence showing that all animal species sleep, Cirelli and Tononi (2008) also indicated that sleep loss has severe negative consequences, including death. In laboratory experiments, prolonged sleep deprivation has been shown to kill rats, flies, and cockroaches. Humans who suffer from genetic insomnia can also die. In less extreme cases, sleep deprivation leads to deterioration of cognitive functions in animals (Horne 1988, 1992). A chronic sleep-restricted state can cause fatigue, daytime sleepiness, clumsiness, and weight gain (Horne 1988). This implies that sleep has an important core function for animals.

Several researchers have suggested that sleep may play a vital role in the normal functioning of the cerebrum. Cirelli and Tononi (2008) hypothesized that sleep can regroup the brain by giving the synapses a chance to return to baseline levels following a whole day of learning. Ramm (1989) showed that during non-REM (rapid eye movement) sleep, there is increased protein synthesis in the brain that contributes to increased neuronal/glial growth and repair. Some animal studies have indicated that REM sleep is necessary for turning off the release of neurotransmitters (i.e., monoamines) and allowing their receptors to recover from desensitization and regain their sensitivity, which in turn allows monoamines to be effective at normal levels (Rotenberg 2006). Thus, if sleep plays a vital role in cerebral recovery, then cerebral function would be expected to be impaired by the loss of sleep. Of course, this is not to say that sleep has no role in regulating body functions. Sleep deprivation has been found to result in several forms of physiological dysfunction, such as aching muscles, dizziness, nausea, headaches, increased blood pressure, increased risk for diabetes, increased risk of fibromyalgia, and obesity. However, the evidence reported so far has yet to prove that sleep is truly restorative for the brain and/or body. Some reports have shown no adverse biochemical, physiological, or hormonal changes following sleep deprivation. Moreover, even though Ramm (1989) has shown that there is increased neuronal/ glial growth and repair during non-REM sleep, the fundamental mechanisms for brain protein turnover have yet to be demonstrated (commented by Horne 1992). At present, although no evidence can directly provide causal inferences regarding the true function of sleep (for an extensive review on why we sleep, see Horne 1988), the evidence nevertheless demonstrates the existence of a close relationship between sleep and the normal functioning of the brain and body.

6.2.2 Sleep Problems and Sleep Disorders

Although adequate sleep seems to serve an important role in normal cerebral functioning, many healthy young adults suffer from sleep loss within the diagnostic boundary of "excessive daytime sleepiness." For example, Levine et al. (1988) reported that 40% of the young adults in their study suffered from chronic partial sleep loss without even being aware of their sleep problems. In contrast, many patients in clinical settings are aware of and adversely affected by their sleep problems, including shortened sleep duration and disturbed sleep. Many of these sleep problems are diagnosed as sleep disorders. According to the International Classification of Sleep Disorders (ICSD), there are four major categories of sleep disorders: dyssomnias, parasomnias, medical or psychiatric sleep disorders, and proposed sleep disorders. Dyssomnias are disorders of the initiation and maintenance of sleep and of excessive sleepiness, such as insomnia and hypersomnia. General complaints related to insomnia include difficulty falling asleep, frequent awakening, early morning awakening, insufficient or total lack of sleep, daytime fatigue, tiredness or sleepiness, lack of concentration, irritability, anxiety, and sometimes depression and forgetfulness. The prevalence of insomnia is relatively high. Approximately 30% of respondents in a variety of adult samples drawn from different countries report one or more of the symptoms of insomnia: difficulty initiating sleep, difficulty maintaining sleep, waking up too early and, in some cases, poor sleep quality (Ancoli-Israel and Roth 1999).

Sleep loss and sleepiness have been shown to contribute significantly to accidents in everyday life situations, such as motor vehicle crashes and work error-related damage (reviewed in Oken, Salinsky, and Elsas 2006; Stepanski 2002). When people become sleepy, they usually experience difficulties in maintaining task performance at an adequate level. Given the existence of so many types of sleep disorders and the fact that even healthy young adults may suffer from partial sleep loss, it is critical to evaluate how and to what extent sleep loss and sleepiness deteriorate cognitive functions. This assessment can be carried out by means of psychological performance tests.

6.2.3 Sleep Deprivation and Task Performance

In laboratory settings, it is often found that after extended wakefulness or sleep deprivation, the typical performance pattern comprises slower, more variable responses and decreases in accuracy, which are concomitant with increases in errors of both commission and omission (Doran, van Dongen, and Dinges 2001). Such performance decrements are often attributed to a general attentional deficit (i.e., arousal decrement), and this proposition has been supported by several behavioral (Jennings, Monk, and van der Molen 2003; Oken, Salinsky, and Elsas 2006; Versace et al. 2006), electrophysiological (Humphrey, Kramer, and Stanny 1994; Morris et al. 1992), and functional brain imaging (Chee et al. 2008) studies. However, even though performance decrements are consistently found following sleep deprivation, the mechanisms mediating the performance decrements may vary depending on the type of task being investigated (for a critical review, see Harrison and Horne 2000).

6.2.3.1 Simple Tasks

The most common tasks used to investigate the effects of sleep deprivation are vigilance tasks, such as the Psychomotor Vigilance Test (PVT; Dinges and Kribbs 1991; Dinges and Powell 1988; Dorrian, Rogers, and Dinges 2005) or Wilkinson Auditory Vigilance Test (WAVT; Wilkinson 1960, 1963). In PVT tasks, subjects are required to respond immediately to the appearance of a rare target (e.g., a red dot) by pressing a button to remove the target from the screen. It has been demonstrated that successive days of sleep restriction (e.g., 4, 5, or 6 hours of sleep per day) or a single night of total sleep deprivation causes a significant decrease in performance of such a vigilance task even by day 2 (e.g., Dawson and Reid 1997; Dinges et al. 1997; Jones et al. 2006; van Dongen et al. 2003). The initial theory based on vigilance task performance proposed that sleep deprivation reduces the nonspecific arousal level of the body but has no specific effects (e.g., Wilkinson 1992). Consistent with this theory, it is commonly thought that sleep deprivation causes a general decrease in arousal, deteriorating basic cognitive functions such as alertness, vigilance, and simple reaction time (Doran, van Dongen, and Dinges 2001). Two hypotheses have been advanced to explain the general deleterious effects of sleep loss on vigilance tasks. The first is the "lapses" hypothesis, which posits normal performance until the occurrence of a lapse (i.e., delayed response or omission) (Williams, Lubin, and Goodnow 1959). The second is the "state instability" hypothesis, which highlights increasing fluctuations in neurocognitive performance with sleep loss (Doran, van Dongen, and Dinges 2001). The neural basis of the impaired vigilance task may involve modifications in a distributed cortico-subcortical network, mainly including fronto-parietal regions and the thalamus, which have been shown to mediate the intensity of attention (Cabeza and Nyberg 2000). Sleep deprivation has been reported to result in changes within this network (Thomas et al. 2000), supporting the view that sleep deprivation degrades general attentional functioning.

However, even short vigilance tasks are inevitably monotonous and lack environmental stimulation, factors that may exacerbate the negative effects of sleep loss (Harrison and Horne 2000; Horne, Anderson, and Wilkinson 1983). In other words, there may be a confounding effect of an additional worsening of performance in such simple tasks owing to lack of interest and tedium. Moreover, vigilance tasks may focus on only one aspect of attentional function. The term *attention* is not a monolithic concept but refers to a constellation of smaller cognitive operations, such as orienting to sensory stimuli, maintaining the alert state, and coordinating and reconfiguring the mental computations needed to perform the complex tasks of daily life (Fernandez-Duque and Posner 1997). Cognitive operations that fall under the last category are switching between tasks and inhibiting proponent responses, as well as other skills usually referred to as executive functions (Baddeley, Chincotta, and Adlamet 2001). Many attentional models have suggested that attention can be divided into separate, but interrelated, subsystems that can be defined both neuroanatomically and functionally (e.g., Posner and Petersen 1990; van Zomeren and Brouwer 1994). For example, Posner and Petersen (1990) proposed two independent but interacting attentional systems: the posterior and anterior systems. The posterior system is involved in directing attention to relevant locations using the component processes of engaging, shifting, and disengaging. These three processes are associated with three brain regions: the parietal lobe (Posner et al. 1984), the thalamus (Rafal and Posner 1987), and the superior colliculus (Posner, Synder, and Davidson 1980). The anterior system, including the prefrontal cortex and the anterior cingulate cortex (ACC), is involved in planning, monitoring, and controlling the posterior system. Thus, to obtain a complete picture of how sleep loss may result in adverse effects on cognitive performance, we should not only use simple tasks that may focus on only one aspect of attention, but also use more complex or higher-level control tasks (Horne 1988, 2000). Moreover, using higher-level control tasks can minimize the confounding factor of low motivation (Horne 2000). In contrast to what is normally observed in simple tasks, the impact of sleep deprivation on higher-level control tasks is more difficult to reverse through the provision of more incentives to increase motivation and/or effort (e.g., Harrison and Horne 2000; Horne and Pettitt 1985; Williams, Lubin, and Goodnow 1959; Wilkinson 1961).

6.2.3.2 Higher-Level Control (Frontal Lobe-Sensitive) Tasks

What kinds of tasks can be classified as higher-level control tasks? Tasks such as verb generation (Barch et al. 2000), dual-task control (D'Esposito et al. 1995), the Stroop-like interference task (Carter et al. 2000), error detection (Carter et al. 1998; Dehaene, Posner, and Tucker 1994; Gehring and Knight 2000; Kiehl, Liddle, and Hopfinger 2000), task switching (Allport, Styles, and Hsieh 1994; Rogers and Monsell 1995), and decision making (Harrison and Horne 1997, 1998, 1999; Horne 1988) are often thought to fall in this category. These tasks, also known as "executive" tasks, have been found to be correlated with prefrontal lobe activity (Baddeley 1990; Norman and Shallice 1986). Therefore, the frontal lobe is thought to be critically involved in the ability to plan or set goals, in supervisory attention processes, in response inhibition, and in action-monitoring functions such as error detection and conflict processing.

Horne (1988, 1993) has suggested that sleep probably provides a specific form of recovery for the cerebral cortex, particularly the prefrontal cortex. Petiau et al. (1998) and Drummond et al. (1999, 2000) observed significant changes in the prefrontal cortex in participants who underwent sleep deprivation. Thomas et al. (2000, 2003) demonstrated that sleep loss reduces glucose metabolism in the prefrontal cortex. Sleep loss associated with diminished frontal activity would be expected to influence the performance of higher-level frontal-sensitive tasks (Gosselin, De Koninck, and Campbell 2005; Harrison and Horne 2000; Jones and Harrison 2001; Killgore, Balkin, and Wesensten 2006). Harrison and Horne (2000) provided an extensive review on the impact of sleep deprivation on decision making and suggested that sleep deprivation may not generally reduce arousal but may instead affect performance on higher-level cognitive tasks that rely on frontal lobe functions (known as the "Harrison–Horne hypothesis"; see also Horne 1988, 1993). The results of several studies have provided convergent evidence showing that sleep loss induces the selective impairment of attention processes, particularly the top-down attentional control processes that rely on the frontal lobe (Chee et al. 2008; Jennings, Monk, and van der Molen 2003; Versace et al. 2006).

Sleep deprivation selectively impairs performance on some, but not all, higher-level control tasks. For example, Jennings, Monk, and van der Molen (2003) found that one night of sleep deprivation does not alter processes of supervisory attention in general, such as preparation for task shifting or response inhibition, but specifically impairs the ability to use preparatory bias to speed performance, which is perceived as an active effort to cope with a challenging task. In line with this view, Versace et al. (2006) also claimed that sleep curtailment selectively attenuates the disengaging and shifting mechanisms involved in the stimulus-induced responses when an invalid cue is presented. Harrison and Horne (2000) further distinguished between two kinds of higher-level control tasks: convergent and divergent thinking tasks. The former tasks, such as anagram tests, do not really evaluate frontal function, and thus the adverse effect of sleep deprivation on this type of task can be masked by increased subjective effort. In contrast, the adverse effects of sleep deprivation on the latter type of tasks, such as the Wisconsin Card Sorting Task (WCST) or simulated battle games, may not be easily attenuated by providing external incentives.

6.3 Error Monitoring: Error Detection and Error Correction

Among the higher-order control tasks, error monitoring may be considered a mostly dynamic and adaptive control task that requires close monitoring of the ongoing activity and post-error modifications and adjustments when errors are detected to achieve the intended goal. As mentioned by Reason (1990)

> To err is human. No matter how well we come to understand the psychological antecedents of errors or how sophisticated are the cognitive "prostheses"—devices to aid memory or decision making—we eventually provide for those in high-risk occupations, errors will still occur. Errors are, as we have seen, the inevitable and usually acceptable price human beings have to pay for their remarkable ability to cope with very difficult informational tasks quickly and, more often than not, effectively. (p. 148)

Thus, the issue of how error detection and post-error remedial actions can be maintained following sleep deprivation is critical. We know from everyday life that sleepiness may not only increase the risk of making incorrect behavioral choices but may also reduce the ability to remedy errors, which can sometimes have catastrophic consequences. Unintentional human error in the workplace is the most frequently (~70%) identified cause of accidents across industries. For example, several internationally well-known disasters have been documented as human errors and took place in industries as diverse as nuclear power (e.g., the Three Mile Island accident), aviation (e.g., pilot errors), space exploration (e.g., the Challenger disaster), and medicine (e.g., medical malpractice). Despite the obvious importance of the topic, the sleep deprivation literature contains very few empirical studies investigating the impact of sleep deprivation on error monitoring (see the series of studies by Hsieh and colleagues described below).

6.3.1 Electrophysiological Correlates of Error Detection: ERN and Pe

To study error monitoring in the laboratory, a number of tasks that require rapid responses are commonly used. These tasks allow for an adequate number of error trials, and they include modified versions of the Eriksen Flankers task (Eriksen and Eriksen 1974), the Simon task (Simon 1969), and the Go/No-Go task. In addition, it is difficult to infer from performance measures alone whether the participant is aware that an error has been made. For this reason, many laboratories use ERPs to complement the performance measures by monitoring the response of the brain following errors. In a conventional Eriksen Flankers task, participants search for a centrally presented target that is flanked on each side by two stimuli that are associated with either the same response as the target (congruent trial; e.g., >>>>>) or the opposite response (incongruent trial; e.g., <<><<). The participant's task is to respond to the target and ignore any distracting information. The commission of an error in this task has been successfully demonstrated to evoke two well-known ERP components: error negativity (Ne; Falkenstein et al. 1990, 1991), also known as error-related negativity (ERN; Coles et al. 1991; Gehring et al. 1990; Gehring et al. 1993), and error positivity (Pe; Botvinick et al. 2001; Falkenstein et al. 2000; Holroyd and Coles 2002) (see Figure 6.1). The ERN is a frontocentral maximum ERP occurring approximately 60–100 milliseconds following an error that is often seen in response-locked averages from tasks that require rapid responses (including go/no-go tasks, flanker tasks, and choice reaction tasks; for a review, see Falkenstein et al. 2000). Regarding the neural basis of ERN, electrophysiological source localization analyses have indicated that ERN is generated by a single source in the medial frontal cortex, most likely the ACC (Dehaene, Posner, and Tucker 1994; Holroyd, Dien, and Coles 1998; van Veen and Carter 2002). Neuroimaging studies also provide evidence that the ERN is generated in the ACC (e.g., Carter et al. 1998; Kiehl, Liddle, and Hopfinger 2000).

6.3.1.1 Functional Significance of ERN

At present, there are several views of the functional significance of the ERN, such as error detection, response conflict detection/monitoring, detection of motivationally or emotionally salient events (especially negative ones), and reinforcement learning.

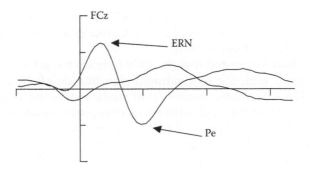

FIGURE 6.1
The response-locked event-related potentials for error and correct trials at FCz, where the error-related negativity was maximal which was followed by error positivity (Pe). The response onset occurred at 0 millisecond and negative is plotted up.

Some researchers have hypothesized that ERN is elicited by the mismatch that occurs when comparing error information with the expected correct response (known as the "error-detection" or "mismatch" theory; Coles et al. 2001; Falkenstein et al. 1991). This theory is supported by evidence showing that subjects exhibited larger ERNs when the error response and the correct response were more dissimilar (Bernstein, Scheffers, and Coles 1995; Falkenstein, Hohnsbein, and Hoormann 1995; Scheffers et al. 1996). Further support comes from evidence that subjects who are more certain of their errors have increased ERN amplitudes regardless of whether they actually make an error (Scheffers and Coles 2000). However, the error account has been questioned in part because a similar, although smaller, negativity is sometimes also seen on correct trials (correct response negativity). Another negativity that some consider to be the same as the ERN is the so-called medial frontal negativity. This is elicited in response to feedback stimuli in a gambling task where participants are asked to choose one of two values and then give feedback about whether they won or lost and what they would have lost or won had they chosen the other value. The negativity under such conditions resembles the feedback ERN and is sensitive to both response correctness (where an error means that choosing the alternative would have resulted in a smaller loss or a bigger gain) and utility (i.e., gain or loss) (Gehring and Willoughby 2002).

Other researchers have suggested that ERN represents the detection of *conflict*, rather than *error* per se, between simultaneous incompatible representations of response-related processing (known as the "conflict-detection" theory; Botvinick et al. 2001; Carter et al. 1998; Ullsperger, Bylsma, and Botvinick 2005; Yeung, Botvinick, and Cohen 2004). The conflict-detection theory focuses on conflict monitoring rather than on error detection per se and suggests that errors are simply a specific example of response conflict that occurs between the current (i.e., erroneous) response and the alternative (i.e., error correcting) response. Conflict monitoring has been demonstrated to localize in or very near the ACC (Dehaene, Posner, and Tucker 1994; Holroyd, Dien, and Coles 1998). Neuroimaging studies (e.g., Carter et al. 1998; Kiehl, Liddle, and Hopfinger 2000) have provided corroborating evidence for the activation of the ACC in association with errors. Researchers supporting this view have also compared the ERN to a negative deflection in the stimulus-locked ERP; that is, the N2 peaks between 200 and 400 milliseconds after stimulus presentation. N2 is most pronounced in trials with high response conflict (e.g., incongruent trials in the Eriksen Flankers task: <<><<). The N2 is thought to reflect the co-activation of the correct and incorrect responses on *correct* trials (Falkenstein, Hoormann, and Hohnsbein 1999; Yeung, Botvinick, and Cohen 2004). Some localization studies have further shown that ERN and N2 have similar scalp topographies and a common neural source (i.e., the caudal ACC) (Carter et al. 1998; van Veen and Carter 2002; Yeung, Botvinick, and Cohen 2004).

Some researchers have suggested that the ERN indexes the activity of a general evaluative system concerned with the motivational significance of the error (Luu, Collins, and Tucker 2000). Direct evidence comes from studies showing that the amplitude of the ERN is modulated by individual differences in negative emotionality (Luu, Collins, and Tucker 2000) and anxiety (Hajcak, McDonald, and Simons 2003). In particular, the amplitude of the ERN has been found to be greater for individuals high in negative emotionality than for individuals low in negative emotionality (Hajcak, McDonald, and Simons 2004; Luu, Collins, and Tucker 2000). Tucker and Luu (2006) further suggested that the ERN reflects the degree of affective distress as ERN amplitude increases with negative emotionality/affect. Additional evidence comes from direct motivational manipulation, which has been demonstrated to modulate the amplitude of the ERN. In these studies, errors associated with a motivationally significant context (i.e., losing 100 points) evoked larger ERN amplitudes compared to other conditions (i.e., losing 5 points) (Hajcak et al. 2005).

The most elaborative theory of the ERN has been referred to as the reinforcement learning theory, which links the ERN to a learning signal generated by the ACC when the consequences of an action are worse than expected; this signal is used to modify performance on the task at hand (Holroyd and Coles 2002; Nieuwenhuis et al. 2004). According to the reinforcement learning theory, the ERN reflects a negative reward prediction error—a signal elicited when the monitoring system has to revise its reward expectations for the worse. The amplitude of the ERN is proportional to the size of the prediction error; that is, the amplitude of the ERN depends on the difference between the actual and expected outcomes of the trial. According to this theory, the neural basis of the ERN reflects the transmission of a reinforcement learning signal to the ACC. This error signal is then carried by the mesencephalic dopamine system and used to train the anterior cingulate motor cortex to optimize performance on the task at hand. In other words, the ERN is generated when a negative temporal difference error is carried by the mesencephalic dopamine system to the anterior cingulate motor areas during or after response generation. The ERN is produced when the system first detects that the consequences of an action are worse than expected. Evidence supporting this theory shows that drug-induced stimulation can modulate the ERN amplitude. Specifically, the administration of the dopamine agonist d-amphetamine results in an increase in the ERN amplitude, whereas the administration of the dopamine antagonist haloperidol results in a decrease in the ERN amplitude (e.g., de Bruijn et al. 2004).

Regardless of which hypothesis is more accurate, the amplitude of the ERN has been demonstrated to be modulated by several factors, such as task difficulty (West and Alain 1999), stimulus or response uncertainty (Pailing and Segalowitz 2004a), error rates (Gehring et al. 1993), the tradeoff between speed and accuracy (Gehring et al. 1993; Gehring et al. 1995; Ullsperger and Szymanowski 2004), time stress (Falkenstein et al. 1990), alcohol intake (Ridderinkhof et al. 2002), and aging (Falkenstein, Hoormann, and Hohnsbein 2001; Mathewson, Dywan, and Segalowitz 2005).

6.3.1.2 Functional Significance of Pe

Following the ERN, a second error-related ERP component, the error positivity (Pe), has been observed to occur between 200 and 400 milliseconds at the Cz site following an error response. The Pe is a late positive deflection at the centro-parietal sites (Falkenstein, Hohnsbein, and Hoormann 1996; Falkenstein et al. 2000; Nieuwenhuis et al. 2001). The source of the Pe has been localized in the rostral ACC and the superior parietal cortex (van Veen and Carter 2002). Compared to the ERN, the functional significance of the Pe is less understood. The Pe has been proposed to be associated with conscious error recognition (Falkenstein et al. 2000; Leuthold and Sommer 1999; Nieuwenhuis et al. 2001), error number (Carbonnell and Falkenstein 2006; Dywan, Mathewson, and Segalowitz 2004; Overbeek, Nieuwenhuis, and Ridderinkhof 2005), or emotional reaction to errors (Falkenstein et al. 2000; van Veen and Carter 2002), and it has also been related to performance adjustments following an error (Hajcak, McDonald, and Simons 2003; Nieuwenhuis et al. 2001). Some researchers have suggested that while the ERN may signal rapid, automatic corrections, the Pe may reflect a slower and more conscious correction system.

6.3.2 Electrophysiological Correlates of Error Correction

As previously mentioned, the complete process of error monitoring includes not only the error detection process but also the post-error remedial actions. The term "post-error remedial actions" refers to the phenomenon in which, after making an error, participants attempt either to correct the error immediately (a behavior also known as short-term adjustment or immediate error correction for the current trial; e.g., Fiehler, Ullsperger, and von Cramon 2004; Hsieh, Cheng, and Tsai 2007; Hsieh, Tsai, and Tsai 2009) or to make long-term adjustments in their response strategies to avoid future errors. Such adjustments may include responding with increased reaction times (also known as "post-error slowing"; e.g., Rabbitt 1966) or with increased accuracy and a lower error rate on the following trial (Laming 1979; Tsai et al. 2005). The immediate error correction rate is calculated as the percentage of errors corrected. Post-error remedial actions are quantified by the difference between task performance in the trials following errors and task performance in the trials following correct responses. For example, if the post-error probability of error is reduced, this means that the probability of an error immediately following an error (i.e., repeated errors) is lower than the probability of an error immediately following a correct response (Laming 1979).

Compared to error detection, fewer psychophysiological studies have delineated the neural implementation of subsequent error corrections (Fiehler, Ullsperger, and von Cramon 2004, 2005; Rodríguez-Fornells, Kurzbuch, and Münte 2002). Most available evidence has indicated that the ERN amplitude may also be related to subsequent error corrections. A study by Gehring et al. (1993) demonstrated a relationship between the ERN and the probability of error correction. In their study, participants were found to slow down after making errors, and this adjustment was larger for errors associated with larger ERNs. Moreover, Falkenstein, Hohnsbein, and Hoormann (1996) and Rodríguez-Fornells, Kurzbuch, and Münte (2002) observed larger ERN amplitudes for corrected than for uncorrected errors. However, a similar earlier study by Falkenstein, Hohnsbein, and Hoormann (1994) failed to find any difference in the ERN amplitudes following corrected and uncorrected errors in response to visual stimuli. A more recent ERP study found that the ERN amplitude can predict compensatory post-error slowing in trials following errors (Debener et al. 2005). Fiehler, Ullsperger, and von Cramon (2005) suggested a relationship between error detection and error correction by proposing that the ERN amplitude reflects the size of the error signal generated by the error detection system. This error signal could then be used as an input to a remedial action system that reduces response speed in trials conducted following an error (see also Fiehler, Ullsperger, and von Cramon 2004; Gehring et al. 1993; Scheffers et al. 1999). Perhaps, one of the strongest pieces of evidence regarding the relationship between error detection and error correction is the recently published neuroimaging investigation by Fiehler, Ullsperger, and von Cramon (2004). This study indicated that cortical areas, specifically the rostral cingulate zone (rostral ACC) and the pre-supplementary motor area, both of which are believed to be involved in error detection, may also play a role in error correction, thus supporting the argument for a common neuroanatomical substrate for error detection and error correction (Fiehler, Ullsperger, and von Cramon 2004). Notably, Gehring and Knight (2000) found that corrective behavior was impaired in individuals with lateral prefrontal damage. They further proposed that the lateral prefrontal cortex interacts with the ACC in monitoring and guiding compensatory systems. Others have also suggested that remedial actions may be reflected by brain activity in the ACC and the adjacent medial frontal cortex (Carter et al. 1998; Garavan et al. 2002; Hester et al. 2005; Hester et al. 2008; Kerns et al. 2004; Kiehl, Liddle, and Hopfinger 2000; Ullsperger and von Cramon 2001; van Veen and Carter 2002), prefrontal cortex, and parietal cortex (Hester et al. 2005; Kerns et al. 2004). The results published thus far indicate that the ERN amplitude is closely related to post-error remedial actions. However, in a series of studies on the effects of sleep deprivation on error monitoring, Hsieh and colleagues failed to observe modulation of the ERN amplitude as a function of post-error remedial actions. Interestingly, they observed that the Pe amplitude was modulated concurrently with the post-error remedial actions (discussed in more detail in a later section of this chapter).

6.3.3 Causes of Errors

Although many researchers have observed that errors are associated with reduced ERN amplitude, the real causes of these errors remain unknown. Some researchers have suggested that errors result from the inadequate selection of actions because of a disruption in the ability to effectively monitor the previous action. According to this theory, a response-locked potential, known as the error preceding positivity, should be present prior to errors. A second theory suggests that stimulus and/or response conflict can account for response errors. The evidence supporting this theory is equivocal. A third theory suggests that errors are the result of hasty responses. However, not all studies have observed significantly faster response times for errors versus correct responses. A fourth theory suggests that errors may be the result of temporary disruption of preparatory attention processes (e.g., Padilla et al. 2006). According to this theory, error trials may be preceded by a reduced contingent negative variation. In summary, there is currently no consensus regarding the causes of errors.

6.4 Sleep Deprivation and Error Monitoring

No matter what actually causes errors, sleep deprivation may increase the risk of committing errors as well as reduce the ability to remediate actions, in line with the frontal lobe hypothesis of sleep loss. A recent functional neuroimaging study (Chee et al. 2008) has shown that response lapses during a visual selective attention task were associated with reduced activation in several brain regions, particularly the fronto-parietal regions that mediate cognitive control, in participants who had undergone one night of sleep deprivation. On the basis of the empirical evidence from several recent behavioral and electrophysiological studies, error monitoring has been added to the list of deleterious effects of extended wakefulness and sleep deprivation on cognitive control. The reduction in the ability to monitor errors following sleep deprivation may result in catastrophic accidents. A famous example is the Exxon Valdez oil tanker accident, America's worst oil spill. The direct cause of this disaster was a human performance error that had been observed and previously brought to the individual's attention. The problem was that the compensatory action was initiated too late to remedy the situation because the severely sleep-deprived mate did not immediately respond to the warning that an error had been made. In this case, sleep deprivation not only increased the chance of making errors but also resulted in inadequate behavioral adjustments following errors. This could reduce the chances of immediate correction or of avoiding future errors and eventually lead to tragic consequences. The key factor in these human errors is the lack of close monitoring of the ongoing activity by attentional control. Given that error monitoring is critical to prevent disasters, it is important to study in depth how it may be deteriorated and how such deterioration may be exacerbated following sleep deprivation. Although various forms of sleep loss may exist, this review focuses on the effects of one night of total sleep deprivation.

6.4.1 Sleep Deprivation and Error Detection*: ERN and Task Difficulty

A series of recent (Hsieh, Cheng, and Tsai 2007; Hsieh, Tsai, and Tsai 2009; Hsieh, Li, and Tsai 2010; Tsai et al. 2005) and previous (Horne and Pettit 1985; Murphy et al. 2006; Scheffers et al. 1999) studies have shown that all components of error monitoring, including error detection and error correction, are impaired following sleep deprivation. These studies have consistently shown that the impairment of error detection by sleep deprivation is reflected by the ERN (e.g., Hsieh, Cheng, and Tsai 2007; Hsieh, Tsai, and Tsai 2009; Hsieh, Li, and Tsai 2010; Scheffers et al. 1999; Tsai et al. 2005). Scheffers et al. (1999) used memory search and visual search tasks and observed that extended wakefulness reduced the amplitude of the ERN evoked by committing errors. Hsieh and colleagues used various versions of the Eriksen Flankers task and found that one night of total sleep deprivation resulted in a reduction in the amplitude of the ERN (Hsieh, Cheng, and Tsai 2007; Hsieh, Li, and Tsai 2010; Tsai et al. 2005) (see Figure 6.2).

Another recent electrophysiological study by Murphy et al. (2006), also using the Eriksen Flankers task, obtained results that were inconsistent with those of Tsai et al. (2005) and of other studies on the decrease in the ERN amplitude following sleep loss. Murphy et al. (2006) observed no effect of extended wakefulness on the amplitude of the ERN. These studies differed in many aspects of their methodologies. They not only manipulated sleep loss differently (one manipulated one night of sleep deprivation (i.e., Tsai et al. 2005), whereas the other manipulated 20 hours of wakefulness time (i.e., Murphy et al. 2006)), but the variations of the Eriksen Flankers task they used also differed. In the study by Tsai et al. (2005), an arrow version of the Eriksen Flankers task (e.g., <<><<) was used, whereas in the study by Murphy et al. (2006), a letter version of the Eriksen Flankers task (e.g., HHSHH) was used. Whether the type of stimuli used in the Eriksen Flankers task caused the difference in the results should be investigated further. Recent functional magnetic resonance imaging studies have indicated that cerebral compensatory mechanisms involving an increase in activity in specific brain regions may appear when performing a more difficult task after sleep deprivation (Drummond et al. 2004, 2005). Therefore, it is possible that the lack of a reduction in the ERN observed in the study by Murphy et al. (2006) may reflect the involvement of more compensatory mechanisms to cope with the increase in task difficulty (e.g., a letter version of the Eriksen Flankers task). This speculation, however, is not supported by subsequent studies (e.g., Hsieh, Cheng, and Tsai 2007; Hsieh, Li, and Tsai 2010), which used a letter version of the Eriksen Flankers task (e.g., HHSHH). In particular, in the study by

---

* Please note that, although we claim here that the reduction in the ERN amplitude reflects error detection deterioration, as mentioned previously, the amplitude of the ERN has been shown to be sensitive not only to error detection per se (Bernstein, Scheffers, and Coles 1995) but also to response conflict (Botvinick et al. 2001; Carter et al. 1998), worse-than-prediction actions (Holroyd and Coles 2002), and emotional/motivational factors (e.g., Boksem et al. 2006; Luu, Collins, and Tucker 2000; Pailing and Segalowitz 2004a; Ullsperger and von Cramon 2001). Thus, future research is needed to clarify which explanation is more pertinent to sleep deprivation.

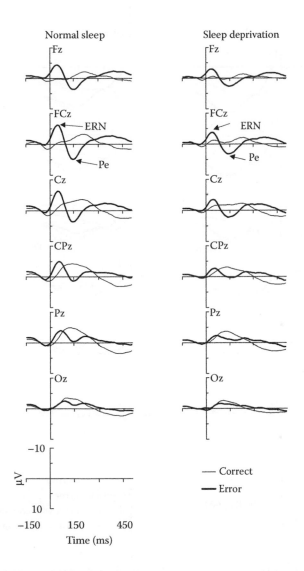

FIGURE 6.2

Grand average response-locked event-related potential waveforms derived from recordings on erroneous (thick line) and correct (thin line) trials in normal sleep and sleep deprivation. The response onset occurred at 0 millisecond and negative is plotted up. Electroencephalography data are presented from electrode sites Fz, FCz, Cz, CPz, Pz, and Oz. (From Tsai, L. L. et al. 2005. *Sleep* 28:707–13. Copyright 2010 by the American Academy of Sleep Medicine. Reprinted by permission.)

Hsieh, Cheng, and Tsai (2007), an even more complicated Eriksen Flankers task was used. That is, rather than just two stimuli being mapped onto two response keys (e.g., "S": press left key; "H": press right key), four stimuli were mapped onto only two response keys (e.g., "S" or "C": press left key; "H" or "K": press right key). Regardless of which version of the Eriksen Flankers task was used in the series of studies by Hsieh and colleagues, a reduced ERN following sleep deprivation was consistently observed (see Figures 6.3 and 6.4). If the inconsistency between the studies by Tsai et al. (2005) and Murphy et al. (2006) was simply a result of the difficulty of the Eriksen Flankers task with letter stimuli, no deficit would have been expected in the later two studies by Hsieh and colleagues (2007, 2010), where the

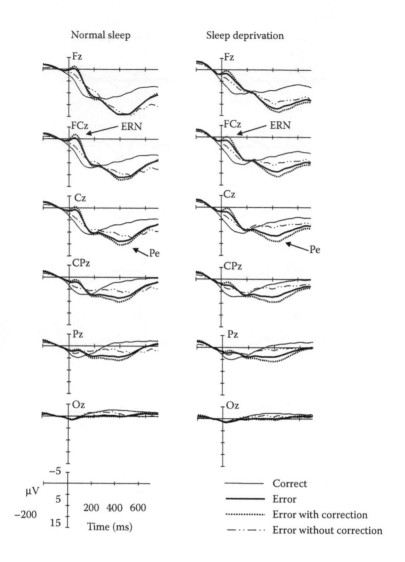

FIGURE 6.3

Grand average response-locked event-related potential waveforms derived from recordings on correct, error, error with correction, and error without correction trials in normal sleep and sleep deprivation at channels Fz, FCz, Cz, CPz, Pz, and Oz. Response onset occurs at 0 millisecond. The arrow represents error-related negativity and Pe. (From Hsieh, S., I. C. Cheng, and L. L. Tsai: Immediate error correction process following sleep deprivation. *Journal of Sleep Research*. 2007. 16:137–47. Copyright Wiley-VCH Verlag GmbH & Co. KGaA. Reproduced with permission.)

more difficult letter version of the Eriksen Flankers task might have recruited even more compensatory mechanisms following sleep deprivation.

6.4.2 Sleep Deprivation and Error Correction: Explicit Instruction to Make Immediate Error Corrections

Thus far, the literature has shown that, in addition to its influence on error detection, as reflected by the ERN, sleep deprivation also influences subsequent error correction (e.g., Murphy et al. 2006; Tsai et al. 2005). For example, Tsai et al. (2005) observed that one night of sleep deprivation impaired post-error remedial actions, that is, impaired the

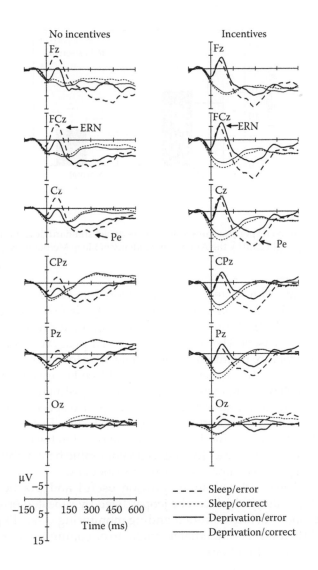

FIGURE 6.4
Averaged response-locked event-related potential (ERP) waveforms for trials with correct and erroneous responses, respectively. The error-related negativity (ERN) is a component of response-locked ERPs recorded at FCz. Pe refers to error positivity. (From Hsieh, S., T. H. Li, and L. L. Tsai. 2010. *Sleep* 33:499–507. Copyright 2010 by the American Academy of Sleep Medicine. Reprinted by permission.)

ability to avoid making errors again, once erroneous responses were made (see Figure 6.5). However, in a follow-up study with an explicit instruction to make immediate error corrections, Hsieh, Tsai, and Tsai (2009) observed that even under conditions of sleep deprivation, participants maintained the ability to adjust their response strategies to avoid making more errors following erroneous responses. That is, error corrective behavior (i.e., subsequent trials' accuracy rate) could effectively attenuate the impact of sleep deprivation on post-error adjustments (see Figure 6.6: upper-right figure). Hsieh, Tsai, and Tsai (2009) further examined whether the maintenance of post-error adjustment after sleep deprivation was dependent on the presence of immediate corrective behavior. They separated

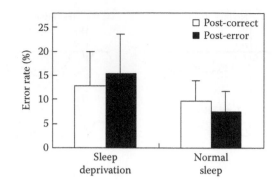

FIGURE 6.5

Post-error remedial actions on response accuracy. Error bars depict standard deviation. (From Tsai, L. L. et al. 2005. *Sleep* 28:707–13. Copyright 2010 by the American Academy of Sleep Medicine. Reprinted by permission.)

the data from the trials immediately following errors into two datasets: one from the trials following corrected errors and a second from the trials following uncorrected errors. The data derived from the trials immediately following correct responses were subtracted from each of the two datasets. The results showed that post-error adjustments involving reducing repeated errors are maintained completely after total sleep deprivation, irrespective of whether error corrective behavior is executed (see Figure 6.6: upper-left figure). In addition, corrective behavior imposes other post-error adjustments involving reducing the number of lapses (omissions) and enhancing the response speed, particularly after total sleep deprivation (see Figure 6.6: bottom two figures). Hsieh, Tsai, and Tsai (2009) further hypothesized that a cerebral mechanism might be involved in the effect of error correction on post-error adjustments because electroencephalographic beta activity is increased following erroneous responses compared to correct responses.

The findings of Hsieh and colleagues provide useful and practical information for increasing workplace safety, which can be jeopardized by repeated errors, particularly in the case of monotonous but attention-demanding monitoring tasks. Explicitly instructing workers to correct their errors immediately upon error commitment might help to maintain post-error adjustment functions.

6.4.3 Sleep Deprivation, Motivational Incentives, and Post-Error Adjustments

Hsieh and colleagues examined the influence of another countermeasure, financial rewards, on the effects of total sleep deprivation on error monitoring (see Hsieh, Li, and Tsai 2010). In contrast to error correction processes that are involved in internal monitoring and explicitly induce self-generated performance feedback, motivational incentives constitute externally provided feedback information. As mentioned, motivational incentives may effectively attenuate the impact of sleep deprivation on simple tasks, but they may not be effective in the context of higher-level control tasks. Nevertheless, because explicit instruction to correct errors has been demonstrated to effectively attenuate the impact of sleep deprivation on post-error adjustments, it is worth examining whether providing external motivational incentives may result in the same effect. Hsieh, Li, and Tsai (2010) conducted a study to address this issue in which they manipulated motivational incentives on a trial-by-trial basis. Participants performed a letter version of the Eriksen Flankers

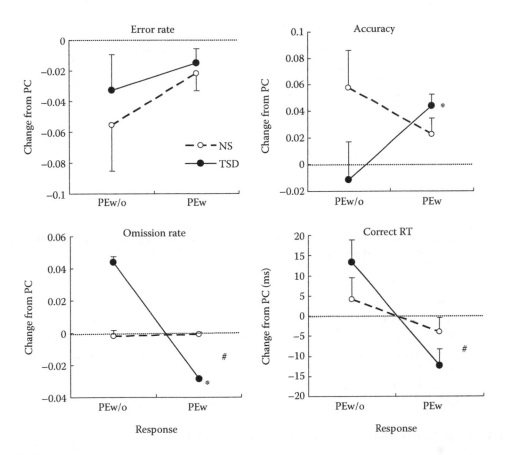

FIGURE 6.6

The mean changes in the error rate, accuracy, and omission rate in the trial following errors (PE) as compared to the trial following the correct response (PC). The mean reaction time (RT) in the correct responses following correct responses was subtracted from the mean RT following errors. $n = 14$, because two participants corrected all the errors committed under the normal sleep (NS) condition. TSD, total sleep deprivation. Error bars depict standard errors. *$P < 0.05$, the effect of interaction between the sleep conditions and response type using two-factor analyses of variance followed by the LSD test for comparisons between trials after corrected errors (PEw) and those after uncorrected errors (PEw/o) under the TSD condition. #$P < 0.05$, main effect of response type. (From Hsieh, S., C. Y. Tsai, and L. L. Tsai: Error correction maintains posterror adjustments after one night of total sleep deprivation. *Journal of Sleep Research*. 2009. 18:159–66. Copyright Wiley-VCH Verlag GmbH & Co. KGaA. Reproduced with permission.)

task in which each trial's response was followed by either a financial reward for a correct response or a financial punishment for an incorrect one. All participants performed the task twice, once on a morning following a normal sleep night and once following a night of sleep deprivation. The two tests were separated by a week, and the sequence of the two sleep conditions was counterbalanced across all subjects.

Hsieh, Li, and Tsai (2010) first examined whether monetary incentives, like explicit error correction instruction, affected post-error behavior adjustments under normal sleep conditions. Significant post-error behavior adjustments were observed in the correct response and error rates under normal sleep conditions. However, although monetary rewards and punishments enhanced cognitive performance under both normal sleep and sleep deprivation conditions and also reduced the effects of total sleep deprivation on the amplitude of the ERN, monetary rewards could not attenuate the effects of total sleep deprivation on

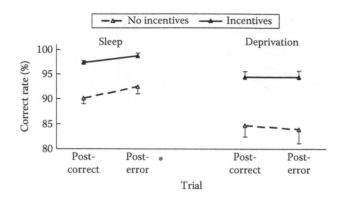

FIGURE 6.7

Post-error accuracy adjustments. The error bars depict the standard error of mean. The effect of the interaction between the trial types and sleep conditions was significant. *$P < 0.05$ versus the post-correct trials under normal sleep condition as evaluated by a posthoc Tukey test. (From Hsieh, S., T. H. Li, and L. L. Tsai. 2010. *Sleep* 33:499–507. Copyright 2010 by the American Academy of Sleep Medicine. Reprinted by permission.)

post-error accuracy adjustments (see Figure 6.7). Thus, the results obtained by Hsieh, Li, and Tsai (2010) show that motivation incentives can selectively reduce the effects of total sleep deprivation on some brain activities (i.e., the ERN amplitude) but do not attenuate the effects of sleep deprivation on performance decrements in tasks that require higher-level control processes. Thus, monetary incentives and sleep deprivation may act through both common and distinct mechanisms to affect cognitive performance.

6.4.4 Sleep Deprivation, Monetary Incentives, and ERN

In the study by Hsieh, Li, and Tsai (2010), which used incentive manipulation, monetary incentives were shown to attenuate the adverse effects of sleep deprivation on the amplitude of the ERN (see Figure 6.4). Despite this physiological change, there was no attenuation of the adverse effects of sleep deprivation on post-error adjustments. The finding of a correlation among sleep deprivation, reward, and the amplitude of the ERN may suggest a common neurophysiological mechanism. First, some research has indicated that one night of sleep deprivation changes dopaminergic brain activity; for example, the specific binding of [11C]raclopride to dopamine D2/D3 receptors in the striatum and thalamus was significantly reduced (Volkow et al. 2008). Furthermore, using positron emission tomography with F-18 deoxyglucose, it was also shown that one night of sleep deprivation changes regional cerebral metabolic activity in the thalamus, basal ganglia, white matter, and cerebellum (Wu et al. 1991). Therefore, the mechanism underlying sleep deprivation may involve a reduction in the activity of dopaminergic projection structures. Second, the basal ganglia have long been recognized as an important structure for the motivational aspects of behavior and reward (Nauta 1986; Schultz, Tremblay, and Hollerman 2000). Accordingly, the effect of monetary incentives may modulate the activity of the dopamine system. Third, a recent theory proposed that the response ERN is produced by the dopamine system for reinforcement learning (Holroyd and Coles 2002). According to this reinforcement learning theory, a response monitoring system located in the basal ganglia evaluates ongoing events and predicts whether they will end in success or failure. The impact of the dopamine signals on the ACC modulates the amplitude of the ERN such that phasic decreases in dopamine activity (indicating that ongoing events are worse than expected) are associated with large ERNs and phasic increases in dopamine activity (indicating that ongoing events are better than expected) are associated with small ERNs (Holroyd and Coles 2002). Therefore, the observation that the reduction in the ERN amplitude following sleep deprivation can be alleviated by reward provides empirical evidence for a neurophysiological mechanism common to sleep deprivation, reward, and the ERN.

6.4.5 Implications of the Pe and Post-Error Remedial Actions

Although research has consistently shown that both the ERN and the Pe are concomitant with error trials, their functional significances may be dissociable. Across the series of studies by Hsieh and colleagues on sleep deprivation, some dissociable changes in ERN and Pe amplitudes in relation to post-error remedial actions have been found. In particular, Hsieh and colleagues have consistently observed that the Pe amplitude changes concurrently with the efficacy of post-error remedial actions. For example, in the study by Tsai et al. (2005), where post-error remedial actions were impaired because of sleep deprivation, the Pe amplitude was also found to be reduced. In contrast, in the study by Hsieh, Cheng, and Tsai (2007), where post-error remedial actions were maintained at a level matching that of normal sleep conditions (owing to the explicit instruction to make immediate error corrections), the Pe amplitude did not change. These results seem to support the hypothesis that the Pe amplitude is related to post-error remedial actions. Hsieh, Li, and Tsai (2010) provided further evidence for this theory by demonstrating a relationship between the Pe amplitude and post-error remedial actions under conditions in which external incentives were provided. Although the incentives alleviated the reduction in the ERN amplitude, they could not alleviate the reduction in the Pe amplitude following sleep deprivation. These results strengthen the hypothesis that the ERN and the Pe reflect different mechanisms involved in error monitoring.

The dissociable effects of the interaction of sleep deprivation and monetary incentives on the ERN and the Pe appear to agree with the functional and neuronal sources of the ERN and the Pe. The ERN has been shown to be generated in the caudal ACC (van Veen and Carter 2002), whereas the Pe has been shown to be generated either in the rostral ACC (van Veen and Carter 2002) or in Brodman area 24 of the ACC (Hermann et al. 2004). Furthermore, the conventional view that the functional significance of the Pe is associated with conscious error recognition (Falkenstein et al. 2000; Leuthold and Sommer 1999; Nieuwenhuis et al. 2001) has been challenged. Rather, the functional significance of the Pe is likely to be related to performance adjustments following an error (Hajcak, McDonald, and Simons 2003; Nieuwenhuis et al. 2001).

6.5 Conclusions and Future Directions

This chapter reviews how sleep deprivation may impair error monitoring, including error detection and error correction, as reflected in the ERN and the Pe. The present review has not only demonstrated the impact of sleep deprivation on error monitoring, but has also provided further information regarding the possible functional significance of the ERN and the Pe. Nevertheless, the literature reviewed here is limited given that few studies directly address these issues. More research is necessary to be able to expand these findings. In addition, the reviewed studies focus solely on the impact of one night of total sleep deprivation.

It is known that many sleep disorders result in sleep fragmentation rather than a total night of sleep loss. Thus, future studies manipulating sleep restriction are warranted. Moreover, shift workers, people with prolonged working hours and on-call workers in health-care settings deserve researchers' attention as fatigue and its role in medical errors are now regarded as a challenge to the provision of quality medical training and care.

Practically, the evidence reviewed in this chapter has shown that sleep deprivation reduces one's ability to detect and/or correct errors as reflected in the amplitude of the ERN, which is important because many workers are prone to partial sleep loss. To prevent the possible catastrophic consequences of human errors due to partial sleep loss, employers may consider taking steps to improve work safety on the basis of the research reviewed in this chapter. These measures could include explicitly instructing workers to correct their errors immediately upon error commitment and/or providing external incentives to motivate accurate responses. Such techniques may help to reduce, although not totally eliminate, the impact of sleep loss.

More effectively, researchers could develop an online detection system that measures the ERN to increase a worker's awareness of his or her current mental state prior to the occurrence of the error. For example, such a system could be activated by the reduction of the ERN amplitude to take control of the situation or to notify the operator about his or her likelihood of committing an error. Developing such a system is pertinent to neuroergonomics research (see also Fedota and Parasuraman 2009; Parasuraman and Rizzo 2008). Parasuraman and colleagues have suggested two ways of using neuroergonomics to contribute to the design of more error-tolerant or resilient systems. One approach is to provide better methods for intelligent error monitoring systems, and the other is to allow for improved feedback to the operator on the system's current state. Schalk et al. (2000) also demonstrated that real-time identification of erroneous trials via the ERN using a brain–computer interface can effectively improve task performance.

Future studies could also emphasize individual differences in error monitoring. Some studies have found that the ERN can be influenced by individual differences in affective style, motivation, or personality (e.g., Luu, Collins, and Tucker 2000; Pailing and Segalowitz 2004b; Tucker et al. 1999). A very recent study has even found that a specific genotype, the 5-HT1A C(–1019)G polymorphism, modulates error detection (Beste et al. 2010). In this genetic study, participants with the CC genotype of the functional 5-HT1A C(–1019)G polymorphism were found to exhibit the strongest Ne and post-error slowing effects. Given this evidence of individual differences in error monitoring, more effort could be devoted to evaluating individual differences in error-monitoring ability and creating specialized training programs to adequately improve particular individuals' error monitoring. In a similar vein, employers could consider assigning individuals to jobs on the basis of their ERN/Pe responses.

References

Allport, A., E. A. Styles, and S. Hsieh. 1994. Shifting intentional set: Exploring the dynamic control of tasks. In *Attention and Performance*, Vol. 15, edited by C. Umiltà and M. Moscovitch, 421–452. Hillsdale, NJ: Lawrence Erlbaum Associates.

Ancoli-Israel, S. and T. Roth. 1999. Characteristics of insomnia in the United States: Results of the 1991 National Sleep Foundation Survey. I. *Sleep* 22 (Suppl. 2): S347–53.

Baddeley, A. D. 1990. *Human Memory: Theory and Practice*. London: Lawrence Erlbaum Associates.

Baddeley, A. D., D. M. Chincotta, and A. Adlam. 2001. Working memory and the control of action: Evidence from task switching. *Journal of Experimental Psychology General* 130:641–57.

Barch, D. M., T. S. Braver, F. W. Sabb, and D. C. Noll. 2000. Anterior cingulated and the monitoring of response conflict: Evidence from an fMRI study of overt verb generation. *Journal of Cognitive Neuroscience* 12:298–309.

Bernstein, P. S., M. K. Scheffers, and M. G. H. Coles. 1995. Where did I go wrong? A psychophysiological analysis of error detection. *Journal of Experimental Psychology: Human Perception and Performance* 21:1312–22.

Beste, C., K. Domschke, V. Kolev, J. Yordanova, A. Baffa, M. Falkenstein, and C. Konrad. 2010. Functional 5-HT1a receptor polymorphism selectively modulates error-specific subprocesses of performance monitoring. *Human Brain Mapping* 31:621–30.

Boksem, M. A., M. Tops, A. E. Wester, T. F. Meijman, and M. M. Lorist. 2006. Error-related ERP components and individual differences in punishment and reward sensitivity. *Brain Research* 1101:92–101.

Botvinick, M. M., T. S. Braver, D. M. Barch, C. S. Carter, and J. D. Cohen. 2001. Conflict monitoring and cognitive control. *Psychological Review* 108:624–52.

Cabeza, R. and L. Nyberg. 2000. Neural basis of learning and memory: Functional neuroimaging evidence. *Current Opinion in Neurology* 13:415–21.

Carbonnell, L. and M. Falkenstein. 2006. Does the error negativity reflect the degree of response conflict? *Brain Research* 1095:124–30.

Carter, C. S., T. S. Braver, D. M. Barch, M. M. Botvinick, D. Noll, and J. D. Cohen. 1998. Anterior cingulated cortex, error detection, and the online monitoring of performance. *Science* 280:747–9.

Carter, C. S., A. M. MacDonald, Jr., M. M. Botvinick, L. L. Ross, V. A. Stenger, D. Noll, and J. D. Cohen. 2000. Parsing executive processes: Strategic vs. evaluative functions of the anterior cingulated cortex. *Proceedings of the National Academy of Sciences of the United States of America* 97:1944–8.

Chee, M. W., J. C. Tan, H. Zheng, S. Parimal, D. H. Weissman, V. Zagorodnov, and D. F. Dinges. 2008. Lapsing during sleep deprivation is associated with distributed changes in brain activation. *Journal of Neuroscience* 28:5519–28.

Cirelli, C. and G. Tononi. 2008. Is sleep essential? *PLoS Biology* 6 (8):e216. doi:10.1371/journal.pbio.0060216.

Coles, M. G. H., W. J. Gehring, G. Gratton, and E. Donchin. 1991. Stimulus-response compatibility and psychophysiology. In *Tutorials in Motor Neuroscience*, Vol. 62, edited by J. Requin and G. E. Stelmach, 27–8. New York: Kluwer Academic Publishers/Plenum Press.

Coles, M. G. H., M. K. Scheffers, and C. B. Holroyd. 2001. Why is there an ERN/Ne on correct trials? Response representations, stimulus-related components, and the theory of error-processing. *Biological Psychology* 56:173–89.

Dawson, D. and K. Reid. 1997. Fatigue, alcohol and performance impairment. *Nature* 388:235.

Debener, S., M. Ullsperger, M. Siegel, K. Fiehler, D. Y. von Cramon, and A. K. Engel. 2005. Trial-by-trial coupling of concurrent electroencephalogram and functional magnetic resonance imaging identifies the dynamics of performance monitoring. *Journal of Neuroscience* 25:11730–7.

de Bruijn, E. R. A., W. Hulstijn, R. J. Verkes, G. S. F. Ruigt, and B. G. C. Sabbe. 2004. Drug-induced stimulation and suppression of action monitoring in healthy volunteers. *Psychopharmacology (Berlin)* 177 (1–2): 151–60.

Dehaene, S., M. I. Posner, and D. M. Tucker. 1994. Localization of a neural system for error detection and compensation. *Psychological Science* 5:303–5.

D'Esposito, M. D., J. A. Detre, D. C. Alsop, R. K. Shin, S. Atlas, and M. Grossman. 1995. The neural basis of the executive system of working memory. *Nature* 378:279–81.

Dinges, D. F. and N. B. Kribbs. 1991. Performing while sleepy: Effects of experimentally-induced sleepiness. In *Sleep, Sleepiness and Performance*, edited by T.H. Monk, 97–128. Chichester, UK: Wiley.

Dinges, D. F. and J. W. Powell. 1988. Sleepiness is more than lapsing. *Sleep Research* 17:84.

Dinges, D. F., F. Pack, K. Williams, K. A. Gillen, J. W. Powell, G. E. Ott, C. Aptowicz, and A. I. Pack. 1997. Cumulative sleepiness, mood disturbance, and psychomotor vigilance performance decrements during a week of sleep restricted to 4-5 hours per night. *Sleep* 20:267–77.

Doran, S. M., H. P. A. van Dongen, and D. F. Dinges. 2001. Sustained attention performance during sleep deprivation: Evidence of state instability. *Archives of Italian Biology* 139:253–67.

Dorrian, J., N. L. Rogers, and D. F. Dinges. 2005. Psychomotor vigilance performance: A neurocognitive assay sensitive to sleep loss. In *Sleep Deprivation: Clinical Issues, Pharmacology and Sleep Loss Effects*, edited by C. Kushida, 39–70. New York: Marcel Dekker.

Drummond, S. P. A., G. G. Brown, J. C. Gillin, J. L. Stricker, E. C. Wong, and R. B. Buxton. 2000. Altered brain response to verbal learning following sleep deprivation. *Nature* 403:655–7.

Drummond, S. P. A., G. G. Brown, J. S. Salamat, and J. C. Gillin. 2004. Increasing task difficulty facilitates the cerebral compensatory response to total sleep deprivation. *Sleep* 27:445–51.

Drummond, S. P. A., G. G. Brown, J. L. Stricker, R. B. Buxton, E. C. Wong, and J. C. Gillin. 1999. Sleep deprivation induced reduction in cortical functional response to serial subtraction. *NeuroReport* 10 (18): 3745–8.

Drummond, S. P. A., M. J. Meloy, M. A. Yanagi, H. J. Orff, and G. G. Brown. 2005. Compensatory recruitment after sleep deprivation and the relationship with performance. *Psychiatry Research* 140:211–23.

Dywan, J., K. J. Mathewson, and S. J. Segalowitz. 2004. Error-related ERP components and source monitoring in older and younger adults. In *Errors, Conflicts, and the Brain. Current Opinions on Performance Monitoring*, edited by M. Ullsperger, and M. Falkenstein, 184–92. Leipzig: Max-Planck Institute for Cognition and Neuroscience.

Eriksen, B. A. and C. W. Eriksen. 1974. Effects of noise letters upon the identification of a target letter in a nonsearch task. *Perception & Psychophysics* 16:143–9.

Falkenstein, M., J. Hohnsbein, and J. Hoormann. 1994. Event-related correlates of errors in reaction tasks. *Perspectives of Event-related Potential Research, EEG Supplement* 44:287–96.

Falkenstein, M., J. Hohnsbein, and J. Hoormann. 1995. Event-related potential correlates of errors in reaction tasks. *Electroencephalography and Clinical Neurophysiology*. Supplement 44:287–96.

Falkenstein, M., J. Hohnsbein, and J. Hoormann. 1996. Differential processing of motor errors. In *Recent Advances in Event-Related Brain Potentials Research*, EEG Supplement No. 45, edited by C. Ogura, Y. Koga, and M. Shimokochi, 579–85. Amsterdam: Elsevier.

Falkenstein, M., J. Hohnsbein, J. Hoormann, and L. Blanke. 1990. Effects of errors in choice reaction tasks on the ERP under focused and divided attention. In *Psychophysiological Brain Research*, edited by C. M. H. Brunia, A. W. K. Gaillard, and A. Kok, 192–5. Tilburg: Tilburg University Press.

Falkenstein, M., J. Hohnsbein, J. Hoormann, and L. Blanke. 1991. Effects of crossmodal divided attention on late ERP components. II. Error processing in choice reaction tasks. *Electroencephalography and Clinical Neurophysiology* 78:447–55.

Falkenstein, M., J. Hoormann, S. Christ, and J. Hohnsbein. 2000. ERP components on reaction errors and their functional significance: A tutorial. *Biological Psychology* 51:87–107.

Falkenstein, M., J. Hoormann, and J. Hohnsbein. 1999. ERP components in Go/Nogo tasks and their relation to inhibition. *Acta Psychologica* 101:267–91.

Falkenstein, M., J. Hoormann, and J. Hohnsbein. 2001. Changes of error-related ERPs with age. *Experimental Brain Research* 138 (2): 258–62.

Fedota, J. R. and R. Parasuraman. 2009. Neuroergonomics and human error. *Theoretical Issues in Ergonomics Science* 11 (5): 402–21.

Fernandez-Duque, D. and M. I. Posner. 1997. Relating the mechanisms of orienting and alerting. *Neuropsychologia* 35 (4): 477–86.

Fiehler, K., M. Ullsperger, and D. Y. von Cramon. 2004. Neural correlates of error detection and error correction: Is there a common neuroanatomical substrate? *European Journal of Neuroscience* 19:3081–7.

Fiehler, K., M. Ullsperger, and D. Y. von Cramon. 2005. Electrophysiological correlates of error correction. *Psychophysiology* 42:72–82.

Garavan, H., T. J. Ross, K. Murphy, R. A. P. Roche, and E. A. Stein. 2002. Dissociable executive functions in the dynamic control of behavior: Inhibition, error detection, and correction. *NeuroImage* 17:1820–9.

Gehring, W. J., M. G. H. Coles, D. E. Meyer, and E. Donchin. 1990. The error-related negativity: An event-related brain potential accompanying errors. *Psychophysiology* 27:S34 (Abstract).

Gehring, W. J., M. G. H. Coles, D. E. Meyer, and E. Donchin. 1995. A brain potential manifestation of error-related processing. In *Perspectives of Event-related Potential Research*, EEG Supplement No. 44, edited by G. Karmos, M. Molnar, V. Csepe, I. Czigler, and J. E. Desmedt, 261–72. Amsterdam: Elsevier.

Gehring, W. J., B. Goss, M. G. H. Coles, D. E. Meyer, and E. Donchin. 1993. A neural system for error detection and compensation. *Psychological Science* 4:385–90.

Gehring, W. J. and R. T. Knight. 2000. Prefrontal-cingulate interactions in action monitoring. *Nature Neuroscience* 3:516–20.

Gehring, W. J. and A. R. Willoughby. 2002. The medial frontal cortex and the rapid processing of monetary gains and losses. *Science* 295 (5563): 2279–82.

Gosselin, A., J. De Koninck, and K. B. Campbell. 2005. Total sleep deprivation and novelty processing: Implications for frontal lobe functioning. *Clinical Neurophysiology* 116:211–22.

Hajcak, G., N. McDonald, and R. F. Simons. 2003. To err is autonomic: Error-related brain potentials, ANS activity, and post-error compensatory behavior. *Psychophysiology* 40:895–903.

Hajcak, G., N. McDonald, and R. F. Simons. 2004. Error-related psychophysiology and negative affect. *Brain and Cognition* 56 (2): 189–97.

Hajcak, G., J. S. Moser, N. Yeung, and R. F. Simons. 2005. On the ERN and the significance of errors. *Psychophysiology* 42 (2): 151–60.

Harrison, Y. and J. A. Horne. 1997. Sleep deprivation affects speech. *Sleep* 20:871–8.

Harrison, Y. and J. A. Horne. 1998. Sleep loss impairs short and novel language tasks having a prefrontal focus. *Journal of Sleep Research* 7:95–100.

Harrison, Y. and J. A. Horne. 1999. One night of sleep loss impairs innovative thinking and flexible decision making. *Organizational Behavior and Human Decision Processes* 78:128–45.

Harrison, Y. and J. A. Horne. 2000. The impact of sleep deprivation on decision making: A review. *Journal of Experimental Psychology: Apply* 6:236–49.

Hermann, M. J., J., Rommler, A. C. Ehlis, A. Heidrich, and A. J. Fallgatter. 2004. Source localization (LOREA) of the error-related negativity (ERN/Ne) and positivity (Pe). *Cognitive Brain Research* 20:294–9.

Hester, R., N. Barre, K. Murphy, T. J. Silk, and J. B. Mattingley. 2008. Human medial frontal cortex activity predicts learning from errors. *Cerebral Cortex* 18:1933–40.

Hester, R., J. J. Foxe, S. Molholm, M. Shpaner, and H. Garavan. 2005. Neural mechanisms involved in error processing: A comparison of errors made with and without awareness. *NeuroImage* 27:602–8.

Holroyd, C. B. and M. G. H. Coles. 2002. The neural basis of human error processing: Reinforcement learning, dopamine, and the error-related negativity. *Psychological Review* 109 (4): 679–709.

Holroyd, C. B., J. Dien, and M. G. H. Coles. 1998. Error-related scalp potentials elicited by hand and foot movements: Evidence for an output-independent error-processing system in humans. *Neuroscience Letters* 242:65–8.

Horne, J. A. 1988. *Why We Sleep: The Functions of Sleep in Humans and Other Mammals.* New York: Oxford University Press.

Horne, J. A. 1992. "Core" and "optional" sleepiness. In *Sleep, Arousal, and Performance,* edited by R. J. Broughton and R. D. Ogilvie, 27–44. Boston: Birkhäuser.

Horne, J. A. 1993. Human sleep, sleep deprivation and behavior: Implications for the prefrontal cortex and psychiatric disorders. *British Journal of Psychiatry* 162:413–9.

Horne, J. A. 2000. Images of lost sleep. *Nature* 403:605–6.

Horne, J. A., N. R. Anderson, and R. T. Wilkinson. 1983. Effects of sleep deprivation on signal detection measures of vigilance: Implications for sleep function. *Sleep* 6:347–58.

Horne, J. A. and A. N. Pettitt. 1985. High incentive effects on vigilance performance during 72 h of total sleep deprivation. *Acta Psychologica* 58:123–39.

Hsieh, S., I. C. Cheng, and L. L. Tsai. 2007. Immediate error correction process following sleep deprivation. *Journal of Sleep Research* 16:137–47.

Hsieh, S., T. H. Li, and L. L. Tsai. 2010. Impact of monetary incentives on cognitive performance and error monitoring following sleep deprivation. *Sleep* 33:499–507.

Hsieh, S., C. Y. Tsai, and L. L. Tsai. 2009. Error correction maintains posterror adjustments after one night of total sleep deprivation. *Journal of Sleep Research* 18:159–66.

Humphrey, D. G., A. F. Kramer, and R. R. Stanny. 1994. Influence of extended wakefulness on automatic and nonautomatic processing. *Human Factors* 36:652–69.

Jennings, J. R., T. H. Monk, and M. W. van der Molen. 2003. Sleep deprivation influences some but not all processes of supervisory attention. *Psychological Science* 14:473–9.

Jones, C. B., J. Dorrian, S. M. Jay, N. Lamond, S. Ferguson, and D. Dawson. 2006. Self-awareness of impairment and the decision to drive after an extended period of wakefulness. *Chornobiology International* 23 (6): 1253–63.

Jones, K. and Y. Harrison. 2001. Frontal lobe function, sleep loss and fragmented sleep. *Sleep Medicine Reviews* 5:463–75.

Kerns, J. G., J. D. Cohen, A. W. MacDonald, III, R. Y. Cho, V. A. Stenger, and C. S. Carter. 2004. Anterior cingulate conflict monitoring and adjustments in control. *Science* 303:1023–6.

Kiehl, K. A., P. F. Liddle, and J. B. Hopfinger. 2000. Error processing and the rostral anterior cingulated: An event-related fMRI study. *Psychophysiology* 33:282–94.

Killgore, W. D. S., T. J. Balkin, and N. J. Wesensten. 2006. Impaired decision making following 49 h of sleep deprivation. *Journal of Sleep Research* 15:7–13.

Laming. D. 1979. Choice reaction performance following an error. *Acta Psychologica* 43:199–224.

Leuthold, H. and W. Sommer. 1999. ERP correlates of error processing in spatial S-R compatibility tasks. *Clinical Neurophysiology* 110:342–57.

Levine, B., T. Roehrs, F. Zorick, and T. Roth. 1988. Daytime sleepiness in young adults. *Sleep* 11:39–46.

Luu, P., P. Collins, and D. M. Tucker. 2000. Mood, personality and self-monitoring: Negative affect and emotionality in relation to frontal lobe mechanisms of error-monitoring. *Journal of Experimental Psychology: General* 129:43–60.

Mathewson, K. J., J. Dywan, and S. J. Segalowitz, 2005. Brain bases of error-related ERPs as influences by age and task. *Biological Psychology* 70:88–104.

Morris, A. M., Y. So, K. A. Lee, A. A. Lash, and C. E. Becker. 1992. The P300 event-related potential. The effects of sleep deprivation. *Journal of Occupational Medicine* 34:1143–52.

Murphy, T. I., M. Richard, H. Masaki, and S. J. Segalowitz. 2006. The effect of sleepiness on performance monitoring: I know what I am doing, but do I care? *Journal of Sleep Research* 15:15–21.

Nauta, H. J. W. 1986. In relationship of the basal ganglia to the limbic system. In *Handbook of Clinical Neurology. Extrapyramidal Disorders*, edited by P. J. Vinken, G. W. Bruyn, and H. L. Klawans, 19–31. Amsterdam: Elsevier.

Nieuwenhuis, S., C. B. Holroyd, N. Mol, and M. G. H. Coles. 2004. Reinforcement-related brain potentials from medial frontal cortex: Origins and functional significance. *Neuroscience and Biobehavioral Reviews* 28:441–8.

Nieuwenhuis, S., K. R. Ridderinkhof, J. Blom, G. P. H. Guido, and A. Kok. 2001. Error-related brain potentials are differentially related to awareness of response errors: Evidence from an antisaccade task. *Psychophysiology* 38:752–60.

Norman, D. A. and T. Shallice 1986. Attention to action: Willed and automatic control of behavior. In *Consciousness and Self-Regulation: Advances in Research and Theory*, edited by R. Davidson, G. Shwartz, and D. Shapiro, 1–18. New York: Plenum Press.

Oken, B. S., M. C. Salinsky, and S. M. Elsas. 2006. Vigilance, alertness, or sustained attention: Physiological basis and measurement. *Clinical Neurophysiology* 117:1885–1901.

Overbeek, T. J. M., S. Nieuwenhuis, and K. R. Ridderinkhof. 2005. Dissociable components of error processing: On the functional significance of the Pe vis-à-vis the ERN/Ne. *Journal of Psychophysiology* 19:319–29.

Padilla, M. L., R. A. Wood, L. A. Hale, and R. T. Knight. 2006. Lapses in a prefrontal-extrastriate preparatory attention network predict mistakes. *Journal of Cognitive Neuroscience* 18 (9): 1477–87.

Pailing, P. E. and S. J. Segalowitz. 2004a. The effects of uncertainty in error monitoring on associated ERPs. *Brain and Cognition* 56:215–33.

Pailing, P. E. and S. J. Segalowitz. 2004b. The error-related negativity as a state and trait measure: Motivation, personality, and ERPs in response to errors. *Psychophysiology* 41:84–95.

Parasuraman, R. and M. Rizzo 2008. *Neuroergonomics: The Brain at Work*. New York: Oxford University Press.

Petiau, C., Y. Harrison, G. Delfiore, C. Degueldre, A. Luxen, G. Franck, J. A. Horne et al. 1998. Modifications of fronto-temproal connectivity during a verb generation task after a 30 hour total sleep deprivation. A PET study. *Journal of Sleep Research* 7 (Suppl. 2): 208.

Posner, M. I. and S. E. Petersen. 1990. The attention system of the human brain. *Annual Review of Neuroscience* 13:25–42.

Posner, M. I., C. R. R. Synder, and B. J. Davidson. 1980. Attention and the detection of signals. *Journal of Experimental Psychology: General* 109:160–74.

Posner, M. I., J. A. Walker, F. J. Friedrich, and R. D. Rafal. 1984. Effects of parietal injury on covert orienting of visual attention. *Journal of Neuroscience* 4:1863–74.

Rabbitt, P. M. A. 1966. Errors and error correction in choice-response tasks. *Journal of Experimental Psychology* 71:264–72.

Rafal, R. and M. I. Posner. 1987. Deficits in human visual spatial attention following thalamic lesions. *Proceedings of the National Academy of Sciences of the United States of America* 84:7349–53.

Rail, R. V., M. C. Nicolau, A. Gamundi, M. Akaârir, S. Aparicio, C. Garau, S. Tejada et al. 2007. The trivial function of sleep. *Sleep Medicine Reviews* 11 (4): 311–25.

Ramm, P. 1989. Mapping of regional cerebral glucose metabolism and protein synthesis during sleep in animals. In *Sleep '88*, edited by J. A. Horne, 79–81. Stuttgart, Germany: Gustav Fischer.

Reason, J. 1979. Actions not as planned: The price of automatization. In *Aspect of Consciousness*, Vol. 1, edited by G. Underwood and R. Stephens, 67–89. London: Academic Press.

Reason, J. 1990. *Human Error*. Cambridge: Cambridge University Press.

Ridderinkhof, R., Y. De Vlugt, A. Bramlage, M. Spaan, M. Elton, J. Snel, and G. P. H. Band. 2002. Alcohol consumption impairs detection of performance errors in mediofrontal cortex. *Science* 298:2209–11.

Rodríguez-Fornells, A., A. R. Kurzbuch, and T. F. Münte. 2002. Time course of error detection and correction in humans: Neurophysiological evidence. *Journal of Neuroscience* 22:9990–6.

Rogers, R. D. and S. Monsell. 1995. Costs of a predictable switch between simple cognitive tasks. *Journal of Experimental Psychology: General* 124:207–31.

Rotenberg, V. S. 2006. REM sleep function and brain monoamine regulation: An application of the search activity concept. In *Sleep and Sleep Disorders: A Neuropsychopharmacological Approach*, edited by M. Lader, D. P. Cardinalli, and S. R. Pandi-Perumal, 27–35. Georgetown, TX and New York: Landes Bioscience/Eurekah.com and Springer Science + Business Media.

Schalk, G., J. R. Wolpaw, D. J. McFarland, and G. Pfurscheller. 2000. EEG-based communication: Presence of an error potential. *Clinical Neurophysiology* 111:2138–44.

Scheffers, M. K. and M. G. Coles, 2000. Performance monitoring in a confusing world: Error-related brain activity, judgments of response accuracy, and types of errors. *Journal of Experimental Psychology: Human Perception and Performance* 26 (1): 141–51.

Scheffers, M. K., M. G. Coles, P. Bernstein, W. J. Gehring, and E. Donchin. 1996. Event-related brain potentials and error-related processing: An analysis of incorrect responses to go and no-go stimuli. *Psychophysiology* 33 (1): 42–53.

Scheffers, M. K., D. G. Humphrey, R. R. Stanny, A. F. Kramer, and M. G. H. Coles. 1999. Error-related processing during a period of extended wakefulness. *Psychophysiology* 36:149–57.

Schultz, W., L. Tremblay, and J. R. Hollerman. 2000. Reward processing in primate orbitofrontal cortex and basal ganglia. *Cerebral Cortex* 10 (3): 272–83.

Simon, J. R. 1969. Reactions toward the source of stimulation. *Journal of Experimental Psychology* 81 (1): 174–6.

Stepanski, E. 2002. The effect of sleep fragmentation on daytime function. *Sleep* 25:268–76.

Thomas, M., H. Sing, G. Belenky, H. Holcomb, H. Mayberg, R. Dannals, H. Wagner, Jr. et al. 2000. Neural basis of alertness and cognitive performance impairments during sleepiness. I. Effects of 24 h of sleep deprivation on waking human regional brain activity. *Journal of Sleep Research* 9 (4): 335–52.

Thomas, M., H. Sing, G. Belenky, H. Holcomb, H. Mayberg, R. Dannals, H. Wagner, Jr. et al. 2003. Neural basis of alertness and cognitive performance impairments during sleepiness. II. Effects of 48 and 72 h of sleep deprivation on waking human regional brain activity. *Thalamus and Related Systems* 2:199–229.

Tsai, L. L., H. Y. Young, S. Hsieh, and C. S. Lee. 2005. Impairment of error monitoring following sleep deprivation. *Sleep* 28:707–13.

Tucker, D. M., A. Hartry-Speiser, L. McDougal, P. Luu, and D. deGrandpre. 1999. Mood and spatial memory: Emotion and right hemisphere contribution to spatial cognition. *Biological Psychology* 50:103–25.

Tucker, D. M. and P. Luu. 2006. Adaptive binding. In *Binding in Human Memory: A Neurocognitive Approach*, edited by H. Zimmer, A. Mecklinger, and U. Lindenberger, 85–114. New York: Oxford University Press.

Ullsperger, M., L. M. Bylsma, and M. M. Botvinick. 2005. The conflict adaptation effect: It's not just priming. *Cognitive, Affective, and Behavioral Neuroscience* 5:467–71.

Ullsperger, M. and F. Szymanowski. 2004. ERP correlates or error relevance. In *Errors, Conflicts, and the Brain: Current Opinions on Performance Monitoring*, edited by M. Ullsperger and M. Falkenstein, 171–7. Leipzig: Max-Planck Institute for Cognition and Neuroscience.

Ullsperger, M. and D. Y. von Cramon. 2001. Subprocesses of performance monitoring: A dissociation of error processing and response competition revealed by event-related fMRI and ERPs. *NeuroImage* 14:1387–401.

van Dongen, H. P. A., G. Maislin, J. M. Mullington, and D. F. Dinges. 2003. The cumulative cost of additional wakefulness: Dose-response effects on neurobehavioral functions and sleep physiology from chronic sleep restriction and total sleep deprivation. *Sleep* 26 (2): 117–26.

van Veen, V. and C. S. Carter. 2002. The timing of action-monitoring processes in the anterior cingulate cortex. *Journal of Cognitive Neuroscience* 14:593–602.

van Zomeren, A. H. and W. H. Brouwer. 1994. *Clinical Neuropsychology of Attention*. New York: Oxford University Press.

Versace, F., C. Cavallero, G. De Min Tona, M. Mozzato, and L. Stegagno. 2006. Effects of sleep reduction on spatial attention. *Biological Psychology* 71:248–55.

Volkow, N. D., G. J. Wang, F. Telang, J. S. Fowler, J. Logan, C. Wong, J. Ma et al. 2008. Sleep deprivation decreases binding of [11C]raclopride to dopamine D2/D3 receptors in the human brain. *Journal of Neuroscience* 28:8454–61.

West, R. and C. Alain. 1999. Event-related neural activity associated with the Stroop task. *Cognitive Brain Research* 8:157–64.

Wilkinson, R. T. 1960. The effect of lack of sleep on visual watch keeping. *Quarterly Journal of Experimental Psychology* 12 (1): 36–40.

Wilkinson, R. T. 1961. Interaction of lack of sleep with knowledge of results, repeated testing, and individual differences. *Journal of Experimental Psychology* 62 (3): 263–71.

Wilkinson, R. T. 1963. After-effect of sleep deprivation. *Journal of Experimental Psychology* 66 (5): 439–42.

Wilkinson, R. T. 1992. The measurement of sleepiness. In *Sleep, Arousal and Performance*, edited by R. J. Broughton and R. D. Ogilvie, 254–65. Boston: Birkhäuser.

Williams, H. L., A. Lubin, and J. Goodnow. 1959. Impaired performance with acute sleep loss. *Psychological Monographs* 73:1–26.

Wu, J. C., J. C. Gillin, M. S. Buchsbaum, T. Hershey, E. Hazlett, N. Sicotte, and W. E. Bunney. 1991. The effect of sleep deprivation on cerebral glucose metabolic rate in normal humans assessed with positron emission tomography. *Sleep* 14:155–62.

Yeung, N., M. M. Botvinick, and J. D. Cohen. 2004. The neural basis of error detection: Conflict monitoring and the error-related negativity. *Psychological Review* 111:939–59.

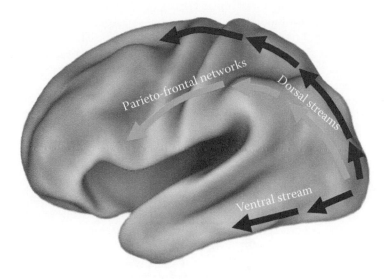

FIGURE 4.1
A schematic diagram of different visual and visuomotor pathways in the brain. The diagram is mapped onto the inflated population-average, landmark, and surface-based (PALS) atlas implemented in CARET software.

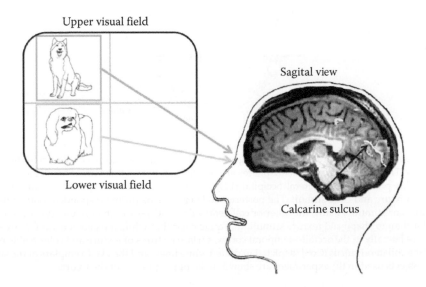

FIGURE 4.2
An illustration of the retinotopic activation in V1 to upper and lower visual field stimulation. The percent blood oxygen level-dependent (BOLD) signal change (%BSC) for lower visual field displays (yellow/orange) is located along the upper bank of the calcarine sulcus (white line), and the %BSC for upper visual field displays (blue/green) is located along the lower bank.

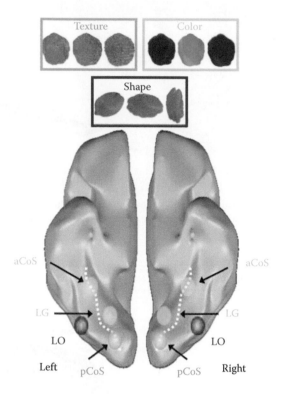

FIGURE 4.3

A schematic representation of areas selective for geometrical and surface features of objects in the ventral perceptual stream. The left and the right hemispheres are shown from below. Brain areas are depicted accordingly to their stimulus preference: the lateral occipital (LO) area (marked in red) responded significantly more to shape than to texture and color stimuli. The posterior collateral sulcus (pCoS) responded more to texture than to shape and color stimuli. Finally, the anterior collateral sulcus (aCoS) and the lingual gyrus (LG) responded more to color than to shape and texture stimuli. It is quite clear that while the geometrical feature of shape is localized more laterally in the occipito-temporal cortex, surface features of texture and color reside more medially within the collateral sulcus (CoS) (depicted in dotted white lines) and the LG. Exemplars of the shape, color, and texture objects used in the experiment are shown in the upper portion of the figure.

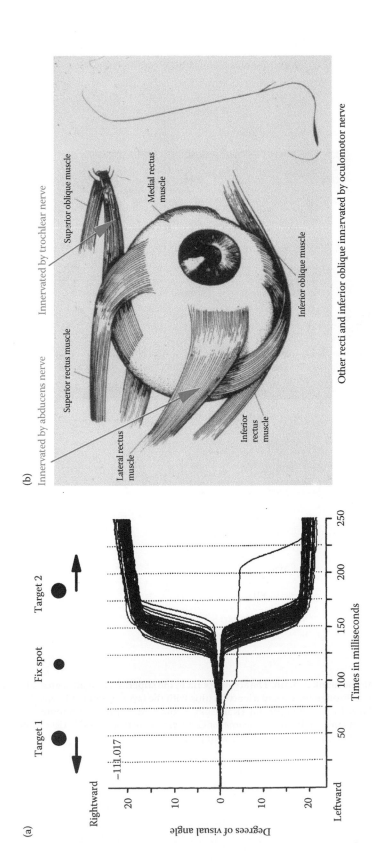

(b)

Innervated by abducens nerve   Innervated by trochlear nerve

Superior oblique muscle

Medial rectus muscle

Superior rectus muscle

Lateral rectus muscle

Inferior rectus muscle

Inferior oblique muscle

Other recti and inferior oblique innervated by oculomotor nerve

(a)

Target 1   Fix spot   Target 2

Rightward

−11j.017

20

10

0

10

20

Leftward

Degrees of visual angle

50   100   150   200   250

Times in milliseconds

FIGURE 5.1

(a) Horizontal eye-movement traces obtained while a monkey performed on a step-ramp task. Following fixation of a central spot it was doused; at the same time, a similar spot appeared either to the right or the left of fixation at an 18-degree eccentricity and was moved peripherally along the horizontal axis at 20 degrees per second. Eye-movement trace collection began when the target was turned on in the periphery. The shorter latencies involved in activating the pursuit system are made evident by the fact that pursuit eye movements for the moving target actually began before the monkey acquired it for foveal viewing with a saccadic eye movement. Pursuit eye movements in this situation began between 75 and 100 milliseconds whereas the saccades were initiated between 125 and 150 milliseconds. (Adapted from Schiller, P. H. and Logothetis, N. K. *Association for Research in Vision and Ophthalmology*, 303, 11, 1987.) (b) The human eye and the six extraocular muscles. As indicated, the lateral rectus is innervated by the abducens nerve, the superior oblique by the trochlear nerve, and the rest by the oculomotor nerve (the sixth, fourth, and third cranial nerves, respectively). (From Sekuler, R. and R. Blake. 1990. In *Perception*, 2nd ed., edited by B. R. Fetterolf and T. Holton, 23–60. New York: McGraw-Hill Publishing.)

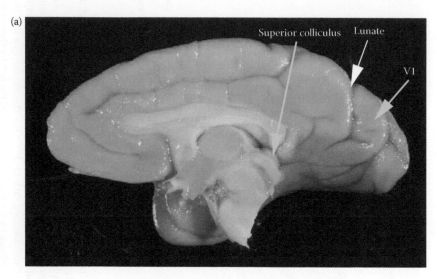

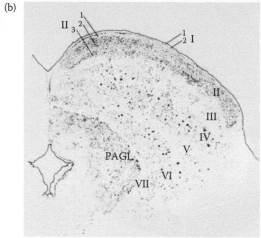

FIGURE 5.3
(a) Midline saggital section through the monkey brain. The arrows point to the superior colliculus, area V1, and the lunate sulcus. (b) Coronal section through the cat superior colliculus with the layers numbered. Layers I and II are called superficial gray and layer III stratum opticum. (Kanaseki, T. and J. M. Sprague: Anatomical organization of pretectal nuclei and tectal laminae in the cat. *Journal of Comparative Neurology*. 1974. 158 (3):319–37. Copyright Wiley-VCH Verlag GmbH & Co. KGaA. Reproduced with permission.)

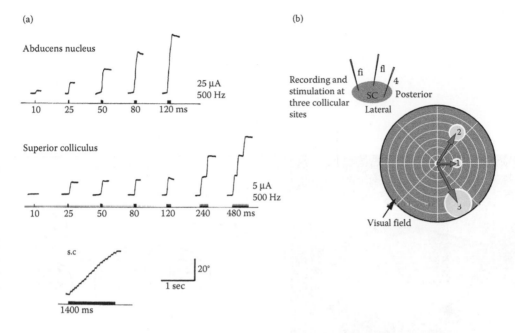

FIGURE 5.4

(a) The effects of electrically stimulating the abducens nucleus and the superior colliculus. Stimulation frequency was held constant at 500 Hertz while burst duration was systematically varied. Stimulation of the abducens nucleus shows increasing saccade size as a function of increasing burst duration. By contrast, stimulation of the superior colliculus at any given site always produces the same direction and amplitude saccade. For long-duration bursts, staircases of saccades are elicited in the superior colliculus; the size of each saccade remains of the same amplitude and direction. (Adapted from Schiller, P. H. and M. Stryker. 1972. *Journal of Neurophysiology* 35 (6): 915–24.) (b) Schematic representation of saccadic eye movements elicited by stimulation of three sites in the superior colliculus. Electrodes are placed in the anterior, medial, and lateral posterior portions of the colliculus (1–3). The location of the receptive fields recorded from these three recording sites is displayed below (yellow disks) as are the effects of electrically stimulating at these sites (red arrows). The stimulation produces a saccadic eye movement that lands the center of gaze at the location where the receptive field had been prior to the movement of the eyes.

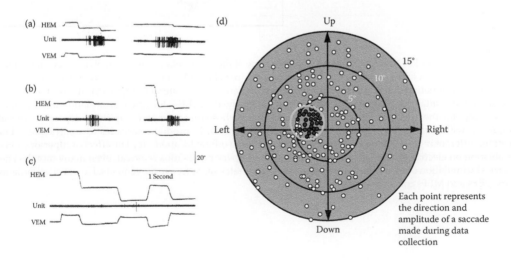

FIGURE 5.5

(a–c) A montage of horizontal and vertical eye movements and action potentials obtained from a collicular cell. The activity is limited to small left and upward eye movements. (d) A polar plot of the direction and amplitude of saccadic eye movements made. The red disks represent eye movements associated with the activity of a single neuron on the colliculus. The white disks show eye movements that were not associated with neuronal activity.

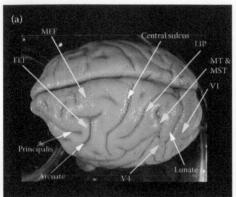
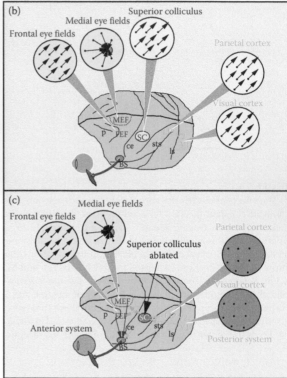

FIGURE 5.6

(a) Top view of a monkey brain. Indicated in blue are some of the areas believed to be involved in eye-movement generation; shown in white are a few of the relevant sulci. (b) Schematic of the saccadic eye movements elicited by electrical stimulation of five areas of the rhesus monkey: area V1, the lateral intraparietal sulcus, the superior colliculus, the frontal eye fields (FEFs), and the medial eye fields (MEFs). Electrical stimulation in all of these areas, except for the MEFs, elicits constant vector saccades whose direction and amplitude depend on the site stimulated within each of these structures. Stimulation of the MEFs produces saccades to a particular orbital location; different regions within this structure code different orbital locations. (c) The effect of superior colliculus ablation on electrical stimulation in the cortex. After superior colliculus removal, even many months later, electrical stimulation of the posterior cortex no longer generates saccadic eye movements. However, stimulation of the FEFs and MEFs continue to be effective.

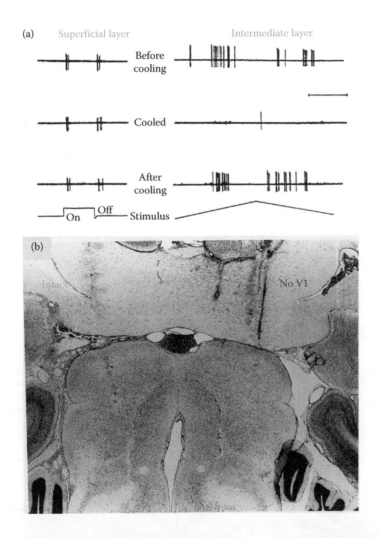

FIGURE 5.7
(a) The effect of inactivating area V1 in the monkey on the responses of neurons in the superficial and the intermediate layers of the superior colliculus to visual stimuli presented in their receptive fields. In the superficial layers, which receive input directly from the retina, V1 cooling has no effect. In the intermediate layers, which receive input from area V1, cooling of V1 eliminates neuronal responses. (b) Coronal section of a monkey superior colliculus. The left hemifield is intact. In the right hemifield, area V1 has been removed. Recordings made several months later show no responses to visual stimuli in the right superior colliculus below the superficial layers. The marker lesions depicted in red were made at the tip of the recording electrode at the sites where visual responses could no longer be elicited.

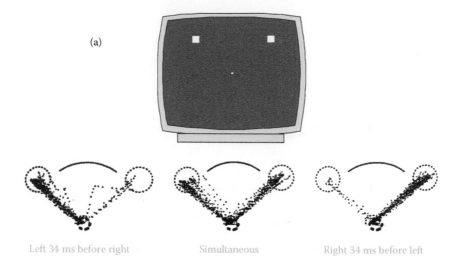

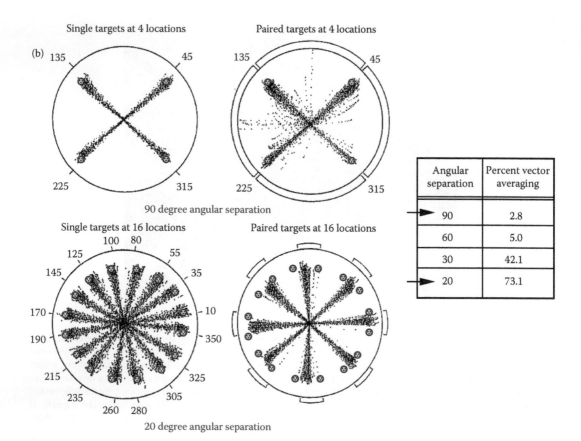

Angular separation	Percent vector averaging
90	2.8
60	5.0
30	42.1
20	73.1

FIGURE 5.8

(a) Traces of eye movements made to two targets that appear either simultaneously (center) or with a temporal offset of 34 milliseconds (left target first on left, right first on right). (b) Traces of eye movements made to single or paired simultaneous targets shown respectively on the left and right. The inset shows the percent of vector-averaged saccades under four angular separation conditions (±4.5° from midpoint between the two targets).

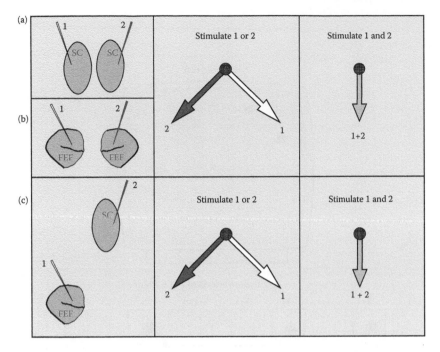

FIGURE 5.9
Shown schematically are the effects of electrically stimulating two sites in the superior colliculus (a), the frontal eye fields (b), and in each of the two structures (c). Shown are the effects of stimulating each site singly and stimulating them simultaneously. Simultaneous stimulation produces vector-averaged saccades.

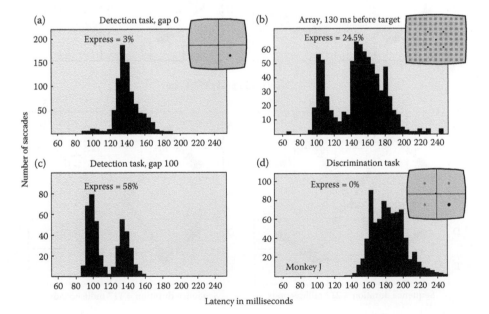

FIGURE 5.11
The distribution of saccadic latencies to visual targets. (a) Following fixation a single target appears in one of two locations; the target appears upon the termination of the central fixation spot. (b) The single target appears in one of two locations 100 milliseconds after the termination of the fixation spot. As a result, a distinct bimodal distribution of saccadic latencies is obtained, the first mode of which is called express saccades. (c) An array of stimuli appears 130 milliseconds prior to the target. The fixation spot terminates upon the appearance of the target. This condition also produces a bimodal distribution of saccadic latencies. (d) A discrimination task is used in which one of the four targets is different from the other three identical stimuli. This condition yields no express saccades and the overall latency is longer than the second mode in the detection task.

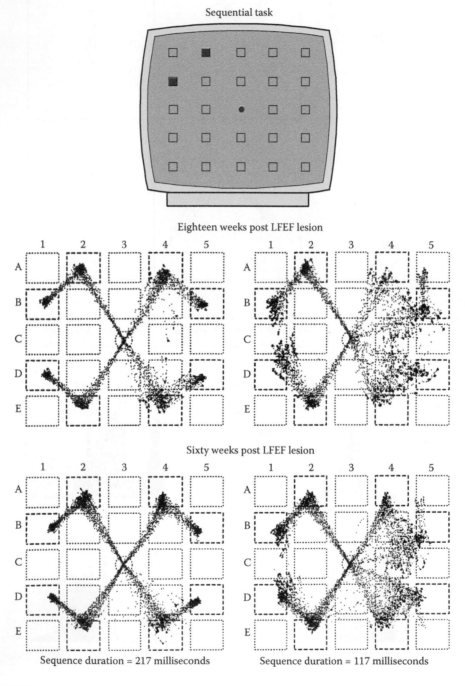

FIGURE 5.14

Eye-movement traces collected when two targets are presented in succession as shown in the top of the figure. Following fixation, two targets were presented successively at four sets of locations with sequence durations of either 217 or 117 milliseconds. Performance is shown 18 and 60 weeks following a left frontal eye field removal. Performance for the shorter sequence is quite poor for rightward saccadic sequences even 60 weeks after the lesion.

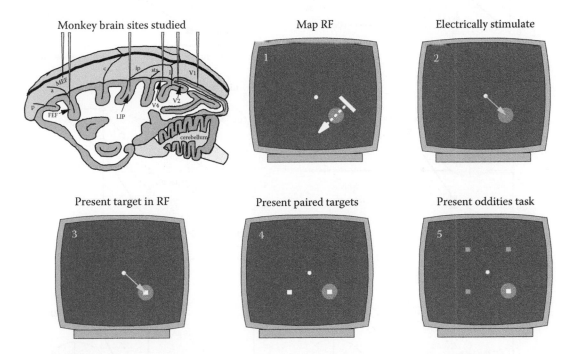

FIGURE 5.15

Experimental procedures for recording, electrically stimulating, and infusing pharmacological agents into various brain areas. The top left figure shows monkey brain and the six areas studied: areas V1, V2, V4, the lateral intraparietal sulcus (LIP), the frontal eye fields (FEFs), and the medial eye fields (MEFs). ce, central sulcus; p, principal sulcus; ip, intraparietal sulcus; sts, superior temporal sulcus; ls, lunate sulcus. The following steps were taken in experimental sessions: (1) The receptive field (RF) of the neurons recorded from was mapped. (2) The motor field (MF) was established by eliciting saccadic eye movements with electrical stimulation. (3) One target was then placed into the RF/MF that elicited saccades with the same vector. (4) Two targets were presented with varied temporal asynchronies with one of them placed into the RF/MF. (5) Four targets were presented, one of which was different from the others in luminance. The luminance, size, wavelength, and shape of the three identical distracters could be systematically varied. Data were collected pairing electrical stimulation with target presentation and examining the effects of infusing pharmacological agents.

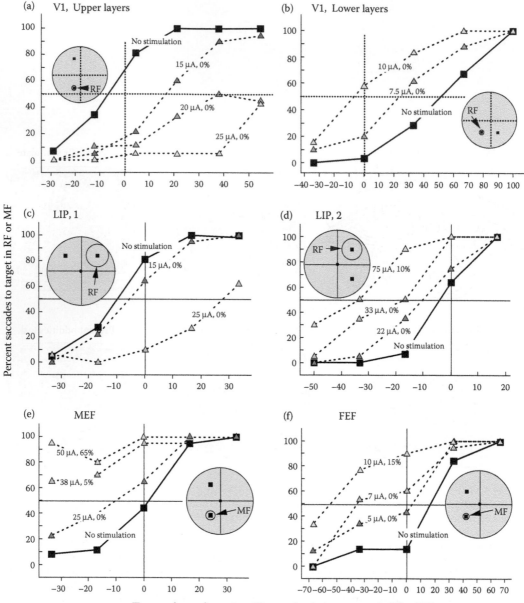

FIGURE 5.16
The effects of electrical stimulation of area V1, the lateral intraparietal sulcus (LIP), the medial eye fields (MEFs), and the frontal eye fields (FEFs) on target selection using the two-target task. Plotted are curves showing the probability with which targets presented in the receptive field are chosen as a function of the temporal asynchrony of the two targets and the current of electrical stimulation used. The current levels used are indicated for each curve. The percent values that follow indicate the percent of saccades generated to electrical stimulation when it was administered in the absence of any target. The insets show the location of the receptive fields and the layout of the targets. RF, receptive field; MF, motor field. (a) Stimulation of the upper layers of V1 produces interference. (b) Stimulation of the lower layers of V1 produces interference. (c) In some regions of the LIP, stimulation produces interference. (d) In other regions of the LIP, facilitation is produced by electrical stimulation. (e) In the MEF, stimulation produces facilitation. (f) In the FEF, stimulation produces facilitation.

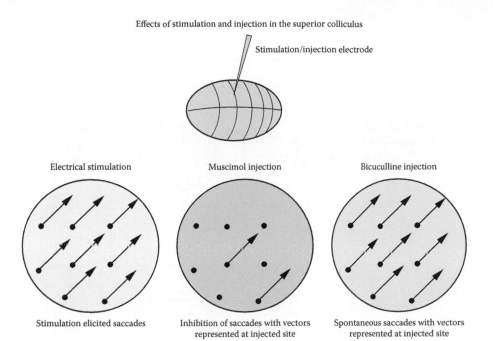

FIGURE 5.17
Schematic of the effects of infusing muscimol or bicuculline into the superior colliculus on eye movements as reported by Hikosaka and Wurtz (1985). At the site of the electrode in the superior colliculus, saccades of a specific vector are elicited at low currents as shown on the left. After muscimol injection, few spontaneous saccades are made with that vector as shown in the center. After bicuculline injection, numerous spontaneous saccades are generated with the vector represented at that site.

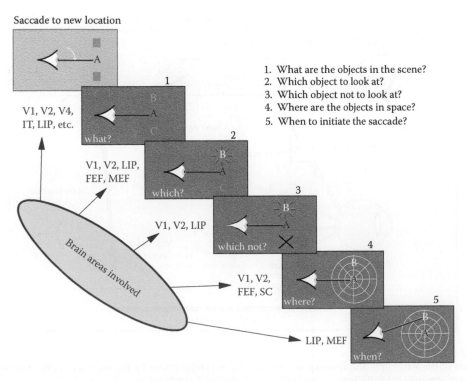

FIGURE 5.20
Schematic representation of the tasks involved in generating a saccadic eye movement.

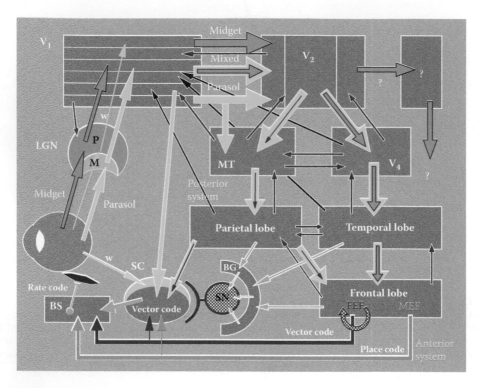

FIGURE 5.21
The neural structures and circuitry involved in the generation of visually guided saccadic eye movements.

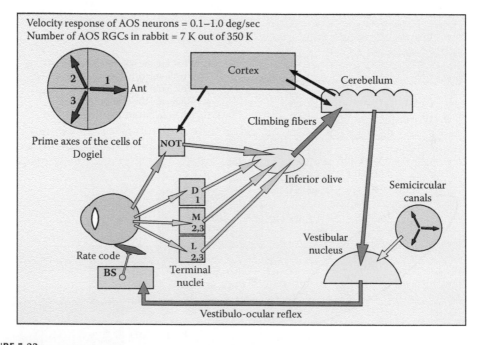

FIGURE 5.23
Diagram of the structures and connections involved in eye stabilization by the accessory optic system. NOT, nucleus of the optic tract; BS, brain stem; D, dorsal; M, medial; L, lateral terminal nuclei.

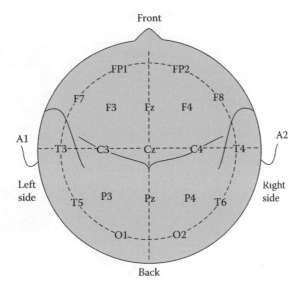

FIGURE 8.1
The international 10–20 system of electrode placement. (From Jasper, H. H. V. 1958. *Electroencephalography and Clinical Neurophysiology* 10: 370–5.)

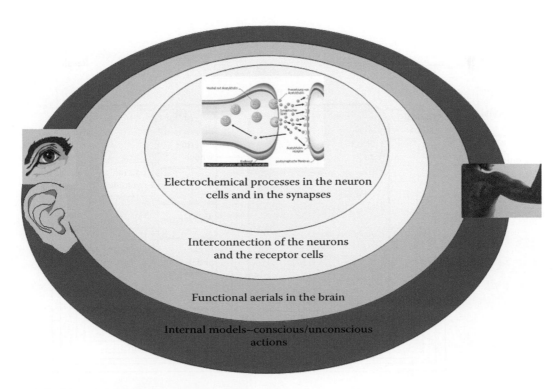

FIGURE 11.1
Shell model of human information processing.

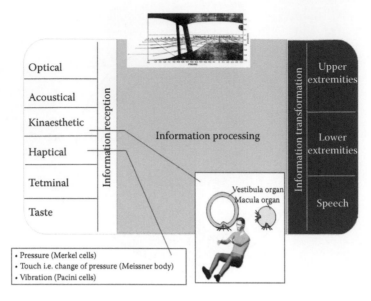

FIGURE 11.2
General model of human information processing.

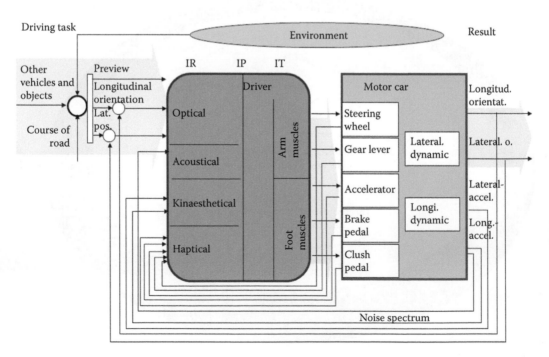

FIGURE 11.3
Closed-loop driver—car.

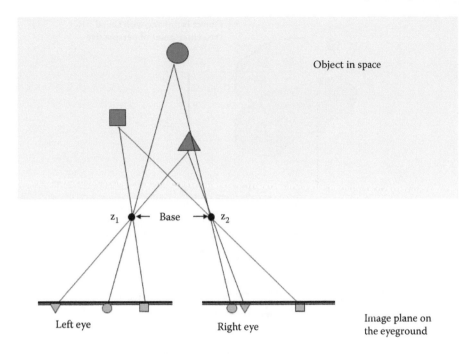

Object in space

z_1 ← Base → z_2

Left eye

Right eye

Image plane on
the eyeground

FIGURE 11.4
Principle of the stereoscopic picture of a spatial constellation at two picture surfaces.

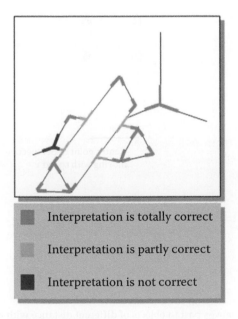

Interpretation is totally correct

Interpretation is partly correct

Interpretation is not correct

FIGURE 11.6
Example of the application of typical angle configurations.

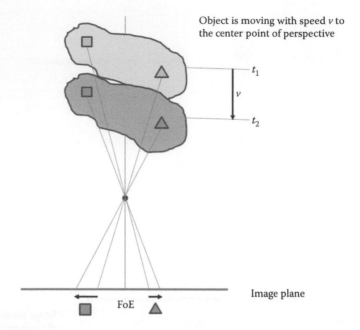

FIGURE 11.7
Motion parallax: Objects with a different distance to the observer, which moves at the same speed, generate pictures of different speed on the image plane (retina) from which conclusions about the distance can be drawn. A unique point (focus of expansion, FoE) is given here on the straight connection between the focus of the central perspective and the point where the motion takes place.

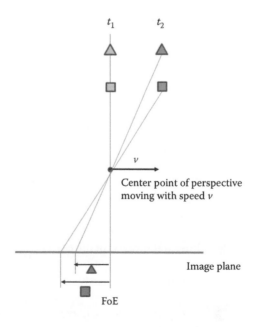

FIGURE 11.8
Motion parallax: The observer moves past in objects of different distance with a speed v (e.g., as with the look from the window of a moving train). The farther away the observed objects are the less they move. The look on a point in the horizon shows no motion (focus of expansion, FoE).

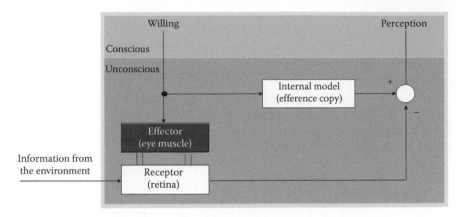

FIGURE 11.14
Reafference principle. (After von Holst, E. 1957. *Studium Generale* 10 (4):232.)

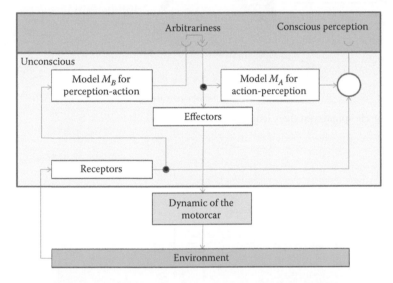

FIGURE 11.16
Behavioral structure of more highly skilled activities in the example of automobile driving.

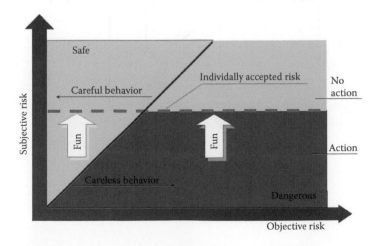

FIGURE 11.19
Example of different combinations of subjective risk estimate, objective risk, and the safety of the action arising from it.

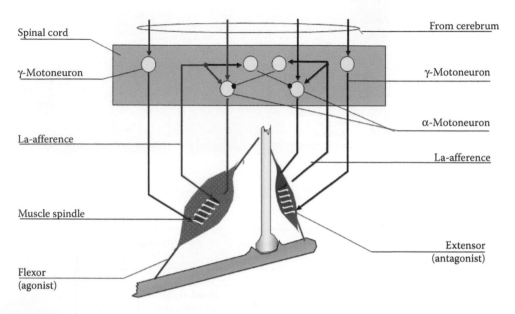

FIGURE 11.20
Control circuit muscle spinal cord (here length servomechanism).

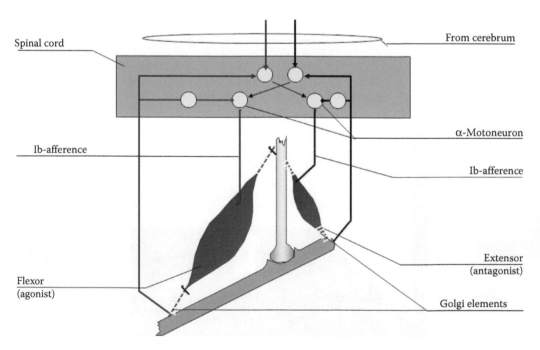

FIGURE 11.21
Control circuit muscle spinal cord (here strength servomechanism).

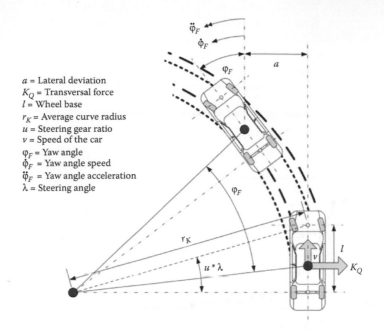

a = Lateral deviation
K_Q = Transversal force
l = Wheel base
r_K = Average curve radius
u = Steering gear ratio
v = Speed of the car
φ_F = Yaw angle
$\dot{\varphi}_F$ = Yaw angle speed
$\ddot{\varphi}_F$ = Yaw angle acceleration
λ = Steering angle

FIGURE 11.22
Geometry of curve driving.

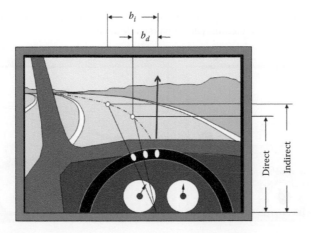

FIGURE 11.23
Point of view of the driver.

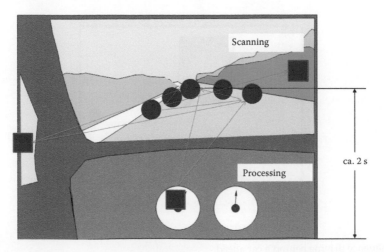

FIGURE 11.24
Glance behavior: By "scanning", the course of the road is received. By "processing", specific areas of interest are glanced.

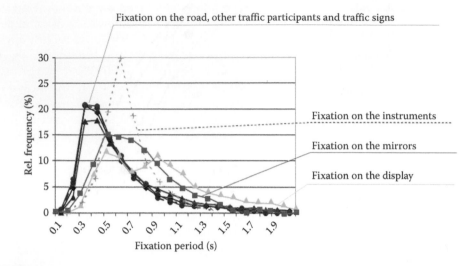

Fixation on the road, other traffic participants and traffic signs

Fixation on the instruments

Fixation on the mirrors

Fixation on the display

FIGURE 11.25
Experimental results of eye tracking experiments. (From Schweigert, M. 2003. Fahrerblickverhalten und Nebenaufgaben Dissertation an der Technischen Universität München.)

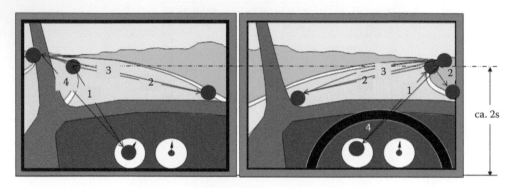

FIGURE 11.26
Typical gaze sequence in a left curve and a right curve.

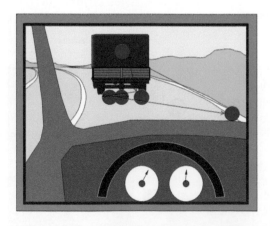

FIGURE 11.27
Typical gaze sequence driving behind a car ahead.

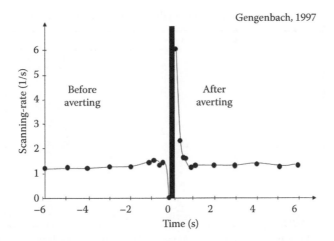

FIGURE 11.28
Scanning rate before and after averting glance from the road.

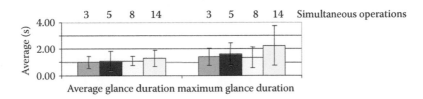

FIGURE 11.29
Glance attention in connection with tertiary tasks.

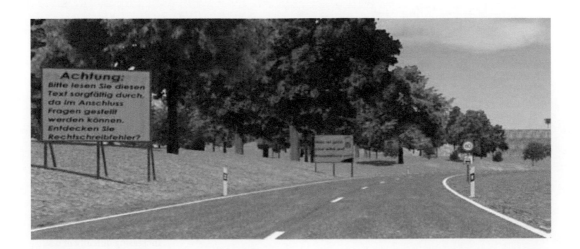

FIGURE 11.30
The advertising board is on the left side; on the right, the tempo limit sign is seen. It is completely cleared and visible at every moment.

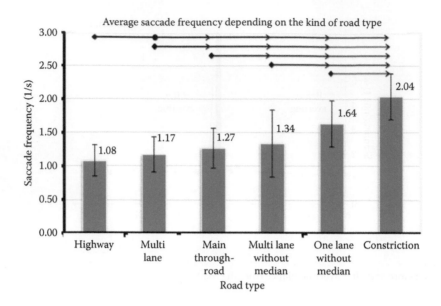

FIGURE 11.31
Mean saccade frequency of all subjects dependent on the heading type.

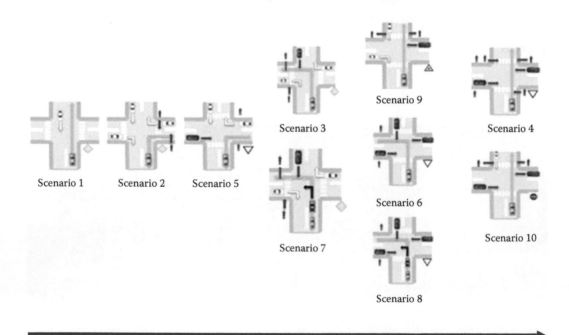

FIGURE 11.32
Investigated intersection situations ordered according to the degree of task difficulty.

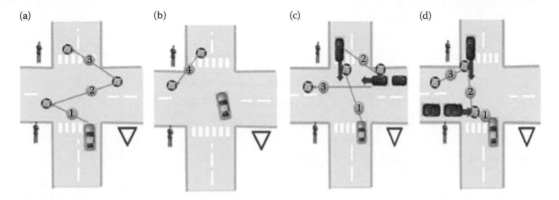

FIGURE 11.33
Typical glance sequence in scenario 6: (a) Drive through if no other road users exist. (b) Bend if no other road users exist. (c) Drive through with oncoming and traffic crossing from the right. (d) Drive through with oncoming and traffic crossing from the left.

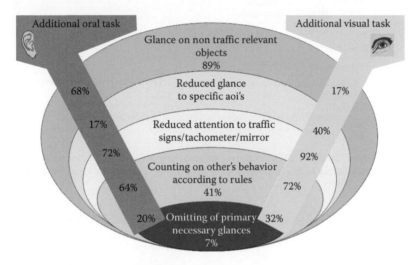

FIGURE 11.34
Percentage of faulty glance behavior. (From Schweigert, M. 2003. Fahrerblickverhalten und Nebenaufgaben Dissertation an der Technischen Universität München.)

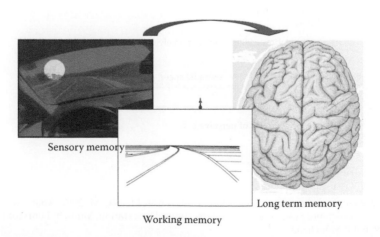

FIGURE 11.35
Stimulation of internal models by external stimuli.

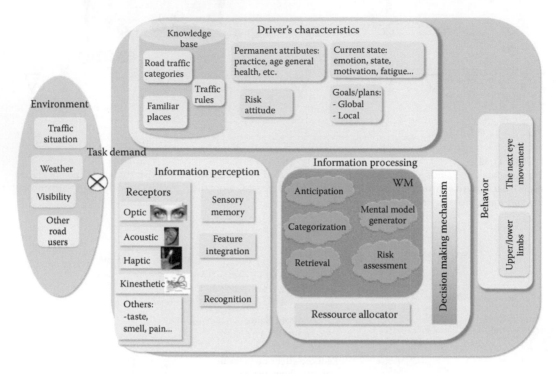

FIGURE 11.36
Multi-agent system. (From Plavšic, M. 2010. Analysis and Modeling of Driver Behavior for Assistance Systems at Road Intersections, Dissertation. Munich: Lehrstuhl für Ergonomie, Technische Universität München.)

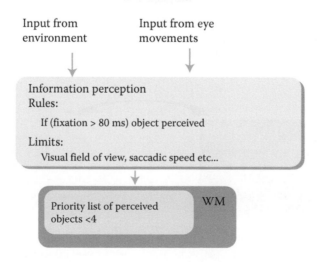

FIGURE 11.37
Modeling example for the information perception agent. (From Plavšic, M. 2010. Analysis and Modeling of Driver Behavior for Assistance Systems at Road Intersections, Dissertation. Munich: Lehrstuhl für Ergonomie, Technische Universität München.)

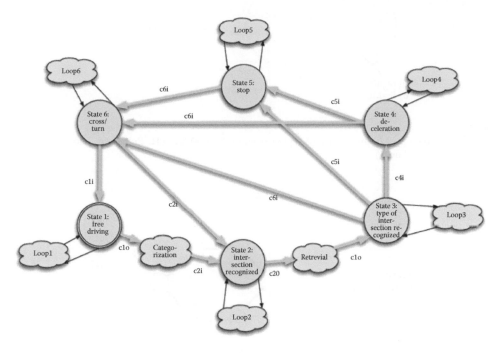

FIGURE 11.38
Temporal and causal distribution of states in an example of crossing the intersection. (From Plavšic, M. 2010. Analysis and Modeling of Driver Behavior for Assistance Systems at Road Intersections, Dissertation. Munich: Lehrstuhl für Ergonomie, Technische Universität München.)

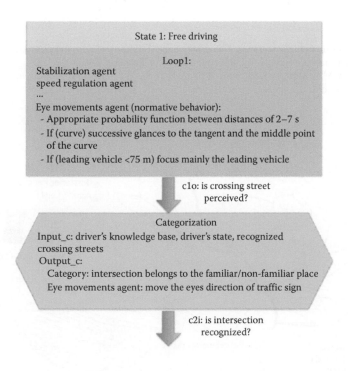

FIGURE 11.39
Cognitive state 1: Free driving. The loop occupies all the agents within one state and is named so because of its repetitiveness. Categorization agent belongs to state 1. (From Plavšic, M. 2010. Analysis and Modeling of Driver Behavior for Assistance Systems at Road Intersections, Dissertation. Munich: Lehrstuhl für Ergonomie, Technische Universität München.)

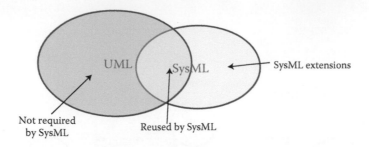

FIGURE 12.2
Relationship between SysML and UML. (Adapted from OMG SysML. 2011. Retrieved october 26, 2011, from http://www.omgsysml.org/.)

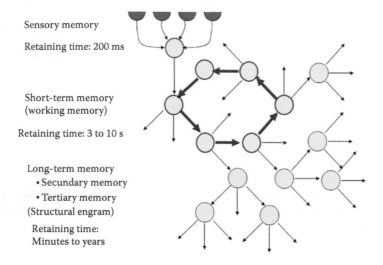

FIGURE 12.3
Extended SysML diagram taxonomy incorporated with considerations of human systems integration. (Extended model based on original framework by Reprinted from *A Practical Guide to SysML: The Systems Modeling Language*. Burlington, MA: Morgan Kaufmann, Friedenthal, S., A. Moore, and R. Steiner, Copyright 2008, with permission from Elsevier.)

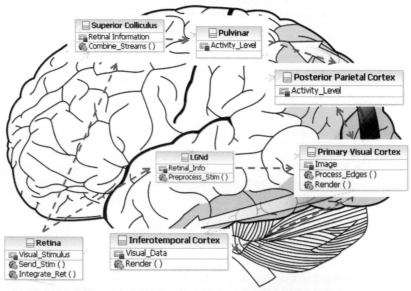

SysML model of dorsal/ventral stream in visual perception

FIGURE 12.4
Generic overview of brain structures related to visual perception represented in SysML.

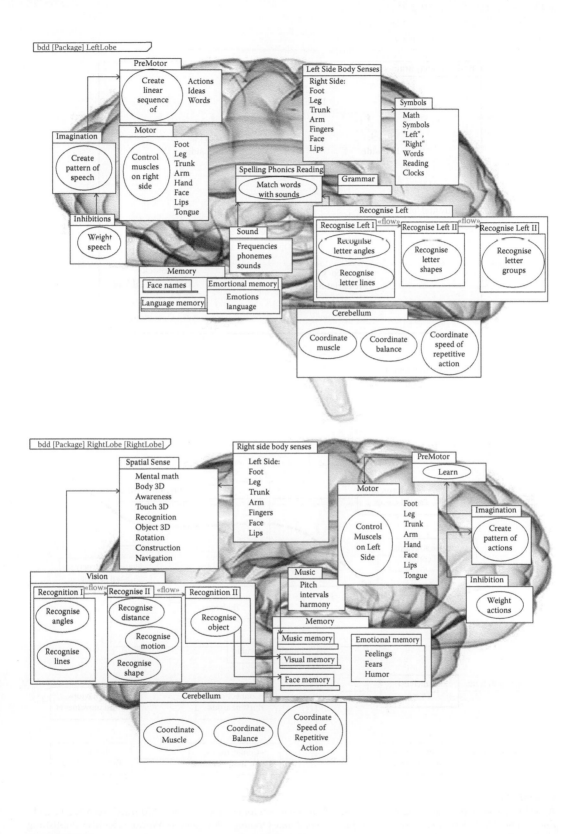

FIGURE 12.5
SysML block definition diagram for the detailed brain left- and right-side structures.

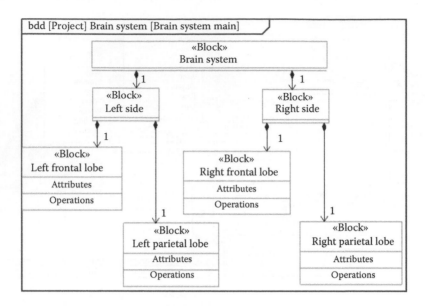

FIGURE 12.6
An example SysML brain subsystem.

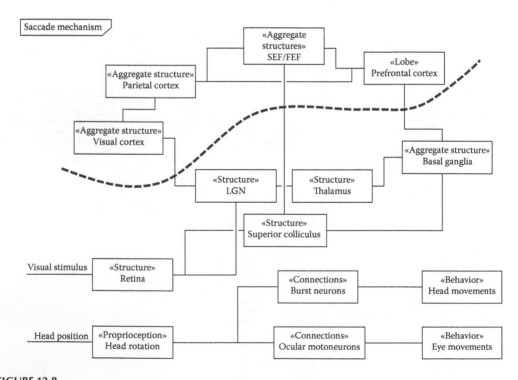

FIGURE 12.8
A SysML package diagram describing the saccade mechanism for eye movements. (Modified from Ng, G. 2009. *Brain-Mind Machinery: Brain-Inspired Computing and Mind Opening*. New Jersey: World Scientific Publishing Company.)

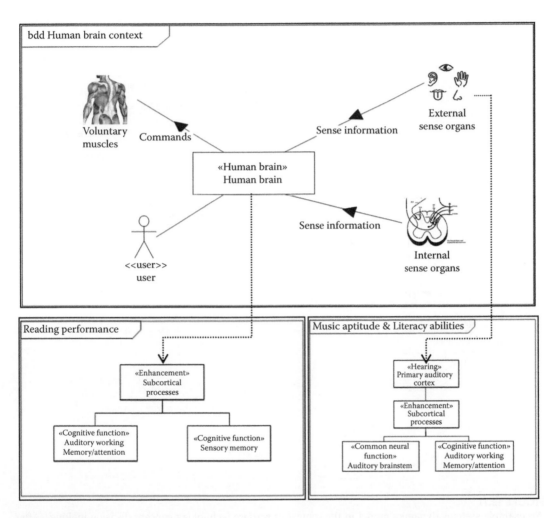

FIGURE 12.10
SysML block definition diagram for example behaviors decomposed by brain structures.

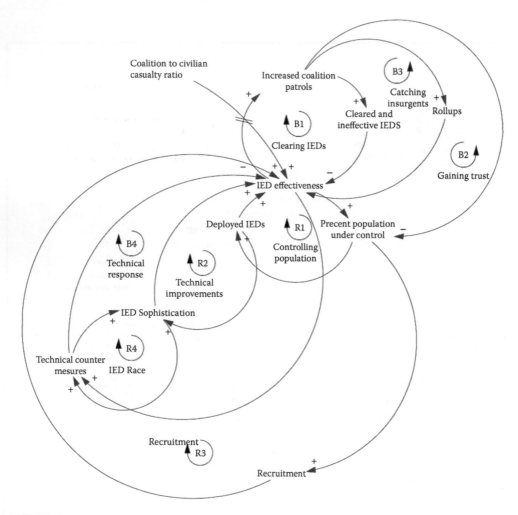

FIGURE 12.11
An example systems dynamics model in the context of warfare technology concept decision making. (After Choucri, N. et al. 2006. Understanding and modeling state stability: Exploiting system dynamics. In *Proceedings of the 2006 Institute of Electronics Engineers Aerospace Conference*, Big Sky, MT, March 4–11, 2006. USA: Institute of Electrical and Electronics Engineers.)

Section II

Neuroadaptive Systems: Challenges and Applications

7

Augmenting Human Performance

Kay M. Stanney

CONTENTS

7.1 Introduction

> Augment: To make (something already developed or well under way) greater, as in size, extent, or quantity; to add an augment to. (*American Heritage Dictionary*)

This chapter examines the general aim of neuroadaptive systems, which are complex adaptive systems consisting of multiple interconnected elements (i.e., human user, computational system, neurophysiological monitoring equipment). These systems aim to use real-time knowledge of human performance and brain function to *augment* system interactions for more efficient and effective operation. Such augmentation should expand or increase the capability of the human operator. Throughout this book, you will read of efforts focused on augmenting human performance in terms of cognitive processes (Chapter 1), executive control and learning (Chapter 2), adaptive behaviors (Chapter 3), object perception (Chapter 4), and visual performance (Chapter 5), as well as overcoming human limitations, such as maladaptive behaviors (Chapter 3) and human error (Chapter 6). Thus, there are multiple human functions that can be augmented to enhance the symbiosis between human and machine. But what does it mean to augment human performance and which aspects of performance should one aim to augment?

In performing or learning any complex skill, multiple dimensions of human performance can be augmented. Over a half-century ago, Bloom defined three domains of human learning: the psychomotor domain (i.e., physical actions and motor skills; what happens in the body), cognitive domain (i.e., knowing; what happens in the mind), and affective domain (i.e., attitudes, feeling, and emotions; what happens in the heart) (see Bloom and Krathwohl 1956). This taxonomy (which is akin to Gagne's knowledge, skills, and attitudes [KSAs]; see Gagne and Briggs 1979; Gagne, Briggs, and Wager 1992) provides a foundation on which to structure augmentations in neuroadaptive systems; specifically, such augmentations can seek to enhance the physical, cognitive, and/or affective state of the human operator. To date, such augmentations have primarily focused on the physical and cognitive states of the user, with few if any focused on overall optimization of all three states (including consideration of the inherent complex interactions between domains). For example, in the psychomotor domain, brain potentials have been coupled with external devices controlled by the physically handicapped (Farwell and Donchin 1988), including individuals with little or no motor function (Pfurtscheller et al. 2000). In the cognitive domain, the Defense Advanced Research Projects Agency's (DARPA's) Augmented Cognition Program (Schmorrow and Stanney 2008) provided a substantial leap forward, demonstrating the ability for sensor-enabled (e.g., electroenchephalography, functional near-infrared imaging, etc.) computational systems to detect a small range of human cognitive states (attention, sensory memory, working memory, and executive function). To fully augment the human state, we next need to increase the dynamic range of, as well as the number of, these couplings. Next-generation neuroadaptive systems promise to close this gap by achieving synergistic cooperation among human physical, cognitive, and affective states. This quest for synergy between human and machine is not new; in fact, it has been pursued through a succession of design eras, each seeking to resolve barriers and better understand the various roles of the human in interactive systems.

7.2 Evolution in System Design

Since the dawn of the information age, system design has become increasingly complicated owing to the advent of new technologies enabling more sophisticated systems to do more, faster than ever feasible before. With greater demands imposed on users of increasingly complex systems, the realities of exceeding the limits of human capabilities become manifest.

> in part because design continually faces new challenges, there are many examples of systems that have either failed entirely or have been adopted despite their inadequacies because of the need for their capabilities. Often the reasons these adopted systems were considered unsuccessful are because they failed to meet the requirements of the human users—they required unreasonable workload, induced psychological and physical stress, or resulted in costly human error. They failed because their developers had inadequate understanding of, or overlooked consideration of, the unique capacities and limitations of people (Pew and Mavor 2007, 12).

For far too long there was little focus on the human operator; the focus was outside the human body and mind (see Figure 7.1) and was instead on system functionality (the more a system could do, the better) and when errors occurred, the tendency was to blame the human (think Florida voting ballot [AskTog 2001]—but before blaming the voter—a quick glance at the ballot design reveals violation of nearly every Gestalt principle!). Such functionality-focused system solutions are limiting because they do not take into consideration human capabilities and limitations and, thus, the benefit of a synergistic coupling between human and machine cannot generally be realized through such a technology-centric approach. System designers need to take into account the complexities of the human user

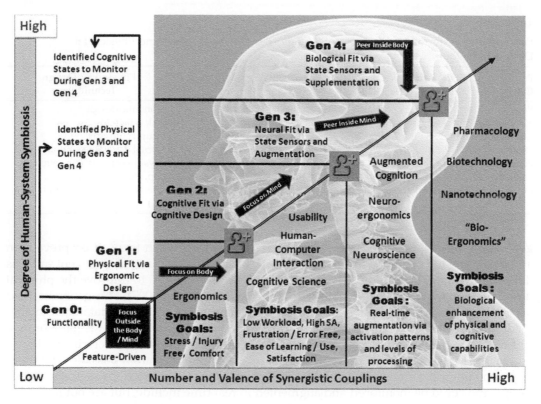

FIGURE 7.1
User-centered design generations.

when designing the interface between the human operator and the computational system. And designers have risen to this challenge; working their way through a succession of "generations" (Boff 2006) that focus on bringing the human and the machine together in ever more synergistic ways.

7.2.1 Physical Fit Generation

Perhaps, it was the frustration of humans continuously bumping up against their physical limitations when using technology, resulting in physical stressors (e.g., work-related musculoskeletal disorders, such as repetitive strain injuries, regional musculoskeletal disorders, soft tissue disorders, etc.), that led to the first user-centered design generation, which focused on the physical fit between the human and the machine; Boff (2006) calls this "Gen One." This first generation was fueled by the science of ergonomics (e.g., anthropometry and biomechanics), which developed design principles and guidelines on how to best match the machine to the physical capabilities and limitations of the human (Kroemer and Grandjean 1997).

In this first generation, designers examined how humans physically interact with machines and equipment—how they sit in front of a computer, how they carry a load, how they reach for and lift an object, and so on—and focused on designing the physical match between the system and the human such that it minimized the physical fatigue, physical stress, physical workload, and potential for injury of the human, while maximizing physical comfort (see Figure 7.1 and Table 7.1). Thus, rather than "augmentation" per se, this

TABLE 7.1

Psychomotor Performance Categories, Self-Reportable Physical States, and Physical Fit
Design Techniques

Psychomotor Performance Categories	Physical States Measurable via Self-Report	Physical Fit Design Techniques
Posture (sitting, standing, slouching, etc.)	Drowsiness	Ergonomic design
Machine control (seeing, manipulating, adjusting, scrolling, typing, feeling, touching, etc.)	Physical fatigue	Break schedules
	Physical stress	Postural supports
	Physical workload	External devices to support
Force application (pushing, pulling, twisting, etc.)	Pain/injury	physical capacity (e.g., strength, grip, etc.)
	Fitness	
Environment (heat acclimation, cold acclimation, etc.)	Heat and cold tolerance	Protective devices (e.g., from heat, etc.)

generation took a proactive (rather than an interactive) approach focused on prevention and designing the system to minimize physical (i.e., bodily) risk factors, and went so far as developing digital human models to support ergonomic analysis to improve the physical design of interactive systems (cf. Ma et al. 2009; Pew and Mavor 2007). This generation did not reach the point where physical state could be monitored and these data used to augment human–system interactions in real time (data on "physical state" was gathered via self-report or checklists in this generation; cf. Booth-Jones et al. 1998; Wictorin, Karlqvist, and Winkel 1993), but it paved the way for making such optimization possible. The types of psychomotor performance (see Table 7.1) that have been supported through ergonomic design and could be monitored and augmented in real time include, but are not limited to (Wilson and Corlett 1998):

- Task position (reaching, grasping, lifting, lowering, lines of sight, etc.)
- Posture (sitting, standing, slouching, etc.)
- Machine control (seeing, manipulating, adjusting, scrolling, typing, feeling, touching, etc.)
- Force application (pushing, pulling, twisting, etc.)
- Environment (heat acclimation, cold acclimation, etc.)

In the physical fit generation, the symbiosis goal was a system that was ergonomically designed, one that minimized stress, fatigue, and injury of the physical body and was a comfortable fit (Stanney et al. 2001). Thus, the outputs of the physical fit generation (see Table 7.1) were a well-designed system from a physical perspective (in terms of size, shape, positioning, lighting, environmental aspects such as heat and noise, etc.), work and rest schedules, postural supports, other such implements that support the anatomical aspects of the human, and protective devices (from heat, cold, etc.).

The physical fit generation resolved physical barriers between the human and the system and provided a better understanding of the physical states that could be monitored in real time, which paves the way for future user-centered design generations to develop means to augment psychomotor performance (see the neural fit generation) or positively modify physical state (see the biological fit generation). While enhancing user-centered design, the physical fit generation was primarily limited to physiological concerns below the neck and thus there was a need to consider cognitive aspects to further enhance the synergy between operator and system (Pew and Mavor 2007).

7.2.2 Cognitive Fit Generation

Once the physical fit between the human and the machine was addressed, designers found that this was not a panacea. As machines became ever more complex, there was a need to examine the cognitive fit between the human and the machine. The second generation— the cognitive fit generation (Boff [2006] calls this "Gen Two")—leveraged the fields of usability engineering, human–computer interaction, and cognitive science, among others, to develop cognitive design principles and guidelines to empower humans to deal with the ever-increasing complexity of machines (Helendar 1987; Klein et al. 1993; Nielsen 1993; Norman 1993; Salvendy 1984; Sheridan and Ferrell 1974). The aim of this generation was to harmoniously integrate the human operator and the computational system to enable effective cognitive interaction (Boff 2006). In this second user-centered design generation, designers examined how humans cognitively interact with machines and equipment— how they perceive, think, and act on information provided by a system—and focused on designing the cognitive match (i.e., what was going on inside the mind) such that it minimized cognitive workload, frustration, and potential for human error, while maximizing situational awareness, ease of learning, ease of use, and user satisfaction (see Figure 7.1 and Table 7.2).

The approach taken by the cognitive fit generation was proactive (rather than interactive); the focus was on designing systems to enhance human information processing and minimize cognitive risk factors (overload, error, loss of situation awareness, etc.; Stanney et al. 2001). This generation went so far as developing cognitive models to support analysis to improve the cognitive design of interactive systems (cf. Card, Moran, and Newell 1983; Pew and Mavor 2007). These models provided a means to evaluate the consistency of a design and ensure methods were available to achieve task goals and recover from human errors. Information on "cognitive states" (e.g., cognitive overload, situation awareness, etc.) was gathered via self-report or observable behavior (cf. Endsley 1995; Hart and Staveland 1988) in this generation. This generation did not, however, reach the point where cognitive

TABLE 7.2

Cognitive Performance Categories, Self-Reportable Cognitive States, and Cognitive Fit Design Techniques

Cognitive Performance Categories	Cognitive States Measurable via Self-Report	Cognitive Fit Design Techniques
Communication (oral comprehension, written comprehension, oral expression, written expression)	Cognitive workload	Cognitive design
	Situational awareness	Task allocation schemes
	Potential for human error	Cognitive models/architectures
Conceptualization (memorization, problem sensitivity, originality, flexibility of ideas, flexibility of closure, selective attention, spatial orientation, visualization)	Ease of learning	
	Ease of use	
	User satisfaction	
Reasoning (inductive reasoning, category flexibility, deductive reasoning, information ordering, mathematical reasoning, number facility)		
Speed-loaded (time sharing, speed of closure, perceptual speed and accuracy, reaction time, choice reaction time)		

state could be monitored and these data used to augment human–system interactions in real time, but, as with the physical fit generation, it provided the foundation on which to achieve such optimization. The types of cognitive performance (see Table 7.2) that have been characterized and supported via cognitive design and could be monitored in real time include, but are not limited to (Fleishman and Quaintance 1984):

- Communication (oral comprehension, written comprehension, oral expression, written expression)
- Conceptualization (memorization, problem sensitivity, originality, flexibility of ideas, flexibility of closure, selective attention, spatial orientation, visualization)
- Reasoning (inductive reasoning, category flexibility, deductive reasoning, information ordering, mathematical reasoning, number facility)
- Speed-loading (time sharing, speed of closure, perceptual speed and accuracy, reaction time, choice reaction time)

In the cognitive fit generation, the symbiosis goal was a system (often times a user interface design) that was well designed from a cognitive perspective, one that minimized cognitive stress, imposed an appropriate level of cognitive workload, maintained situation awareness, and was effective, efficient, and satisfying to use (Nielsen 1993; Norman 1993; Stanney et al. 2001). Thus, the outputs of the cognitive fit generation were a well-designed system from a cognitive perspective (in terms of visibility, effective conceptual models, consistency, reduced uncertainty, transparency, aesthetics, minimalistic design, error recovery, etc.), task allocation schemes that address cognitive workload, and cognitive models/architectures (Bryne 2008) that could be used to direct cognitive design or support automated systems (see Table 7.2).

The cognitive fit generation addressed cognitive barriers between the human operator and the computational system and provided a better understanding of the cognitive states that could be monitored in real time, which paves the way for future user-centered design generations to develop means to augment cognitive performance (see the neural fit generation) or effectively utilize cognition enhancers (see biological fit generation). The cognitive fit generation, as with the physical fit generation, however, took an observational approach—the behavior of the human operator was characterized through such techniques as cognitive task analysis (Crandall, Klein, and Hoffman 2006) and predictions were made on how best to design a system to avoid overload, frustration, human error, and so on. These generations did not peer inside the mind and body so that the state of the human could be more fully characterized and augmented in real time. The neural fit generation overcame the limitations of outside-looking-in observational approaches by developing cognitive sensors that acquire physiological and neurophysiological parameters that can be reliably associated with specific cognitive and/or physical states in real time while an individual is engaged with an interactive system.

7.2.3 Neural Fit Generation

Gen Three—the neural fit generation—"is characterized by a marked shift from building better work environments (and user interface designs) toward enabling humans to work better" (Boff 2006, 393). This generation is leveraging the fields of augmented cognition, neuroergonomic, cognitive neuroscience, among others, to develop a tightly coupled neural fit between the human and the computational system. The neural fit generation focuses on truly integrating the human and the system by peering inside the mind during system interaction (see Figure 7.1). Specifically, this generation seeks an interactive solution, where human cognitive and physical states are monitored in real time and adaptive augmentation strategies are interactively triggered to enhance human capabilities (Stanney et al. 2009). This generation was the next logical progression from the physical and cognitive fit generations, as it sought to identify not just how to measure but how to "augment" human performance to enhance the capabilities of the human operator, which are often exceeded by increasingly complicated computational system designs. To determine how best to augment, one can look to the resulting outputs of cognitive performance, which result in new cognitive states (see Table 7.3), such as new levels of task proficiency/knowledge, or altered levels of workload, engagement, distraction, arousal, awareness, confusion, stress, bias, and so on. (Berka et al. 2004; Berka et al. 2007). These cognitive states can be measured in real time by several different types of physiological sensors (see the review by Stanney et al. 2009). For example, electroencephalography has been shown to reflect subtle shifts in sensory memory, working memory, attention, and executive function, alertness/vigilance, engagement, cognitive load, and workload. Functional near-infrared sensors have been used to detect various cognitive states, including sensory memory, working memory load, general workload, and loss of concentration. Variations in galvanic skin response levels have been associated with shifts in arousal, attention, working memory, cognition, attention, emotion, engagement, anxiety, and stress. Oculomotor and cardiovascular measures have also been associated with variations in cognitive states. Development of real-time cognitive state sensors is evolving and new; more reliable solutions are anticipated over the next decade.

The challenge with all cognitive state measures is to gather the state data in real time and use these data to drive adaptive changes that augment human cognitive performance. The general objectives of such augmentation are (at least) twofold: (1) to accelerate gains in task proficiency and/or knowledge and (2) to enhance cognitive state such that

TABLE 7.3

Cognitive Performance Elements and Related Cognitive States That Could Be Monitored and Trigger Augmentations

Cognitive Performance to Augment	Cognitive States to Monitor in Real Time	Real-Time Augmentation Techniques
Same as cognitive fit generation (see Table 7.2)	Skill proficiency Knowledge Workload Cognitive load Alertness/vigilance Disengagement Distraction Arousal Awareness Confusion Loss of concentration Cognitive stress Cognitive bias Sensory memory Working memory Attention Executive function	Adaptations of presentation (modality augmentation, cuing, decluttering, and context-sensitive help, etc.) Adaptations of schedule (pacing, sequencing, etc.) Adaptation of system autonomy (task delegation)

performance or learning is improved. Depending on the type of cognitive actions required during system interaction, the operator may start to experience any one of the cognitive states summarized in Table 7.3 (e.g., cognitive overload, distraction, confusion, etc.), which could hinder task performance and/or learning. In augmented applications, such changes in cognitive state are monitored in real time and then, as needed, augmentations of cognitive performance are triggered to address human limitations (e.g., real-time physiological assessment of workload, engagement, distraction, etc. are coupled with adaptive techniques to assist with focusing attention, supporting working memory, etc.; Schmorrow and Stanney 2008). Adaptive techniques (Fuchs et al. 2007; Stanney et al. 2009) can involve adaptations of information presentation (e.g., changing the modality, cuing, decluttering, and context-sensitive help), adaptations of information schedule (e.g., pacing and sequencing), or adaptation of system autonomy (e.g., task delegation), among others (see Table 7.3). These techniques are used to augment human capabilities, thereby leading to gains in task proficiency or acceleration of learning.

Not only cognitive performance but also psychomotor performance could be augmented. To achieve this, an understanding of the resulting outputs from psychomotor performance must be considered; specifically how psychomotor performance changes the physical state of the human operator. Many types of physical state changes can occur (see Table 7.1), such as heightened levels of drowsiness, physical fatigue, physical stress, physical workload, pain, injury, reduced fitness, heat and cold intolerance, and so on (Karsh, Holden, and Alper 2006). For example, as a work shift progresses, an operator is likely to become more physically fatigued and may become drowsy. Depending on the type of physical actions required of the musculoskeletal system during the shift, the operator may start to experience pain or injury from overuse. In augmented applications, these changes in physical state would be monitored in real time and then, as needed, augmentations of psychomotor performance would be instantiated (e.g., real-time physiological assessment of physical fatigue* and drowsiness† could be coupled with external devices to assist with task position, posture, machine control, and force application as required; physiological heat strain of an environment could be monitored in real time and heat acclimation techniques triggered when needed [Walker, Dawson, and Ackland 2001]).

Thus, with the neural fit generation, system designers are no longer bound to making inferences based on overt behaviors and subjective responses; they can identify the neural bases of such cognitive functions as perceiving, attending, remembering, and deciding and such physical functions as reaching, grasping, manipulating, and holding. Through understanding of brain functions, the requisite KSAs for a given system can be precisely specified, neural signatures of learning processes and outcomes can be developed, adaptive augmentations can be triggered to enhance human performance, and so on. Better understanding of such brain functions can quantify constraints on human capabilities and, as past generations have, inform design guidelines that collectively lead to enhanced design of even the most complex of systems; but it can also support real-time adaptations that interactively augment human capabilities. Thus, the symbiosis goal of the neural fit generation is real-time augmentation of human cognitive and physical capabilities based on neural activation patterns and levels of processing. Such couplings

---

* For example, a reduction of electroencephalograph peak alpha frequency has been found to be an indicator of physical fatigue (Ng and Raveendran 2007).
† For example, visual measures, such as PERCentage of eyelid CLOSure (PERCLOS), have been found to be highly reliable and valid measures of alertness level (Dinges et al. 1998).

seek to augment rather than alter the human state, the latter of which is the objective of the biological fit generation.

7.2.4 Biological Fit Generation

Gen Four—the biological fit generation—focuses on biologically modifying human physical and/or cognitive capabilities to enhance human performance (Boff 2006). This generation can leverage the fields of pharmacology, biotechnology, nanotechnology, and "bio-ergonomics," among others, to identify how best to achieve a biological fit that maximizes human effectiveness. The biological fit generation seeks to truly integrate the human and the system by peering inside the body during system interaction (see Figure 7.1). Specifically, this generation seeks an interactive solution, where human cognitive and physical states are monitored in real time and adaptive supplementations are interactively triggered to enhance human capabilities. Currently, this generation generally focuses on using pharmacology and biotechnology to modify effects of disease, aging, or injury (Solomon, Noll, and Mordkoff 2009); however, "the armed forces seek sustained vigilance and cognitive superiority in military operations and continue to be at the forefront of testing and implementing safe and effective psycho-pharmacological agents" (Boff 2006, 395). Thus, this generation aims to reach beyond medicinal specialties to enhance operational performance and learning.

From a physical perspective, advances in real-time blood and tissue chemistry analysis for monitoring astronaut health and physiological changes from microgravity and radiation exposure (Dogariu, Goltsov, and Scully 2008; Fan et al. 2008; Merrill 2009) could be used to determine the current physical state of an individual, trigger supplementation, and assess their effectiveness in overcoming drowsiness, fatigue, stress, and other physical states (see Table 7.1). In terms of supplementation, performance-enhancing drugs and supplements—commonly used by athletes—could be used to enhance physical performance in operational environments, such as stimulants (e.g., caffeine) that induce temporary improvements in physical function (e.g., enhanced alertness, wakefulness, and locomotion, etc., decreased fatigue), painkillers (e.g., over-the-counter drugs such as NSAIDs like Ibuprofen and acetaminophen) that mask pain so an individual can continue to perform beyond their usual pain thresholds, nutrachemicals (i.e., dietary supplements, vitamins, minerals, amino acids, etc.) that have been shown to enhance performance in athletes, such as creatine, which has been shown to enhance anaerobic training, strength, and performance, as well as other drugs (Academy of Medical Sciences 2008; National Research Council 2008; Tokish, Kocher, and Hawkins 2008).

From a cognitive perspective, cognitive enhancers could be used to alter the cognitive state of an individual such that they are optimally receptive to learning. Cognition enhancers have been defined as "drugs able to facilitate attentional abilities and acquisition, storage and retrieval of information, and to attenuate the impairment of cognitive functions associated with head traumas, stroke, age and age-related pathologies" (Gualtieri et al. 2002, 125). Specifically, nootropics are drugs, supplements, nutraceuticals, and functional foods that are potentially capable of enhancing one or more of the following cognitive processes in healthy humans: short- and long-term memory, attention, mental concentration, working memory, learning potential, motivation, and reaction time. Such enhancers could, thus, be used to enhance learning and performance by augmenting an individual's biological state, rendering them more cognitively receptive to learning (Lanni et al. 2008). The use of such biological enhancers to augment physical capabilities and cognitive processes in healthy humans is being explored, with the potential to enhance performance and learning not only under normal circumstances but also under highly demanding training regimens, such as those used to train military warfighters or emergency medical personnel (Stanney, Costello, and Kennedy 2007). Table 7.4 provides a summary of potential benefits associated with the use of biological state enhancers during operational performance and learning.

As with the neural fit generation, the biological fit generation seeks an interactive solution that takes the outcomes of real-time physiological and neurophysiological monitors of cognitive and/or physical states and triggers pharmacological aids that overcome human limitations. Thus, the symbiosis goal of the biological fit generation is modification (i.e., biological enhancement) of the actual state of the human to achieve optimal human performance. It is important to note that this focus on altering human capabilities comes with ethical concerns that question the rectitude of tampering with the fundamentals of human nature (Boff 2006).

TABLE 7.4

Biological Enhancers That Target Modifications of Human Cognitive and Physical Performance Capabilities

Biological Enhancer	Targeted Modifications of Human Capabilities
Stimulants (e.g., caffeine)	Induce temporary improvements in physical function (e.g., enhance alertness, wakefulness, locomotion; decrease fatigue)
Painkillers (e.g., NSAIDs)	Mask pain so an individual can continue to perform beyond their usual pain thresholds
Nutrachemicals (e.g., dietary supplements, vitamins, minerals, amino acids, etc.)	Enhance anaerobic and aerobic physical performance (e.g., enhance speed and strength)
Neurohormones, herbs, nutrients, brain boosting drugs (e.g., Ritalin, Provigil, Inderal)	Enhance one or more parts of an individual's memory (e.g., spatial, working, episodic procedural), as well as enhance learning and cognitive speed[a]
Stimulants, alertness-enhancing compounds (e.g., Modafinil, Dextroamphetamine, Zolpidem), antidepressants	Increase attention and concentration; impulse control
Stimulants, alertness-enhancing compounds	Mitigate negative cognitive affects of sleep and malnutrition
Anti-oxidant vitamins, naturally occurring hormones (e.g., Dehydroepiandrosterone—DHEA)	Potentially prevent deterioration of cells brought about by natural aging; may prevent gradual cognitive degeneration that begins in middle age

Source: Adapted from Academy of Medical Sciences *Brain Science, Addiction and Drugs*, An Academy of Medical Sciences Working Group Report, chaired by Professor Sir Gabriel Horn, Academy of Medical Sciences, London, England, 2008; Caldwell, J. A., Dextroamphetamine and modafinil are effective countermeasures for fatigue in the operational environment, in *Strategies to Maintain Combat Readiness during Extended Deployments—A Human Systems Approach. Meeting Proceedings RTO-MP-HFM-124*, paper 31, pp. 31-1–31-16, RTO, Neuilly-sur-Seine, France, 2005, http://www.rto.nato.int/abstracts.asp; National Research Council, *Emerging Cognitive Neuroscience and Related Technologies*, The National Academies Press, Washington, DC, 2008; Stanney, K. M., A. Costello, and R. S. Kennedy. 2007. *Technology* 11: 83–105; Tokish, J. M., M. S. Kocher, and R. J. Hawkins. 2008. *American Journal of Sports Medicine* 32 (6): 1543–53.

[a] For example, recent studies suggest that Ritalin may boost the ability to focus on tasks and enhance the speed of learning by increasing the activity of the neurotransmitter dopamine inside the brain (Tye et al. 2010).

7.3 Collective Human State

Through a succession of user-centered design generations, each era has sought to realize ever-greater levels of human–system symbiosis through a growing number and heightened valence of physical, cognitive, neural, and biological synergistic couplings (see Figure 7.1). Some generations (physical fit and cognitive fit) work from the outside, characterizing human performance by its outcomes and designing to overcome human limitations. Other generations (neural fit and biological fit) work from the inside, characterizing, in real time, human physical and cognitive states and triggering adaptations that augment or modify human capabilities. Neuroadaptive systems can integrate the synergistic tactics of each of these generations, leveraging the benefits of the one before it and adding yet another dimension of synergistic coupling (see Figure 7.1). Collectively these couplings can characterize, in real time, human performance, brain function, and human biology and use this knowledge of collective "human state" to augment human–system interactions for more efficient and effective operation. The resulting level of human–system symbiosis should lead to unprecedented levels of productivity and user engagement.

Any such efforts to enhance human performance must take into consideration the interactions between human physical, cognitive, and affective states and their collective influence on the overall human state. For example, the physical state of drowsiness is known to affect the cognitive state of alertness and associated cognitive performance. Those who have been sleep deprived show decrements in many aspects of cognitive performance, including simple task performance (e.g., reaction time, vigilance, attention, etc.), as well as complex cognitive task performance (e.g., working memory, verbal fluency and speech articulation, language, logical reasoning, creative and flexible thinking and planning, decision making, and judgment; Thomas et al. 2000, 2003). Beyond performance decrements, the physiological basis of drowsiness can be demonstrated as a decrease in saccadic velocity, which is a measure of oculomotor response that could be measured and monitored in real time. The neural basis of drowsiness, which could also be measured and monitored in real time, presents itself as decreased brain activity and function, specifically decreases in the prefrontal cortex and thalamus, with larger reductions in activity in the distributed cortico-thalamic network mediating attention and higher-order cognitive processes. Such changes in neural activity could be preceded by or associated with blood composition changes; specifically, increased plasma levels of adrenaline, adrenocorticotropic hormone, and corticosterone could indicate drowsiness (Meerlo, Sgoifo, and Suchecki 2008). These physiological, neurophysiological, and blood-level indicators of drowsiness could collectively be monitored in real time and when issues are identified could, in turn, trigger augmentation and/or supplementation. In terms of augmentation, visual highlighting, auditory cuing, omnidirectional attention funneling, and other such techniques could be used to direct attention in drowsy individuals (Biocca et al. 2006), and recent studies suggest that exposure to pictorial scenes of nature could be used to restore directed attention when fatigued, perhaps by increasing glucose levels (Tang and Posner 2009). In terms of supplementation, caffeine could be administered, as it has been shown to have beneficial effects on alertness (Kamimori et al. 2000; McLellan, Kamimori, Bell, et al. 2005; McLellan, Kamimori, Voss, et al. 2005), as well as maintain performance in sleep-deprived individuals, such as military personnel (Lieberman and Tharion 2002; McLellan, Kamimori, Bell, et al. 2005; McLellan, Kamimori, Voss, et al. 2005). It is essential to consider such interactive effects between human states as well as to look beyond psychomotor and cognitive performance to affective performance because affective states (e.g., anxiety, depression, stress, certain emotions) can profoundly affect cognitive performance (Ashby, Isen, and Turken 1999). Further, it is important to realize that it may not be possible to enhance all aspects of psychomotor, cognitive, and affective performance, as one area could be enhanced at the expense of impairing another (Academy of Medical Sciences 2008).

7.4 Conclusions

With each successive user-centered design generation, we have come ever closer to the ultimate neuroadaptive system—one that constitutes a closed-loop system in which human–system interactions are driven by synergistic cooperation among a multi-tier of neural and biological sensors of physical, cognitive, and affective states, which taken together define the current "human state" and in turn drive augmentation and/or modification of this state, as needed, to achieve optimized human performance. Thus, while the efforts of today focus on augmenting individual components of human performance, such as attention, object recognition, cognitive function, and muscular performance, as well as overcoming human limitations, such as mental fatigue, sleep deprivation, and human error, the neuroadaptive systems of tomorrow will aim to collectively optimize all measurable dimensions of human performance. Such neuroadaptive systems promise to not only resolve the barriers between the human and the computational system but also achieve ever-higher levels of human and machine symbiosis, thereby leading to unprecedented levels of productivity and engagement.

Acknowledgments

This material is based on work supported in part by the Office of Naval Research (ONR) under SBIR contract N00014-08-C-0186 and the Defense Advanced Research Projects Agency (DARPA) under contract W31P4Q-07-C-0214. Any opinions, findings and conclusions, or recommendations expressed in this material are those of the author and do not necessarily reflect the views or the endorsement of ONR or DARPA. I am indebted to Lee Kollmorgen, who opened my mind to the world beyond WIMPs and its vast potential; to Dylan Schmorrow, for his visionary genius that inspired many of the ideas in this paper, and to Kenneth Boff, who mused with me on the topics in this paper several years ago.

References

Academy of Medical Sciences. 2008. *Brain Science, Addiction and Drugs.* An Academy of Medical Sciences Working Group Report, chaired by Professor Sir Gabriel Horn. London, England: Academy of Medical Sciences.

Ashby, F. G., A. M. Isen, and A. U. Turken. 1999. A neuropsychological theory of positive affect and its influence on cognition. *Psychological Review* 106 (3): 529–50.

AskTog. 2001. The butterfly ballot: Anatomy of a disaster, January 2001. Accessed March 1, 2010. http://www.asktog.com/columns/042ButterflyBallot.html.

Berka, C., D. J. Levendowski, M. Cvetinovic, M. M. Petrovic, G. F. Davis, M. N. Lumicao, V. T. Zivkovic, M. V. Popvic, and R. E. Olmstead. 2004. Real-time analysis of EEG indices of alertness, cognition and memory acquired with a wireless EEG headset. *International Journal of Human-Computer Interaction* 17 (2): 151–70.

Berka, C., D. J. Levendowski, M. N. Lumicao, A. Yau, G. Davis, V. T. Zivkovic, R. E. Olmstead, P. D. Tremoulet, and P. L. Craven. 2007. EEG correlates of task engagement and mental workload in vigilance, learning, and memory tasks. *Aviation Space and Environmental Medicine* 78 (5, Suppl.): B231–44.

Biocca, F., A. Tang, C. Owen, and X. Fan. 2006. Attention funnel: Omnidirectional 3D cursor for mobile augmented reality platforms In *CHI 2006 Proceedings*, 1115–22. Montréal, Québec, Canada April 22–27, 2006.

Bloom, B. S. and D. R. Krathwohl. 1956. *Taxonomy of Educational Objectives: The Classification of Educational Goals, by a Committee of College and University Examiners. Handbook I: Cognitive Domain*. New York, NY: Longmans, Green.

Boff, K. R. 2006. Revolutions and shifting paradigms in human factors and ergonomics. *Applied Ergonomics* 37 (4): 391–9.

Booth-Jones, A. D., G. K. Lemasters, P. Succop, M. R. Atterbury, and A. Bhattacharya. 1998. Reliability of questionnaire information measuring musculoskeletal symptoms and work histories. *American Industrial Hygiene Association Journal* 59 (1): 20–4.

Bryne, M. D. 2008. Cognitive architecture. In *Handbook of Human-Computer Interaction*, 2nd ed., edited by J. Jacko and A. Sears, 93–113. Mahwah, NJ: Lawrence Erlbaum Associates.

Caldwell, J. A. 2005. Dextroamphetamine and modafinil are effective countermeasures for fatigue in the operational environment. In *Strategies to Maintain Combat Readiness during Extended Deployments—A Human Systems Approach. Meeting Proceedings RTO-MP-HFM-124*, paper 31, pp. 31-1–31-16. Neuilly-sur-Seine, France: RTO. http://www.rto.nato.int/abstracts.asp.

Card, S. K., T. P. Moran, and A. Newell. 1983. *The Psychology of Human-Computer Interaction*. Hillsdale, NJ: Lawrence Erlbaum Associates.

Crandall, B., G. Klein, and R. R. Hoffman. 2006. *Working Minds: A Practitioner's Guide to Cognitive Task Analysis*. Cambridge MA: MIT Press.

Dinges, D. F., M. Mallis, G. Maislin, and J. W. Powell. 1998. Evaluation of techniques for ocular measurement as an index of fatigue and the basis for alertness management. *Technical Report 808 762*. Department of Transportation Highway Safety Publication, Washington, DC.

Dogariu, A., A. Goltsov, and M. O. Scully. 2008. Real-time blood analysis using coherent anti-stokes Raman scattering. In *Conference on Lasers and Electro-Optics/Quantum Electronics and Laser Science Conference and Photonic Applications Systems Technologies, Optical Society of America Technical Digest* (CD), San Jose, California, paper JWC4.

Endsley, M. R. 1995. Measurement of situation awareness in dynamic systems. *Human Factors* 37 (1): 65–84.

Fan, R., O. Vermesh, A. Srivastava, B. K. H. Yen, L. Qin, H. Ahmad, G. A. Kwong et al. 2008. Integrated barcode chips for rapid, multiplexed analysis of proteins in microliter quantities of blood. *Nature Biotechnology* 26: 1373–8.

Farwell, L. A. and E. Donchin. 1988. Talking off the top of your head: Toward a mental prosthesis utilizing event-related potentials. *Electroencephalography and Clinical Neurophysiology* 70: 510–23.

Fleishman, E. A. and M. K. Quaintance. 1984. *Taxonomies of Human Performance: The Description of Human Tasks*. Boston, MA: Academic Press.

Fuchs, S., K. S. Hale, K. M. Stanney, J. Juhnke, and D. Schmorrow. 2007. Enhancing mitigation in augmented cognition. *Journal of Cognitive Engineering and Decision Making* 1: 309–26.

Gagne, R., L. Briggs, and W. Wager. 1992. *Principles of Instructional Design*, 4th ed. Fort Worth, TX: Harcourt Brace Jovanovich College.

Gagne, R. M. and L. J. Briggs. 1979. *Principles of Instructional Design*, 2nd ed. New York, NY: Holt, Rinehart, and Winston, Inc.

Gualtieri, F., D. Manetti, M. N. Romanelli, and C. Ghelardini. 2002. Design and study of piracetam-like nootropics, controversial members of the problematic class of cognition enhancing drugs. *Current Pharmaceutical Design* 8: 125–8.

Hart, S. G., and L. E. Staveland. 1988. Development of NASA-TLX (Task Load Index): Results of empirical and theoretical research. In *Human Mental Workload*, edited by P. A. Hancock and N. Meshkati, 139–83. North-Holland: Elsevier Science.

Helendar, M. 1987. *Handbook of Human Computer Interaction*. Amsterdam: Elsevier Press.

Kamimori, G. H., D. M. Penetar, D. Headley, D. R. Thorne, R. Otterstetter, and G. Belenky. 2000. Effect of three caffeine doses on plasma catecholamines and alertness during prolonged wakefulness. *European Journal of Clinical Pharmacology* 56: 537–44.

Karsh, B.-T., R. J. Holden, and S. J. Alper. 2006. A human factors engineering paradigm for patient safety: Designing to support the performance of the healthcare professional. *Quality and Safety in Health Care* 15 (Suppl.): i59–65.

Klein, G.A., J. Orasanu, R. Calderwood, and C. E. Zsambok. 1993. *Decision Making in Action: Models and Methods*. Norwood, NJ: Ablex Publishing Corporation.

Kroemer, K. H. E., and E. Grandjean. 1997. *Fitting the Task to the Human: A Textbook of Occupational Ergonomics*, 5th ed. New York: Taylor & Francis.

Lanni, C., S. C. Lenzken, A. Pascale, I. Del Vecchioa, M. Racchia, F. Pistoiaa, and S. Govoni. 2008. Cognition enhancers between treating and doping the mind. *Pharmacological Research* 57 (3): 196–213.

Lieberman, H. R. and W. J. Tharion. 2002. Effects of caffeine, sleep loss, and stress on cognitive performance and mood during U.S. Navy SEAL training. *Psychopharmacology* 164: 250–61.

Ma, L., W. Zhang, D. Chablat, F. Bennis, and F. Guillaume. 2009. Multi-objective optimisation method for posture prediction and analysis with consideration of fatigue effect and its application case. *Computers and Industrial Engineering* 57 (4): 1235–46.

McLellan, T. M., G. H. Kamimori, D. G. Bell, I. F. Smith, D. Johnson, and G. Belenky. 2005. Caffeine maintains vigilance and marksmanship in simulated urban operations with sleep deprivation. *Aviation, Space, and Environmental Medicine* 76: 39–45.

McLellan, T. M., G. H. Kamimori, D. M. Voss, D. G. Bell, K. G. Cole, and D. Johnson. 2005. Caffeine maintains vigilance and improves run times in simulated night operations for Special Forces. *Aviation, Space, and Environmental Medicine* 76: 647–54.

Meerlo, P., A. Sgoifo, and D. Suchecki. 2008. Restricted and disrupted sleep: Effects on autonomic function, neuroendocrine stress systems and stress responsivity. *Sleep Medicine Reviews* 12 (3): 197–210.

Merrill, M. 2009. Monitoring technology being developed for astronauts could benefit patients on Earth. *Healthcare IT News*. Accessed February 22, 2010. http://www.healthcareitnews.com/news/monitoring-technology-being-developed-astronauts-could-benefit-patients-earth.

National Research Council. 2008. *Emerging Cognitive Neuroscience and Related Technologies*. Washington, DC: The National Academies Press.

Ng, S. C. and P. Raveendran. 2007. EEG peak alpha frequency as an indicator for physical fatigue. In *Proceedings of the 11th Mediterranean Conference on Medical and Biomedical Engineering and Computing*, edited by T. Jarm, P. Kramar, and A. Zupanic, pp. 517–20. Berlin and Heidelberg: Springer.

Nielsen, J. 1993. *Usability Engineering*. Boston: Academic Press.

Norman, D. A. 1993. *Things That Make Us Smart*. New York: Addison Wesley.

Pew, R. W. and A. S. Mavor, eds. 2007. *Human-System Integration in the System Development Process: A New Look*. Washington, DC: The National Academies Press. Accessed January 6, 2010. http://books.nap.edu/openbook.php?isbn=0309107202andpage=354.

Pfurtscheller, G., C. Guger, G. Muller, G. Krausz, and C. Neurper. 2000. Brain oscillations control hand orthosis in a tetraplegic. *Neuroscience Letters* 292: 211–4.

Salvendy, G., ed. 1984. *Human-Computer Interaction*. North-Holland: Elsevier Science Publishers.

Schmorrow, D. D. and K. M. Stanney. 2008. *Augmented Cognition: A Practitioner's Guide*. Santa Monica, CA: Human Factors and Ergonomics Society.

Sheridan, T. B. and W. R. Ferrell. 1974. *Man-Machine Systems*. Cambridge, MA: MIT Press.

Solomon, L. M., R. C. Noll, and D. S. Mordkoff. 2009. Cognitive enhancements in human beings. *Gender Medicine* 6 (2): 338–44.

Stanney, K. M., A. Costello, and R. S. Kennedy. 2007. Advanced training systems: Benefits, limitations, and some policy considerations. *Technology* 11: 83–105.

Stanney, K. M., D. D. Schmorrow, M. Johnston, S. Fuchs, D. Jones, K. Hale, A. Ahmad, and P. Young. 2009. Augmented cognition: An overview. In *Reviews of Human Factors and Ergonomics*, Vol. 5, edited by F. T. Durso, 195–224. Santa Monica, CA: Human Factors and Ergonomics Society.

Stanney, K. M., M. J. Smith, P. Carayon, and G. Salvendy, 2001. Human-computer interaction. In *Handbook of Industrial Engineering*, 3rd ed, edited by G. Salvendy, 1192–236. New York: John Wiley.

Tang, Y.-Y. and M. I. Posner. 2009. Attention training and attention state training. *Trends in Cognitive Science* 13 (5): 222–7.

Thomas, M., H. Sing, G. Belenky, H. Holcomb, H. Mayberg, R. Dannals, H. Wagner et al. 2000. Neural basis of alertness and cognitive performance impairments during sleepiness. I. Effects of 24 h of sleep deprivation on waking human regional brain activity. *Journal of Sleep Research* 9 (4): 335–52.

Thomas, M., H. Sing, G. Belenky, H. Holcomb, H. Mayberg, R. Dannals, H. Wagner et al. 2003. Neural basis of alertness and cognitive performance impairments during sleepiness. II. Effects of 48 and 72 h of sleep deprivation on waking human regional brain activity. *Thalamus and Related Systems* 2 (3): 199–229.

Tokish, J. M., M. S. Kocher, and R. J. Hawkins. 2008. Ergogenic aids: A review of basic science, performance, side effects, and status in sports. *American Journal of Sports Medicine* 32 (6): 1543–53.

Tye, K. M., L. D. Tye, J. J. Cone, E. F. Hekkelman, P. H. Janak, and A. Bonci. 2010. Methylphenidate facilitates learning-induced amygdala plasticity. *Nature Neuroscience* 13: 475–81.

Walker, S. M., B. Dawson, and T. R. Ackland. 2001. Performance enhancement in rally car drivers via heat acclimation and race simulation. *Comparative Biochemistry and Physiology Part A* 128: 701–7.

Wictorin, C., L. Karlqvist, and J. Winkel. 1993. Validity of self-reported exposures to work postures and manual handling. *Scandinavian Journal of Work, Environment and Health* 19: 208–14.

Wilson, J. R. and E. N. Corlett. 1998. *Evaluation of Human Work: A Practical Ergonomics Methodology*. London, England: Taylor & Francis.

8

Electroencephalographic Metrics of Workload and Learner Engagement

Carryl L. Baldwin, Joseph T. Coyne, and James Christensen

CONTENTS

8.1 Overview of Topic

At the heart of neuroergonomics are sensor technologies available to measure activity within the brain. A number of different sensor technologies are available that provide either direct or indirect indices of the brain's activity. These include measures taken from the brain such as electroencephalographic (EEG) activity, functional near-infrared imaging, transcranial Doppler sonography, magnetoencephalography, functional magnetic resonance imaging, and indirect physiological measures of brain activity related to sympathetic/parasympathetic nervous system activity such as pupillometry, heart rate, heart rate variability, and electrodermal activity including skin conductance and galvanic skin response. The advantages of each of these methods can be assessed along three criteria including spatial resolution, temporal resolution, and ease of use (Parasuraman and Wilson 2008). Of these sensor technologies, EEG has been the most widely used for real-time assessment because of its fine-grained temporal resolution and ease of use. For this reason, the present chapter will focus primarily on advances made with respect to the use of EEG metrics for assessing workload and engagement.

EEG activity has a long history of use for indexing changes in neuronal activity associated with changes in the amount of effort expended by an individual while performing a given task or set of tasks and for providing an index of an individual's overall arousal or alertness level (Gevins and Smith 2003, 2007). EEG is sensitive to changes in working memory demand (Gevins and Smith 1999) and may be sensitive to increases in perceptual demand that are not detectable by behavioral measures—specifically event-related potential (ERP) components as discussed in more detail later (Baldwin and Coyne 2005; Isreal et al. 1980). It is this level of sensitivity to both a person's state of arousal and level of engagement that makes it well suited to be an index of learner engagement. Further, EEG provides an objective, relatively unobtrusive metric that makes it well suited for use in advanced interfaces that may use assessment of online learner engagement to drive adaptive training protocols. These training protocols can be adaptive to fit the learners' current level of knowledge and other characteristics such as cognitive style, how challenging the learner finds the material (referred to here as workload), and engagement in the learning process. Mental workload, for the current purpose, will be used synonymously with working memory demands, which is most heavily influenced by how mentally challenging the learner finds the material (Parasuraman and Caggiano 2005). In this use of the term, workload is synonymous with the level of mental effort and attentional resources the learner must devote to the learning task. We use the term engagement to represent both the ability and willingness to expend resources toward the task goal. In this use of the term, the assumption is that the ability to expend resources is impacted by factors such as arousal, alertness, and fatigue, whereas willingness to devote resources is impacted by the learners' attitude toward the task (i.e., approach versus avoidance) (e.g., Fairclough et al., in press; Fairclough and Venables 2006; Jung and Reid 2009). This chapter focuses on the many important issues involved in using EEG as an index of mental workload and learner engagement.

We begin with an introduction into the nature of EEG. We briefly discuss its history, what it represents and an overview of standard assessment methodologies that will assist those inexperienced with EEG recordings and analysis in understanding subsequent sections of the chapter.

8.2 Introduction to EEG Methods

EEG recordings date back at least 80 years to the work of Hans Berger published in 1929 where he observed an inverse relationship between task difficulty and 8–12 Hz activity in the alpha band (see reviews in Gevins and Smith 2007; Luck 2005). In the decades since, EEG has gained widespread clinical and experimental application. EEG is used in clinical applications to both diagnose and treat a wide range of conditions such as brain tumors, strokes, epilepsy, severe head injuries, and sleep disturbances (see Nunez and Srinivasan 2006). EEG is also used in numerous experimental applications for assessment of fatigue (Caldwell, Hall, and Erickson 2002; Gevins and Smith 1999), mental workload (Berka et al. 2004; Noel, Bauer, and Lanning 2005), and task engagement (Berka et al. 2007; Gevins and Smith 2003; Kerick, Hatfield, and Allender 2007) as well as hemispheric asymmetry

(Davidson et al. 1990; Smith, McEvoy, and Gevins 1999) and a host of other applications. In the next few sections, we will describe some key aspects of EEG methodology, beginning with a description of what scalp-recorded EEG is and what it is not.

8.2.1 What EEG Is and Is Not

EEG recorded at the scalp is a culmination or average of underlying synaptic activity. Activity at the level of the action potential is generally too small to be detectable at the scalp. In fact, to register synaptic activity at the scalp a number of neural columns must be synchronously active. Because of the conductive nature of the structures and fluids in the brain, scalp-recorded EEG is thought to be most reflective of the structures directly beneath the recording electrode, but is also influenced by activity in adjacent structures, resulting in poor spatial localization. Any activity recorded at the scalp is reflective of the summation of synaptic activity throughout this conductive organ. It is also easily contaminated by heart, eye, and craniofacial muscle activity, which may be of larger magnitude than even a strong synchronous level of synaptic activity.

EEG activity recorded at the scalp does have very high temporal resolution. Its millisecond (ms) level of sensitivity makes it well suited for answering questions regarding the time course of various cognitive and emotional events as well as for applications involving real-time and near-real-time technologies.

8.2.2 Recording Sites and the International 10/20 System

The international 10/20 system (Jasper 1958) was the first systematic method of electrode placement published and it remains the most widely used system for EEG recording. As indicated in Figure 8.1, it is based on measuring the distance between the inion (most prominent protrusion of the occipital bone) and the nasion (top of the nose) and then

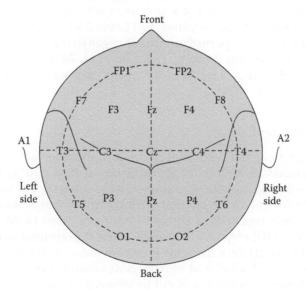

FIGURE 8.1
(**See color insert.**) The international 10–20 system of electrode placement. (From Jasper, H. H. V. 1958. *Electroencephalography and Clinical Neurophysiology* 10: 370–5.)

dividing this distance in steps of 10% and 20%. In a similar manner, the distance from the left and right pre-auricular points (the depression on the side of the head just in front of the middle of each pinnae) is also divided into equal sections. Sites located along imaginary lines between these locations are identified by a letter and, generally, a number. The letter roughly corresponds to the underlying cerebral lobe (i.e., F = frontal, T = temporal, and P = parietal). There is no "central lobe," but the letter C is used to connote the top and center of the head. Then, following the initial letter is a number. Sites on the right side of the head are indicated by even numbers whereas sites on the left side of the head are labeled with odd numbers. Sites falling directly along the center line (between the nasion and inion) are indicated by use of the letter "z" rather than a number. For example, two sites that will be referred to later on are Fz, a site located over the frontal lobe along the midline, and Pz, another midline site located over the parietal lobe. F3 is a site left of the midline over the frontal lobe, whereas F4 is a frontal site situated right of the midline and so on.

8.2.3 Spectral Analysis

Analysis of the spectral components or the amount (power) present for brain electrical oscillations at different spectral frequencies is a well-established EEG technique (Klimesch 1999; Makeig, Debener, et al. 2004; Makeig, Delorme, et al. 2004; Sauseng et al. 2005). It dates back to the pioneering days of Hans Berger and continues today, spurred on by powerful advances in software and computing capabilities. The relative amount of spectral power (i.e., particularly in specific bands as discussed below) has been used to examine the level of mental workload demanded by a wide variety of tasks. For example, theta band power increases and alpha band power decreases during the processing of sentences (Freunberger et al. 2011), and during high-load working memory tasks relative to low-load tasks (Gevins and Smith 2000).

Others have advocated methods distinct from changes in spectral power. For example, Klimesch et al. (2008) (see also Klimesch 1999) suggest examining event-related synchronization and desynchronization of alpha and theta activity as indices of workload and engagement (see also Knyazev, Savostyanov, and Levin 2006). Still others have used examination of event-related spectral perturbation or changes in the frequency power spectrum time-locked to particular events (Makeig, Debener, et al. 2004). The advances in spectral analysis are, perhaps, rivaled only by the major advances observed in its more fine-grained counterpart—ERP analysis.

8.2.4 Event-Related Potentials

ERPs provide a glimpse at the cortico-electrical activity associated with the onset of a discrete event. Analyzed at the level of the millisecond (ms), ERP is the activity associated with a stimulus-locked average of a number of the same type of event. The averaging process is thought to control for the random cortical activity that is not associated with the discrete event. Note that tremendous advances have also been made in single-trial ERP analysis. In single-trial ERP, response to a single event is examined rather than averaging over a number of discrete trials of the same type of event, at a cost of increased noise (e.g., Bryce et al. 2011; De Lucia, Michel, and Murray 2010; Goldman et al. 2009; Stahl, Gibbons, and Miller 2010). Though this work will not be covered in the current discussion, it has potential application as a method of classifying online learner engagement once many of the challenges to real-world application of these techniques (as discussed below) can be resolved. For now, even more traditional averaging approaches to ERP component analysis have limited applicability to online adaptive training platforms because of the obvious need to average cortical responses across some period of time and examine changes relative to the running average.

8.2.5 Minimal versus Dense-Array EEG

The choice of whether to use a minimal (1–9 sites) versus a dense (64+ sites) electrode array is basically one of need and application. The more electrode sites used the more information obtained. To conduct independent components analysis or use source localization analyses in conjunction with magnetic resonance images, some minimum number (at least 26 but generally 64–256) of electrode sites are required. Conversely, if the target application of the research is field or home use, it is unlikely that individuals will have the time, practical capabilities, or inclination to apply an extensive number of electrodes, let alone being tolerant of the additional cost.

Imagine the field soldier seeking an additional self-paced computer-based training program. Now, suppose a neuroadaptive interface incorporating EEG metrics is available to improve the effectiveness and/or efficiency of the training program. It is highly unlikely that the soldier would have the technical knowledge and patience necessary to apply a 64+-electrode array. Conversely, it is quite likely that a simple instructional video with supporting documentation could be developed that would provide the soldier with enough knowledge to apply a 3-electrode array with accompanying ground and reference sites. The gaming industry is developing entertainment technologies that work on the assumption that people are willing and can learn to apply a few electrodes adequately enough to drive applications.

The choice of how many electrodes to use will depend on the intended application. The more electrodes utilized the more information that can be obtained but the lengthier and more complicated the application process required. We now turn focus to a brief review of some of the main spectral bands shown, in previous investigations, to be sensitive to workload and engagement.

8.3 EEG and Workload

Two primary spectral bands have been examined extensively in previous literature owing to their sensitivity to workload and engagement. These two bands are alpha (~7.5–13 Hz), and in particular parietal alpha (alpha activity recorded at and around Pz; see Figure 8.1), and frontal midline (e.g., Fz) theta (~4–7.5 Hz). Activity in the alpha range has often been found to decrease with increasing task difficulty, whereas the converse is observed for activity in the theta range, particularly at frontal midline electrode sites (Gevins et al. 1997).

Pope, Bogart, and Bartolome (1995) have demonstrated successful workload engagement classification using an algorithmic formulation of spectral bands. They examined several candidate formulas and concluded that, for their purposes, a formula consisting of (beta/(alpha + theta)) led to the best engagement classification. They used a modification of the multi-attribute task battery (MAT-B) developed by Comstock and Arnegard (1992) where the tracking task changed from manual to automated depending on the participant's engagement index (EI). Their results were replicated and extended by Freeman et al. (1999) demonstrating an additional benefit for automation changes driven by threshold changes derived from a baseline EI. That is, when the participant's EI crossed a threshold the automation would be engaged or disengaged. This threshold-based method proved even more effective than basing the automation changes on ascending or descending EI numbers over a 2-s period, the method utilized by Pope, Bogart, and Bartolome (1995). Freeman and colleagues again replicated and extended the effective use of the EI as an index of operator workload in a visual search (Freeman et al. 2004) and a compensatory tracking task (Freeman et al. 2000). Others have extended its use in learning tasks.

Chaouachi et al. (2010) examined the relationship between the EI (determined by Pope, Bogart, and Bartolome [1995]) and affect in computerized learning task. Emotions have been shown to be integrally related to cognitive tasks such as problem solving and decision making (Bechara and Damasio 2005; Damasio 1998) and to a person's decision to allocate resources to a given task (Fairclough et al., in press). Chaouachi et al. (2010) found a strong relationship between emotion and the EEG EI. They observed that the EI was highest when learners were experiencing positive emotions and high arousal levels. Interestingly, the second highest level of EI was observed when learners were experiencing negative emotions combined with high arousal levels, which the authors described as a state of confusion or frustration. Further, a strong relationship was observed between the EI and performance. Learners whose EI during the learning task was above their baseline EI tended to perform significantly better than those whose EI during the task was lower than their baseline level. These results in combination with those of Pope, Bogart, and Bartolome (1995) and Freeman and colleagues (1999, 2004) indicate that the EI shows strong promise as a useful metric of learner engagement for real-time applications.

Still other investigators have found success with alternative algorithms. Fairclough et al. (in press) used a combination of frontal theta and frontal asymmetry as a metric of operator engagement. Positive emotions are known to be associated with greater left hemisphere activation whereas negative emotions are associated with greater right hemisphere activation (Davidson 2004). Further, frontal asymmetry has been shown to be related to both emotion and willingness to allocate resources to a task. Increased left frontal activation has been associated with a motivational approach (a tendency to devote resources to a task) whereas right frontal activation has been associated with an avoidance approach (a tendency to disengage from a task) (Coan and Allen 2004; Coan, Allen, and McKnight 2006). Fairclough et al. (in press) found that frontal asymmetry provided a sensitive index of operator engagement. They observed that excessive task demand was associated with frontal asymmetry, and specifically greater right hemisphere activation (an avoidance approach), while providing a financial incentive, increased left hemisphere activation, particularly in the more challenging condition. Frontal theta activity increased in response to increases in task demand only to the extent that successful performance was possible. In the excessive demand condition, increases in frontal theta activity were not observed. In sum, parietal alpha power, frontal theta power, frontal asymmetry, and the EI appear to be promising metrics for real-time applications. We now turn attention to ERP components.

ERP components have frequently been used to index operator engagement, though generally for offline analysis rather than real-time applications. Two components that have demonstrated effective offline workload classification are the N1 and the P300. The N1 is a negative wave deflection occurring approximately 100 milliseconds after stimulus onset. The P300 is a positive wave deflection occurring approximately 300 milliseconds after the stimulus event of interest. Kramer, Sirevaag, and Braune (1987) found the N1 component in response to an irrelevant auditory probe task (participants were instructed to ignore the tones) to be sensitive to increased pilot workload stemming from more difficult portions of a flight path. Baldwin and Coyne (2005) found the P300 component in response to visual probes to be sensitive to increased task difficulty stemming from driving through dense fog relative to clear visibility conditions in a driving simulation. Many other examples can be provided for successful use of the N1 and P300 components for classifying workload. However, as previously mentioned, the need for averaging large numbers of trials to obtain acceptable signals has limited these applications to offline analyses. To work as a means of driving an adaptive training platform, metrics that provide successful classification of learner engagement in real time are needed.

8.4 Working Memory and Learner Engagement

Learning is clearly different from performing a task that one is familiar with. Theoretically, one could use many different pedagogical approaches to assessing the difficulty inherent in learning new material. One method that appears particularly relevant is the cognitive load theory (CLT). CLT asserts that learning is essentially the act of organizing information from working memory into long-term memory (Paas, van Gog, and Sweller 2010; Sweller 1988). As it is well documented that working memory capacity is limited (Baddeley and Hitch 1974; Daneman and Carpenter 1980; Kahneman 1973; Wickens 1984), learning is hindered whenever the task of learning exceeds the learner's working memory capacity.

More specifically, CLT is a model of learning that describes the learning process in terms of human information processing, particularly working memory and long-term memory. A core principle of CLT is that learning places demands on working memory (Sweller 1988, 2006). As working memory is limited by capacity (Kahneman 1973; Miller 1956), learning is integrally tied to both the working memory capacity of the learner and the working memory demand of the instruction and instructional material. The positive correlation between working memory capacity and successful learning is particularly evident in student mastery of scientific concepts (Al-Ahmadi and Oraif 2009; Eun Sook and Reid 2009).

Long-term memory, conversely, is relatively unlimited. Thus, many pedagogical techniques, including CLT, emphasize how information from working memory is organized and grouped together (into schemata) and stored in long-term memory (Ausubel 2000). The goal of training is to facilitate this transfer with minimal expenditure of working memory. Further, rather than mere rote memorization, meaningful learning involves assisting the learner in integrating the new material with what he or she already knows.

If assimilated in a meaningful way in long-term memory, the individual is able to access the information more easily later, which in turn reduces the burden placed upon the working memory system during the retrieval process. CLT places great emphasis on managing demands of the working memory, or cognitive load, of the learning/training process. Using the terminology expressed previously, CLT emphasizes reducing the workload of the learning process.

CLT proposes three specific types of cognitive load that have additive effects. In other words, the sum total of the workload demands placed on each type must not exceed the learner's working memory resources. The first type is called *intrinsic cognitive load* and it refers to the difficulty imposed by the material or task to be learned. For example, scientific concepts are thought to have higher intrinsic load relative to other types of information. Intrinsic cognitive load is heavily influenced by the elemental interactivity of the material—how many interacting elements must be maintained in working memory at any given time. Complex material tends to have high elemental interactivity. Instructional design can do little to change the intrinsic cognitive load of the material or task to be learned. Training should include meaningful ways to link the new concepts and information to what the learner already knows. As expertise develops, schemas are formed and elements become grouped together, enabling the individual to deal with more elements simultaneously and allowing them to overcome the working memory bottleneck. This process reflects learning and the dynamic nature of intrinsic cognitive load within CLT. The number of elements that make up intrinsic load are based upon the individual's ability to group them together.

The second form of cognitive load is *extraneous cognitive load*. It is here that the crux of instructional design is placed. Extraneous load refers to the format and methods used to present the information. For example, material can be presented in the form of text, graphics, through verbal lecture or active exploration. Effective instructional designs place minimal extraneous cognitive load on the learner. This is particularly important when the material contains high intrinsic load. CLT places an emphasis on reducing extraneous load as a method of reducing overall cognitive load, thus facilitating learning.

The third type is *germane cognitive load*. It is essentially the process of creating and organizing information into schema. Germane load is the result of the instructional design (Paas, Renkl, and Sweller 2003). It promotes the development of accurate mental models of the task and relevant schemas as well as facilitation of the transition from controlled to automatic processing that accompanies expertise. It can be compared to Ausubel's (2000) construct of concept learning and concept assimilation, where information is used to form a new concept or schema or is assimilated into an existing one, respectively. Germane load is influenced by the manner, modality, and sequence in which the material is presented and by the learning activities involved. Differential sensitivity has been observed between various measures for each type of load (DeLeeuw and Mayer 2008). For example, DeLeeuw and Mayer (2008) observed that subjective ratings were more sensitive to the intrinsic difficulty of the material to be learned whereas response time was more sensitive to the extraneous load of the learning environment. Though little, if any, work has been done in determining whether different neurophysiological metrics are more sensitive to different types of cognitive load, it is reasonable to think such a relationship might be found.

The goal of training within the framework of cognitive load theory focuses on minimizing extraneous cognitive load through instructional design. This increases the probability that the cognitive resources and working memory capacity of the learner are not being exceeded so that learning can take place. Reducing extraneous cognitive load frees more resources for germane cognitive load, thus facilitating the development of schema acquisition and a shift toward automatic processing and expertise.

Coyne et al. (2009) have incorporated CLT principles with the multiple resource theory (Wickens 1984) in a model of adaptive training illustrated in Figure 8.2.

As illustrated in the model, the adaptive training screen (driven by workload and engagement as classified by neurophysiological metrics such as EEG) can influence presentation of the training material in several ways. Firstly, though it cannot alter the inherent difficulty or intrinsic load of the material to be learned, it can alter the rate at which the new conceptual elements are presented. Secondly, it can use CLT principles, such as worked examples, integration of information, and use of multiple modalities without increasing redundancy to reduce extraneous load. Finally, it can facilitate germane load by assessing what the learner already knows and constructing conflict matrices. These matrices can then be used to present tailored learning examples, thus facilitating schema formation and concept assimilation.

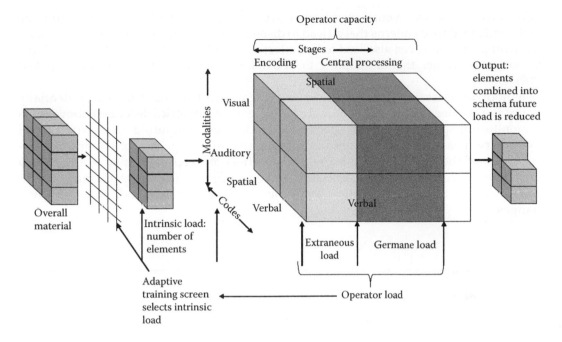

FIGURE 8.2
Adaptive training model.

For example, if the goal is to teach the recognition of different forms of military tanks, the rate at which new information is presented can be driven by the workload the learner is exhibiting in the learning task. This alters the intrinsic load rate. Next, worked examples identifying the name and class of tank could be presented by providing visual images of the tanks to be learned while verbal descriptions of the distinguishing aspects of specific tanks are presented. Multiple modalities are used and the learner does not waste effort (extraneous load is reduced) searching back and forth between the visual image and a written description somewhere else on the screen or page. Finally, as the learner begins to recognize some examples of certain classes of tanks, this information is used to populate a confusion matrix. New items are compared to features that the learner already knows and training materials emphasize the similarities and differences between the new and learned items adaptively, thus facilitating germane load.

8.5 EEG, Workload, and Engagement

To facilitate optimal learning, the trainee should be challenged but not overloaded. If the mental workload of the learner is too low (underload), then at best slower than necessary rates of learning will transpire. The learner exposed to periodic episodes of underload for short durations may simply become bored and disengage from the learning task. More frequent exposure to underload is likely to result in complete disengagement from the learning task, and self-regulated avoidance.

Conversely, excessive mental workload or overload leads to frustration, low confidence levels, and avoidance patterns that all lead to disengagement in the learning task. Overload in learning situations can also lead to less effective learning strategies such as use of rote memorization rather than attempting to understand difficult concepts (Jung and Reid 2009).

Methods of assessing both workload and engagement in real time can potentially ensure the learner is kept in an optimal zone of learning. Metrics described above, such as monitoring spectral power at specific electrode sites, computing an EI, and frontal asymmetry measures could be used in combination to change the format and presentation rate of the material to be learned in an effort to keep the leaner at a relatively constant and acceptable level of workload and engagement. These metrics may need to be on different time scales to allow assessment of both transient and longer duration changes.

8.6 Theoretical Frameworks for Adaptive Interfaces

To date, consensus has yet to be reached regarding the best approach for examining spectral changes in EEG recordings (see discussions in Klimesch et al. 2008; Makeig, Debener, et al. 2004). Although as previously discussed, spectral power changes in alpha and theta band activity have been demonstrated to be sensitive indices of mental workload in many applications (Gevins and Smith, 1999, 2007), others have argued for examination of spectral changes associated with particular working memory processes, task locked to particular events, or as relative changes in synchronization or desynchronization. Rather than debate these issues here, we provide a theoretical framework for candidate neurophysiological metrics.

Learner engagement or workload can change on a moment-by-moment basis (referred to as *phasic* changes) or across longer periods of time (*tonic* changes on the order of 10+ minutes). Tonic and phasic changes are indexed not only on different time scales but also by different metrics or algorithmic derivations (Baldwin et al. 2010; Beatty 1982; Coyne et al. 2010; Kahneman 1973). For example, tonic changes in metrics such as average pupil diameter and EEG have been shown to be associated with general alertness and fatigue (see discussion in Beatty 1982; Caldwell, Hall, and Erickson 2002; Gevins and Smith 1999). Conversely, phasic changes in both pupil diameter (Beatty 1982; Marshall 2007) and EEG (Wilson and Russell 2003a, 2007) have been shown to be sensitive to transient short-duration changes in workload.

Simultaneous monitoring of spectral changes stemming both from relatively long-term or tonic changes in levels of engagement as well as from more rapid phasic changes, such as from event-related spectral perturbations, show promise for operational neuroergonomics. For example, Sauseng et al. (2005) observed that event-related synchronization of alpha range activity distinguishes between retention and active manipulation of visuospatial information in working memory. Huang et al. (2008) have observed tonic changes in alpha bandwidth activity coupled with phasic changes in multiple bandwidths during periods of high visuomotor tracking error. We reason that an effective classifier would need to be sensitive to both tonic and phasic changes in the learner.

8.7 Classification Strategies

Developing classification strategies for indexing cognitive state in real time has been an area of great interest in the research community and several candidate methods have demonstrated varying degrees of success in different applications. As previously mentioned, several linear classification strategies primarily based on spectral power have shown promise as have several EEG-derived algorithms.

The EI, determined by Pope, Bogart, and Bartolome, described previously as (beta/ (alpha + theta)), can be computed in real time by calculating a running average over a 2-second window. This index has been described as a metric of an individual's level of workload while performing a task. The EI has been successful as a means of providing adaptive aiding leading to improved overall performance in a vigilance task (Mikulka, Scerbo, and Freeman 2002) and a complex tracking task (Freeman et al. 2000).

Another linear EEG algorithm that has been used successfully in real-time applications for processing cognitive state is the eXecutive Load Index (XLI) (DuRousseau and Mannucci 2005). XLI is calculated by computing the ratio of ((delta + theta)/alpha) over a moving 2-second window, with the change determined by comparing the value to the previous 20-second running average.

Researchers at Advanced Brain Monitoring (ABM, Carlsbad, CA) have also developed several cognitive state classification algorithms based upon linear and quadratic discriminant function analysis (Berka et al. 2007). Specifically, they have developed classifiers for both workload and engagement. Their EEG index for engagement tracks the demands for sensory processing and attentional resources, whereas the index for workload tracks the level of cognitive demand and is considered to be a correlate of executive function. Their EEG algorithms are derived for each individual on the basis of performance on a set of baseline tasks. Their metrics are proprietary and thus cannot be specified here, but they have documented their success in classifying operator state in a series of basic cognitive tasks including mental arithmetic and a digit span task. In addition to these linear classification strategies, nonlinear classification strategies have shown considerable promise.

Researchers at the Wright-Patterson Air Force Research Laboratory (Ohio) have demonstrated considerable success in classifying operator state using nonlinear classifiers (Wilson and Russell, 2003a,b, 2007). Specifically, they have used an artificial neural network (ANN) to classify operator mental workload in a complex laboratory task and during an unmanned aerial vehicle (UAV) simulation. Their ANN derives its classification from EEG, as well as additional metrics such as electrooculographic, and heart rate data. They trained the ANN on neurophysiological data obtained while individual operators performed either an easy or a challenging version of the task. Subsequently, the individually trained ANN was able to successfully classify high versus low workload with 85%–90% accuracy. Even higher classification rates were obtained when a feature extraction process was implemented, such that in a two-stage process the most relevant classification features for each individual were calculated and, then, only those rated as strong classifiers were used in the second stage of ANN classification. Their ANN classification was successfully implemented in an adaptive automation UAV paradigm. When the ANN classified workload as high, the UAV speed decreased and, conversely, when it was low, the UAV speed increased. Using this adaptive automation paradigm, performance on the UAV task was significantly better than in a nonadaptive version of the task.

Despite these successes, this work has been limited to binary (high/low) classification. In order to be useful in a learning application, any such classification system will need to be capable of finer-grained assessment of workload. Separate detection of underload and overload is needed as well as indices of both phasic and tonic changes in workload and engagement.

8.8 Prestimulus Alpha

One promising method of assessing phasic learner engagement changes in a predictive manner comes from investigations of transient changes in alpha activity occurring prior to the onset of a stimulus (Baldwin et al. 2010). This metric is referred to as *prestimulus alpha* because it is spectral power in the time frame (usually on the order of 1 second) just prior to the onset of the stimulus or event of interest.

Prestimulus alpha can be thought of as a phasic index of a learner's engagement in the task on a moment-by-moment basis. Alpha activity tends to increase as a learner becomes less engaged (Gevins and Smith 2003). In a limited number of recent investigations, increases in prestimulus alpha activity have been demonstrated to be predictive of when engagement may have temporarily decreased to a point where errors are more probable (Baldwin et al. 2010; Ergenoglu et al. 2004; Mazaheri et al. 2009).

For example, using magnetoencephalographic recordings, Mazaheri et al. (2009) demonstrated that elevated occipital alpha activity prior to the onset of a visual stimulus predicted whether or not participants would make an error in an upcoming trial. Using EEG, Ergenoglu et al. (2004) observed significantly elevated alpha activity in a 1-second prestimulus period when participants missed near-threshold visual stimuli relative to when they were detected. Baldwin et al. (2010) found that fast alpha activity (10–13 Hz) at Pz 1 second before targets were presented differed as a function of the type of error that would be made (i.e., misses versus false alarms) and task difficulty. Prestimulus alpha shows promise as a candidate metric for online monitoring of phasic changes in learner engagement and workload.

8.9 Challenges

Attempts to develop effective algorithms of accurately classifying workload and engagement have proved challenging for real-world applications. Particularly challenging is the task of developing metrics that adequately classify the level of engagement for the same individual across subsequent days or across individuals within the same day (Noel, Bauer, and Lanning 2005).

In one on-going collaborative investigation, researchers under the direction of C. L. Baldwin at George Mason University and J. T. Coyne at the Naval Research Laboratory are investigating the classification capabilities of ANNs trained on EEG and pupilometry metrics obtained while participants are performing a set of working memory tasks. Specifically, Penaranda, a graduate student at George Mason, is examining the capabilities of ANNs trained on one task versus a combination of tasks to classify workload on a different task. This within and across-task classification approach may improve our current understanding of the generalizability of classification approaches. This is particularly important for developing neuroadaptive training platforms. In training paradigms, one does not have the ability to work with individuals who have reached asymptote performance levels. By the very nature of the training environment the learner's skill level will be changing. The learner may begin to use different strategies as his or her knowledge develops. Strategy changes could potentially lead to dramatic changes in neurophysiological metrics that would need to be registered and appropriately classified by the adaptive platform. Compounding the challenge of developing workload classifiers that are generalizable across tasks is the presence of individual difference factors.

8.9.1 Individual Differences

A number of individual factors impact the electrophysiological signals that can be used to drive adaptive interfaces. Age is one of these factors. Some of the general changes associated with increased age have been documented. For example, as discussed earlier, increased working memory demand is generally associated with increased frontal midline theta activity. However, this pattern may not be evident in older adults (McEvoy et al. 2001). Upper alpha power tends to decrease and theta power tends to increase from childhood to adulthood and then the pattern tends to reverse again in advanced age (Klimesch 1999). These same bandwidths are influenced both by temporary states, such as fatigue, and by longer duration conditions, such as neurological disorders.

Many pharmaceutical and illicit drugs alter electrophysiological activity. For example, marijuana use tends to decrease amplitude of ERP components and decrease global theta band activity (Ilan, Smith, and Gevins 2004). Individual difference factors such as these are compounded by known artifacts registered in the physiological signals.

8.9.2 Artifact

Continually problematic is the amount of artifact that can contaminate neurophysiological sensors. For example, muscle movement, heart rate, eye movements and blinks, to name a few, have the potential to mask EEG task-related signals. Developing methods of dealing with these artifacts online is an ongoing challenge. Several eye-movement correction algorithms have been developed (e.g., Gratton, Coles, and Donchin 1983; also see Wilson and Russell 2003a) and used with varying degrees of success. However, improving methods of signal amplification, filtering, and the analog to digital conversions required to extract physiological signals from the background of noise are active areas of research critical to the successful implementation of real-time cognitive state gauges.

8.10 Alternative Applications

The present discussion has been framed primarily with respect to developing neuroadaptive training platforms. However, it should be pointed out that the theoretical background and methods discussed here are relevant to a much wider range of applications. Many are well known and discussed in detail elsewhere, such as adaptive automation (Byrne and Parasuraman 1996). One emerging application of particular interest and relevance is using neuroadaptive interfaces for augmenting team cognition. This application would involve much the same approach as used in developing a training platform; however, the unique features of a distributed teaming environment present both advantages and disadvantages.

The advent of distributed teaming and remote collaboration technologies presents significant challenges for personnel who must work effectively despite differences in geographical location, rank, experience, and so on. For example, current U.S. Air Force operations can involve remotely piloted aircraft that are controlled by teams spread across the globe, with communication typically limited to voice or text chat. With only these communication tools, a significant proportion of the cues necessary for natural social interaction are eliminated (Birdwhistell 1970), which may have negative implications for team situation awareness (Wellens 1993).

Effective teaming could be facilitated in such environments by the provision of EEG workload metrics to team members or supervisors. In a face-to-face team problem-solving task, Stevens et al. (2009) found that distinct patterns of EEG activity were associated with different team activities, and that workload was frequently unevenly distributed across teammates. This suggests that better workload balancing within a team may be achievable by supporting team processes with additional "team state" information (Funke and Knott 2010). This could be achieved, for example, by using a color-coded workload indicator (e.g., "green" for low workload, "yellow" for moderate, and "red" for high; Funke and Knott 2010). The simplicity of such a display could help avoid some of the distracting potential of more complex or realistic teammate representations noted by Wellens (1993), while still supporting team adaptability. Another significant benefit of adopting this approach to the application of workload metrics is that the workload measures could serve as a team decision aid, rather than as an obligatory trigger for workload mitigation technologies as in adaptive automation (Funke and Knott 2010). This builds on human capacities for adaptive behavior, while mitigating the potential interference associated with incorrect workload detections. Imperfect workload monitoring or classification is, therefore, not necessarily a significant detriment to performance in this application; humans have been proven capable of properly calibrating their trust of an imperfect aid (McGuirl and Sarter 2006). As long as the accuracy of the system is sufficient to improve performance despite imperfections, it will be of value to distributed teams.

8.11 The Road Ahead: Research Needs

There are many opportunities and challenges in the burgeoning arena of developing translational applications of neuroadaptive training platforms. Some of these are discussed here. Perhaps first and foremost, there is a continuing need to identify neurophysiological metrics that are sensitive to particular aspects of learning, across different time domains and across different tasks. Understanding the neurological basis for these metrics and why they are sensitive to specific aspects will be another ongoing challenge and opportunity for research for many years to come.

As described, to date little success has been made toward the goal of developing generalized algorithms that can classify workload and engagement in the same individual across different tasks, the same individual across different days, nor much less different individuals across either the same or different days. Work in these areas is currently going on in several laboratories. Progress in any of these areas will do much for increasing the feasibility of translational applications.

Specific to the task of learning, previous researchers (e.g., DeLeeuw and Mayer 2008) have found that different metrics are sensitive to different types of cognitive load (i.e., intrinsic, extraneous, and germane). Similarly, different neurophysiological metrics at different time scales have been shown to be sensitive to different aspects of mental workload (Baldwin and Coyne 2005; Baldwin et al. 2010; Griesmayr et al. 2009; Sauseng et al. 2009). Thus, it is reasonable to think that different neurophysiological metrics may be more or less sensitive to different types of cognitive load (i.e., intrinsic, extraneous, and germane). However, as mentioned, to date little, if any, research has examined this possibility and it remains an opportunity for advancing work in neuroadaptive training applications and evaluation.

In sum, tremendous progress has been made toward identifying sensitive neurophysiological indices of workload and engagement. Several EEG metrics have been used in previous investigations to accurately classify workload and drive adaptive interfaces. EEG metrics have also been used successfully in a limited number of investigations to classify both task difficulty (i.e., workload) and a learner's engagement (i.e., an approach or avoidance strategy) in the task. Despite the many challenges to developing effective neuroadaptive training platforms, they hold considerable promise as a means of improving computer-based learning.

References

Al-Ahmadi, F. and F. Oraif. 2009. Working memory capacity, confidence and scientific thinking. *Research in Science & Technological Education* 27 (2): 225–43.

Ausubel, D. P. 2000. *The Acquisition and Retention of Knowledge: A Cognitive View.* Dordrecht, The Netherlands: Kluwer Academic.

Baddeley, A. D. and G. Hitch. 1974. Working memory. In *The Psychology of Learning and Motivation,* Vol. 8, edited by G. H. Bower, 47–89. Orlando, FL: Academic Press.

Baldwin, C. L. and J. T. Coyne. 2005. Dissociable aspects of mental workload: Examinations of the P300 ERP component and performance assessments. *Psychologia* 48: 102–19.

Baldwin, C. L., J. T. Coyne, D. Roberts, J. Barrow, A. Cole, C. Sibley, B. Tayor, and G. Buzzell. 2010. Prestimulus alpha as a precursor to errors in a UAV target orientation detection task. In *Advances in Human Factors, Ergonomics, and Safety in Manufacturing and Service Industries,* edited by W. Karwowski and G. Salvendy. London: CRC Press/Taylor & Francis.

Beatty, J. 1982. Phasic not tonic pupillary responses vary with auditory vigilance performance. *Psychophysiology* 19 (2): 167–72.

Bechara, A. and Damasio, A. R. 2005. The somatic marker hypothesis: A neural theory of economic decision. *Games and Economic Behavior* 52 (2): 336–72.

Berka, C., D. J. Levendowski, M. M. Cvetinovic, M. M. Petrovic, G. Davis, M. N. Lumicao, M. N.,V. T. Zivkovic, M. V. Popovic, and R. E. Olmstead. 2004. Real-time analysis of EEG indexes of alertness, cognition, and memory acquired with a wireless EEG headset. *International Journal of Human-Computer Interaction* 17 (2): 151–70.

Berka, C., D. J. Levendowski, M. N. Lumicao, A. Yau, G. Davis, V. T. Zivkovic, R. E. Olmstead, P. D. Tremoulet, and P. L. Craven. 2007. EEG correlates of task engagement and mental workload in vigilance, learning, and memory tasks. *Aviation, Space, and Environmental Medicine* 78 (5 Suppl.): B231–44.

Birdwhistell, R. 1970. *Kinesics and Context*. Philadelphia, PA: University of Pennsylvania Press.

Bryce, D., D. Szucs, F. Soltesz, and D. Whitebread. 2011. The development of inhibitory control: An averaged and single-trial Lateralized Readiness Potential study. *NeuroImage* 57 (3): 671–85.

Byrne, E. A. and R. Parasuraman. 1996. Psychophysiology and adaptive automation. *Biological Psychology* 42: 249–68.

Caldwell, J. A., K. K. Hall, and B. S. Erickson. 2002. EEG data collected from helicopter pilots in flight are sufficiently sensitive to detect increased fatigue from sleep deprivation. *The International Journal of Aviation Psychology* 12 (1): 19–32.

Chaouachi, M., P. Chalfoun, I. Jraidi, and C. Frasson. 2010. Affect and mental engagement: Towards adaptability for intelligent systems. In *Proceedings of the Twenty-Third International Florida Artificial Intelligence Research Society (FLAIRS) Conference*, Daytona Beach, FL, May 19–21, 2010. USA: AAAI Press. http://www.aaai.org/ocs/index.php/FLAIRS/2010/paper/view/1319/1776.

Coan, J. A. and J. J. B. Allen. 2004. Frontal EEG asymmetry as a moderator and mediator of emotion. *Biological Psychology* 67 (1–2): 7–50.

Coan, J. A., J. J. B. Allen, and P. E. McKnight. 2006. A capability model of individual differences in frontal EEG asymmetry. *Biological Psychology* 72 (2): 198–207.

Comstock, J. R. and R. J. Arnegard. 1992. *The Multi-Attribute Task Battery for Human Operator Workload and Strategic Behavior Research* (NASA Technical Memorandum No. No. 104174). Hampton, VA: NASA Langley Research Center.

Coyne, J. T., C. L. Baldwin, A. Cole, C. Sibley, and D. M. Roberts. 2009. Applying real time physiological measures of cognitive load to improve training. In *Proceedings of the 5th International Conference on Foundations of Augmented Cognition (FAC '09)—Neuroergonomics and Operational Neuroscience held jointly with Human Computer Interaction International 2009*, San Diego, CA, July 19–24, 2009. Berlin and Heidelberg: Springer-Verlag.

Coyne, J. T., C. L. Baldwin, A. Cole, C. Sibley, and D. Roberts. 2009. Applying real time physiological measures of cognitive load to improve training. Lecture Notes in Computer Science, Volume 5638/2009, 469–478. Berlin: Springer.

Damasio, A. R. 1998. Emotion in the perspective of an integrated nervous system. *Brain Research Reviews* 26 (2–3): 83–6.

Daneman, M. and P. A. Carpenter. 1980. Individual differences in working memory and reading. *Journal of Verbal Learning & Verbal Behavior* 19 (4): 450–66.

Davidson, R. J. 2004. What does the prefrontal cortex "do" in affect: Perspectives on frontal EEG asymmetry research. *Biological Psychology* 67 (1–2): 219–34.

Davidson, R. J., J. P. Chapman, L. J. Chapman, and J. B. Henriques. 1990. Asymmetrical brain electrical activity discriminates between psychometrically-matched verbal and spatial cognitive tasks. *Psychophysiology* 27 (5): 528–43.

De Lucia, M., C. M. Michel, and M. M. Murray. 2010. Comparing ICA-based and single-trial topographic ERP analyses. *Brain Topography* 23 (2): 119–27.

DeLeeuw, K. E. and R. E. Mayer. 2008. A comparison of three measures of cognitive load: Evidence for separable measures of intrinsic, extraneous, and germane load. *Journal of Educational Psychology* 100 (1): 223–34.

DuRousseau, D. R. and M. A. Mannucci. 2005. eXecutive Load Index (XLI): Spaital-frequency EEG tracks moment-to-moment changes in high-order attentional resources. In *Foundations of Augmented Cognition*, edited by D. Schmorrow, 245–51. Mahwah, NJ: Lawrence Erlbaum Associates.

Ergenoglu, T., T. Demiralp, Z. Bayraktaroglu, M. Ergen, H. Beydagi, and Y. Uresin. 2004. Alpha rhythm of the EEG modulates visual detection performance in humans. *Cognitive Brain Research* 20 (3): 376–83.

Eun Sook, J. and N. Reid. 2009. Working memory and attitudes. *Research in Science & Technological Education* 27 (2): 205–23.

Fairclough, S. H., K. Gilleade, K. C. Ewing, and J. Roberts. In press. Capturing user engagement via psychophysiology: measures and mechanisms for biocybernetic adaptation. *International Journal of Autonomous and Adaptive Communications Systems*. http://web.me.com/shfairclough/

Stephen_Fairclough_Research/Publications_physiological_computing_mental_effort_stephen_fairclough_files/IJAACS_2010_Fairclough.pdf

Fairclough, S. H. and L. Venables. 2006. Prediction of subjective states from psychophysiology: A multivariate approach. *Biological Psychology* 71 (1): 100–10.

Freeman, F. G., P. J. Mikulka, L. J. Prinzel, and M. W. Scerbo. 1999. Evaluation of an adaptive automation system using three EEG indices with a visual tracking task. *Biological Psychology* 50 (1): 61–76.

Freeman, F. G., P. J. Mikulka, M. W. Scerbo, L. J. Prinzel, and K. Clouatre. 2000. Evaluation of a psychophysiologically controlled adaptive automation system, using performance on a tracking task. *Applied Psychophysiology and Biofeedback* 25 (2): 103–15.

Freeman, F. G., P. J. Mikulka, M. W. Scerbo, and L. Scott. 2004. An evaluation of an adaptive automation system using a cognitive vigilance task. *Biological Psychology* 67 (3): 283–97.

Freunberger, R., M. Werkle-Bergner, B. Griesmayr, U. Lindenberger, and W. Klimesch. 2011. Brain oscillatory correlates of working memory constraints. *Brain Research* 1375: 93–102.

Funke, G. J. and B. A. Knott. 2010. Conceptualization and measurement of team workload. *Invited Colloquium, Air Operations Division, Defence Science and Technology Organisation (DSTO)*, May 2010. Australia: Fishermen's Bend.

Gevins, A. and M. E. Smith. 1999. Detecting transient cognitive impairment with EEG pattern recognition methods. *Aviation, Space, and Environmental Medicine* 70 (10): 1018–24.

Gevins, A. and M. E. Smith. 2000. Neurophysiological measures of working memory and individual differences in cognitive ability and cognitive style. *Cerebral Cortex* 10 (9): 829–39.

Gevins, A. and M. E. Smith. 2003. Neurophysiological measures of cognitive workload during human-computer interaction. *Theoretical Issues in Ergonomics Science* 4 (1): 113–31.

Gevins, A. and M. E. Smith. 2007. Electroencephalography (EEG) in neuroergonomics. In *Neuroergonomics: The Brain at Work*, edited by R. Parasuraman and M. Rizzo, 15–31. Oxford: Oxford University Press.

Gevins, A., M. Smith, L. McEvoy, and D. Yu. 1997. High-resolution EEG mapping of cortical activation related to working memory: Effects of task difficulty, type of processing, and practice. *Cerebral Cortex* 7 (4): 374–85.

Goldman, R. I., C.-Y. Wei, M. G. Philiastides, A. D. Gerson, D. Friedman, T. R. Brown, and P. Sajda. 2009. Single-trial discrimination for integrating simultaneous EEG and fMRI: Identifying cortical areas contributing to trial-to-trial variability in the auditory oddball task. *NeuroImage* 47 (1): 136–47.

Gratton, G., M. G. H. Coles, and E. Donchin. 1983. A new method for off-line removal of ocular artifact. *Electroencephalography and Clinical Neurophysiology* 55: 468–84.

Griesmayr, B., W. R. Gruber, W. Klimesch, and P. Sauseng. 2009. Human frontal midline theta and its synchronization to gamma oscillations during verbal working memory. *Psychophysiology* 46: S145.

Huang, R. S., T. P. Jung, A. Delorme, and S. Makeig. 2008. Tonic and phasic electroencephalographic dynamics during continuous compensatory tracking. *Neuroimage* 39 (4): 1896–909.

Isreal, J. B., G. L. Chesney, C. D. Wickens, and E. Donchin, E. 1980. P300 and tracking difficulty: Evidence for multiple resources in dual-task performance. *Psychophysiology* 17 (3): 259–73.

Jasper, H. H. V. 1958. The ten twenty electrode system of the International Federation. *Electroencephalography and Clinical Neurophysiology* 10: 370–5.

Jung, E. S. and N. Reid. 2009. Working memory and attitudes. *Research in Science & Technological Education* 27 (2): 205–23.

Kahneman, D. 1973. *Attention and Effort*. Englewood Cliffs, NJ: Prentice Hall.

Kerick, S. E., B. D. Hatfield, and L. E. Allender. 2007. Event-related cortical dynamics of soldiers during shooting as a function of varied task demand. *Aviation, Space, and Environmental Medicine*, 78 (5): B153–64.

Klimesch, W. 1999. EEG alpha and theta oscillations reflect cognitive and memory performance: A review and analysis. *Brain Research Reviews* 29 (2–3): 169–95.

Klimesch, W., R. Freunberger, P. Sauseng, and W. Gruber. 2008. A short review of slow phase synchronization and memory: Evidence for control processes in different memory systems? *Brain Research*, 1235: 31–44.

Knyazev, G. G., A. N. Savostyanov, and E. A. Levin. 2006. Alpha synchronization and anxiety: Implications for inhibition vs. alertness hypotheses. *International Journal of Psychophysiology* 59 (2): 151–8.

Kramer, A. F., E. J. Sirevaag, and R. Braune. 1987. A psychophysiological assessment of operator workload during simulated flight missions. *Human Factors* 29: 145–60.

Ilan, A. B., M. E. Smith, and A. Gevins. 2004. Effects of marijuana on neurophysiological signals of working and episodic memory. *Psychopharmacology* 176 (2): 214–22.

Luck, S. J. 2005. *An Introduction to the Event-Related Potential Technique.* Cambridge, Massachusetts: MIT Press.

Makeig, S., S. Debener, J. Onton, and A. Delorme. 2004. Mining event-related brain dynamics. *Trends in Cognitive Sciences* 8 (5): 204–10.

Makeig, S., A. Delorme, M. Westerfield, T. P. Jung, J. Townsend, E. Courchesne, and T. J. Sejnowski. 2004. Electroencephalographic brain dynamics following manually responded visual targets. *Plos Biology* 2 (6): 747–62.

Marshall, S. P. 2007. Identifying cognitive state from eye metrics. *Aviation Space and Environmental Medicine* 78 (5): B165–75.

Mazaheri, A., I. L. C. Nieuwenhuis, H. van Dijk, and O. Jensen. 2009. Prestimulus alpha and mu activity predicts failure to inhibit motor responses. *Human Brain Mapping* 30 (6): 1791–800.

McEvoy, L. K., E. Pellouchoud, M. E. Smith, and A. Gevins. 2001. Neurophysiological signals of working memory in normal aging. *Cognitive Brain Research* 11 (3): 363–76.

McGuirl, J. M. and N. B. Sarter. 2006. Supporting trust calibration and the effective use of decision aids by presenting dynamic system confidence information. *Human Factors* 48 (4): 656–65.

Mikulka, P. J., M. W. Scerbo, and F. G. Freeman. 2002. Effects of a biocybernetic system on vigilance performance. *Human Factors* 44: 654–64.

Miller, G. A. 1956. The magical number seven, plus or minus two: Some limits on our capacity for processing information. *Psychological Review* 63: 81–97.

Noel, J. B., K. W. Bauer, and J. W. Lanning. 2005. Improving pilot mental workload classification through feature exploitation and combination: A feasibility study. *Computers & Operations Research* 32 (10): 2713–30.

Nunez, P. L. and R. Srinivasan. 2006. *Electrical Fields of the Brain*, 2nd ed. Oxford: Oxford University Press.

Paas, F., A. Renkl, and J. Sweller. 2003. Cognitive load theory and instructional design: Recent developments. *Educational Psychologist* 38 (1): 1–4.

Paas, F., T. van Gog, and J. Sweller. 2010. Cognitive load theory: New conceptualizations, specifications, and integrated research perspectives. *Educational Psychology Review* 22 (2): 115–21.

Parasuraman, R. and D. Caggiano. 2005. Neural and genetic assays of mental workload. In *Quantifying Human Information Processing*, edited by D. McBride and D. Schmorrow, 123–55. Lanham, MD: Rowman and Littlefield.

Parasuraman, R. and G. F. Wilson. 2008. Putting the brain to work: Neuroergonomics past, present, and future. *Human Factors* 50: 468–74.

Pope, A. T., E. H. Bogart, and D. S. Bartolome. 1995. Biocybernetic system evaluates indices of operator engagement in automated task. *Biological Psychology* 40 (1): 187–95.

Sauseng, P., W. Klimesch, M. Doppelmayr, T. Pecherstorfer, R. Freunberger, and S. Hanslmayr. 2005. EEG alpha synchronization and functional coupling during top-down processing in a working memory task. *Human Brain Mapping* 26 (2): 148–55.

Sauseng, P., W. Klimesch, K. F. Heise, W. R. Gruber, E. Holz, A. A. Karim, M. Glennon, C. Gerloff, N. Birbaumer, and F. C. Hummel. 2009. Brain oscillatory substrates of visual short-term memory capacity. *Current Biology* 19 (21): 1846–52.

Smith, M. E., L. K. McEvoy, and A. Gevins. 1999. Neurophysiological indices of strategy development and skill acquisition. *Cognitive Brain Research* 7 (3): 389–404.

Stahl, J., H. Gibbons, and J. Miller. 2010. Modeling single-trial LRP waveforms using gamma functions. *Psychophysiology* 47 (1): 43–56.

Stevens, R. H., T. Galloway, C. Berka, and M. Sprang. 2009. Can neurophysiologic synchronies provide a platform for adapting team performance? In *Foundations of Augmented Cognition*, edited by D. D. Schmorrow, I. V. Estabrooke, and M. Grootjen. *Lecture Notes in Computer Science*, Vol. 5638, pp. 658–67. Heidelberg, Germany: Springer.

Sweller, J. 1988. Cognitive load during problem solving: Effects on learning. *Cognitive Science: A Multidisciplinary Journal* 12 (2): 257–85.

Sweller, J. 2006. Discussion of "emerging topics in cognitive load research: Using learner and information characteristics in the design of powerful learning environments". *Applied Cognitive Psychology* 20 (3): 353–7.

Wellens, A. R. 1993. Group situation awareness and distributed decision making: From military to civilian applications. In *Individual and Group Decision Making: Current Issues*, edited by J. Castellan, 267–91. Hillsdale, NJ: Lawrence Erlbaum Associates.

Wickens, C. D. 1984. Processing resources in attention. In *Varieties of Attention*, edited by R. Parasuraman and R. Davies, 63–101. Orlando, FL: Academic Press.

Wilson, G. F. and C. A. Russell. 2003a. Operator functional state classification using multiple psychophysiological features in an air traffic control task. *Human Factors* 45 (3): 381–9.

Wilson, G. F. and C. A. Russell. 2003b. Real-time assessment of mental workload using physiological measures and artificial neural networks. *Human Factors* 45: 635–43.

Wilson, G. F. and C. A. Russell. 2007. Performance enhancement in an uninhabited air vehicle task using psychophysiologically determined adaptive aiding. *Human Factors* 49 (6): 1005–18.

9

Brain–Computer Interfaces: Effects on Brain Activation and Behavior

Sonja C. Kleih, Steve Lukito, and Andrea Kübler

CONTENTS

9.1 Introduction

Brain–computer interfaces (BCI) allow real-time interaction between brain activity and machine devices by converting brain signals into commands for output devices (see Figure 9.1) such as communication aids and neuroprostheses (Millán et al. 2010). The control of BCI devices can be achieved through noninvasive approaches, that is, through

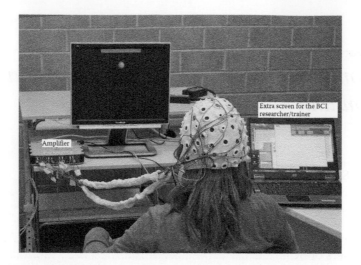

FIGURE 9.1
Participant using a brain–computer interface (BCI) system based on electroencephalography (EEG). The EEG is assessed with an electrode cap; brain signals are amplified and analyzed. The task, which indicates what activity the user is supposed to produce, and the feedback are provided to the user on the computer screen. A separate screen allows the BCI researcher or trainer to observe the brain activity of the BCI user. (This picture displays a potential BCI setup used at the Fondazione Santa Lucia, Rome, Italy.)

measuring electrical activity [electroencephalography (EEG)], or magnetical activity [magnetencephalography (MEG)], or hemodynamic responses of the brain. Slow cortical potentials (SCPs), sensorimotor rhythms (SMRs), event-related potentials (ERPs), and steady-state visual evoked potentials (SSVEPs) are the main input signals for EEG based BCIs. For the detection of hemodynamic responses technologies such as functional magnetic resonance imaging (fMRI) and functional near-infrared spectroscopy (fNIRS) are used. Invasive BCIs, on the other hand, rely on recording of intracortical signals.

In this chapter, we will mainly focus on noninvasive BCIs and attempt to provide readers with important results and recent findings that have been achieved throughout approximately two decades of BCI research. We begin by presenting the potential BCI user groups, that is, patients in the locked-in state, patients diagnosed with amyotrophic lateral sclerosis (ALS), stroke, spinal cord injury (SCI), attention deficit hyperactivity disorder (ADHD), and epilepsy (Section 9.2). The user group list is by no means exhaustive and its contents will possibly expand in the future.

Various input signals of BCI and a brief summary of the imaging technology and neurophysiological signal recording used to obtain the BCI input signals are presented in Section 9.3. Particular attention is given here to the noninvasive P300 ERP-based and the SMR-based BCIs. Both these signals are known for their robustness for detection and analysis and their theiromnipresence in healthy subjects and patients alike (Kübler et al. 2005; Nijboer, Furdea, et al. 2008; Nijboer, Sellers, et al. 2008; Pfurtscheller, Guger, et al. 2000; Pfurtscheller, Neuper, et al. 2000; Pfurtscheller et al. 2006; Vaughan et al. 2006). Specifically for SMR-based BCI, users can learn to actively regulate their SMR signals through motor imagery, provided they receive online feedback and are positively reinforced for correct responses (operant conditioning). Novel BCIs that use input signals depending on feedback other than visual signals, for example, auditory and vibrotactile (Cincotti et al. 2007; Furdea et al. 2009; Halder et al. 2010; Hong et al. 2009), are also described in this section, alongside the currently developed hybrid BCIs that integrate several signals (Allison et al. 2010; Brunner et al. 2010; Pfurtscheller et al. 2010).

Section 9.4 contains details of various assistive devices that have been adapted for use with BCIs in research. These assistive devices include communication devices such as the "Thought Translation Device" (TTD) and the "P300 Speller" for the locked-in patients (Birbaumer et al. 1999; Kübler, Kotchoubey, et al. 2001); neuroprosthesis and orthosis for facilitating grasping function and object manipulation in the environment (Krusienski, Cox, and Shih 2010; Müller-Putz et al. 2005; Pfurtscheller, Müller, and Korisek 2002); power wheelchair and domotic appliances; and BCIs intended for artistic expression (Kübler et al. 2008; Moore 2003; Münßinger et al. 2010), gaming applications (Finke, Lenhardt, and Ritter 2009; Tangermann et al. 2008), and Internet browsing (Bensch et al. 2007; Mugler et al. 2008; Mugler et al. 2010).

Also in Section 9.4 is a brief discussion of neuroadaptation and how neuroadaptation allows control of BCI devices through the neurofeedback principle. We present evidence, primarily from invasive studies with non-human primates, of BCI-induced neuroplasticity for neuroprosthetic control. Recent evidence and critical appraisal of the BCI as a neurorehabilitation tool is presented alongside discussion of the possible role that BCI can play in the context of the current treatment of choice for stroke rehabilitation. Promising results from BCI neurofeedback training in epilepsy (Strehl et al. 2005; Tan et al. 2009) and ADHD are presented in the last part of this section (Strehl et al. 2007), together with a seminal work by deCharms et al. (2005) in application of real-time fMRI (rtfMRI) BCI for neurorehabilitation of chronic pain and the role of BCI in the treatment of emotion dysregulation (Caria et al. 2007; Ruiz et al. 2008).

In spite of the numerous progresses that have been achieved in BCI, there is work to be done in bringing an easy-to-use BCI system out of the laboratories and into the end users' home. Section 9.5 lists some clinical and practical issues that have been encountered during research together with exemplary works that provide solution for these problems. Last but not least, we present an ethical discussion on the use of BCI in locked-in patients. Overall, tremendous research effort is invested to achieve the goals of the BCI such that we are confident that the BCI community will be able to provide ready-to-use systems for a broad variety of potential users in the near future.

9.2 Potential Users of BCIs

BCIs for communication were developed with the goal of enabling motor-disabled people to communicate and, thereby, interact with their environment. The target population of severely motor-disabled people consisted of mostly those with the locked-in syndrome (LIS). Patients with LIS are conscious and awake but show extremely limited expressions owing to severe motor impairment (Laureys et al. 2005). The locked-in state can occur as a final stage of ALS, a neurodegenerative disease that initially manifests as muscle weakness (Rowland and Shneider 2001). Within 3–5 years, first and second motor neurons and also other cortical and subcortical neurons degenerate, resulting in an increasing state of paralysis in the patients. At the end stage of ALS, patients become completely locked-in and have no residual muscle movements including those of the eyes (Kübler and Birbaumer 2008). Patients can only survive if they decide to be artificially ventilated.

LIS can also be caused by a stroke in the brainstem (pons). In the worst case, the pontine stroke leaves the patient with vertical eye movement only (Bauer, Gerstenbrand, and Rumpl 1979; Smith and Delargy 2005). Most often the LIS is of cerebrovascular origin such that thrombotic occlusion of the arteria basilaris leads to infarction in the ventral pons (Katz et al. 1992; Patterson and Grabois 1986). As a result, pyramidal and corticobulbar tracts are interrupted and, in turn, so are both the supranuclear and postnuclear oculomotor fibers. Where residual motor function other than vertical eye movement is preserved, the LIS is referred to as incomplete, and where no movement and thus no communication is possible, the LIS is referred to as total (Bauer, Gerstenbrand, and Rumpl 1979). Higher cortical areas or subcortical areas besides the brainstem are not affected.

Paralysis and motor impairments may also occur as a result of SCI or stroke with varying degrees of paralysis depending on the lesion site (McDonald and Sadowsky 2002). Eighty percent of strokes are caused by cerebral infarction that can be of cardiembolic, atherothrombotic, or lacunar origins. Infarcts can occur in cortical and subcortical structures, which can cause both physical impairment and higher cortical deficits (Bamford 1992; Hoffmann et al. 1997). Possible causes of SCI are traumatic or nontraumatic injuries caused by, for example, accidents in traffic, criminal assaults, or sports and leisure related activities (DeVivo et al. 2006). Nontraumatic causes, which present the majority of cases, can be the result of heterogeneous antecedents including developmental or degenerative diseases (McDonald and Sadowsky 2002), and can lead to tetraplegia or paraplegia that impairs mobility to an extreme extent.

Other potential BCI user groups are people with epilepsy or ADHD. Characterized by paroxysmal burst of excessive electrical activity in the brain (ICD-10; World Health Organization 2004), epilepsy requires anticonvulsant medication or, when intractable, removal of epileptic foci through surgery. Symptoms of ADHD include inattention, hyperactivity, impulsivity (American Psychiatric Association 2000). Medication such as methylphenidate and amphetamine are prescribed for children diagnosed with ADHD, although with much controversy (Mayes, Bagwell, and Erkulwater 2008). Neurofeedback intervention has thus been suggested as a noninvasive method for symptom reduction in both disorders (Lubar 1998; Monastra et al. 2005; Strehl et al. 2007).

9.3 Recording Techniques and Input Signals for BCIs

Different BCIs rely on distinct input signals that can be obtained from several brain imaging and neurophysiological recording techniques and, subsequently, classified with a variety of computational approaches. This section describes the currently available BCIs based on noninvasive signals (e.g., EEG, MEG, fMRI, and fNIRS) and invasive signals (e.g., electrocorticography (ECoG)). Brief descriptions of input signals such as SCP, SMR, P300 ERP, and SSVEPs for EEG-based BCI are given. Here, we mostly focused on SMR and the P300 ERP as input signals for an EEG-based BCI (Kleih et al. 2011), because of their known robustness with regard to signal detection and analysis, their presence in the majority of subjects—healthy and neurologically affected volunteers alike—and their potential for achieving high information transfer rates allowing for fast BCI control. We begin the following section with SCP input because of its historic importance with regard to communication with patients.

9.3.1 BCIs with EEG Input Signals: SCPs, SMRs, and ERPs

The EEG records electrical potentials produced by primary current within the apical dendrites of the pyramidal neurons of the cerebral cortex. BCI users can control their EEG signals, for example, the SCP and the SMR, by means of feedback training and operant conditioning. SCPs are shifts of the depolarization level of the apical dendrites in cortical layers I and II caused by synchronous firing of the cortical pyramidal neurons as a result of intracortical and thalamocortical inputs. Negative SCPs lead to facilitation of neuronal firing whereas positive SCPs increase the excitation threshold. It has long been shown that SCPs can be brought under voluntary control by means of neurofeedback and that this leads to change in behavior (Lutzenberger et al. 1979, 1982). To achieve regulation of SCPs, users are provided with a cursor (on a computer screen) whose vertical movement corresponds to the SCP amplitude. Regulation of SCP allows for binary responses that can be used as input for BCI (Birbaumer et al. 1999; Kübler, Neumann, et al. 2001). The SCP BCI is a firmly established method for communication and multiple testings of SCP BCI in patients with LIS indicated performance of up to 94% accuracy (Birbaumer et al. 1999; Kübler et al. 2004; Neumann and Birbaumer 2003). As their name suggests, SCPs occur from a few hundred milliseconds up to several seconds, which restricts the amount of information transferred per time unit. Despite its slowness SCP BCI was used at the patients' home, even without the presence of researchers, to communicate messages of considerable length (Birbaumer et al. 1999; Neumann et al. 2003).

While the SCP BCI feeds back the EEG amplitude in the time domain, SMRs are fed back in the frequency domain and are frequently used as input signal because they can be controlled by motor imagery. The SMRs are rhythms of the alpha band from 8 to 12 Hz (μ rhythm) and the beta band from 18 to 25 Hz over the sensorimotor cortex (SMC; M1/S1) (McFarland et al. 2000). In a state of relaxation the SMR is synchronized, and thus of high amplitude (event-related synchronization [ERS]). It desynchronizes and the amplitude decreases during planning, imagining, and executing motor acts (event-related desynchronization [ERD]) (Pfurtscheller 1992; Pfurtscheller and Neuper 2005). Similarly to the SCP signal, SMR regulation can be achieved by means of operant learning. Most SMR BCI users' initial performance is already above chance because strategies for SMR regulation of the signal are readily at hand and require feedback for further "fine-tuning" only (Blankertz et al. 2010; Guger et al. 2003; Nijboer, Furdea, et al. 2008).

In a typical SMR training setup, volunteers imagine right- and left-hand, feet, or tongue movements following corresponding visual cues presented on a computer screen. To use the elicited EEG activity as a feedback in an SMR BCI, data needs to be classified for each frequency and EEG channel (Blankertz et al. 2008; Graimann et al. 2002; Lotte et al. 2007; Pfurtscheller and Lopes da Silva 2005). Each trial of motor imagery needs to be bandpass filtered; samples need to be squared and subsequently averaged over trials and sample points. Highest contrasting ERD (event-related band power decrease)/ERS (event-related band power increase) patterns associated with a maximum value of variance r^2 (see Figure 9.2) are subsequently chosen as input signal for the SMR-based BCI (McFarland and Wolpaw 2008).

With regard to SMR BCI performance, Blankertz et al. (2008) reported that 13 of 14 healthy BCI novices achieved an average online accuracy of 82% in their first motor-imagery training session. Either imagery of foot movement was contrasted with that of one hand (left/right) or the imagery of the left hand was contrasted with that of the right hand. Remarkably, only in one of these subjects no distinguishable brain activity could be found (Blankertz et al. 2008). Likewise Pfurtscheller et al. (2008) found classification accuracies

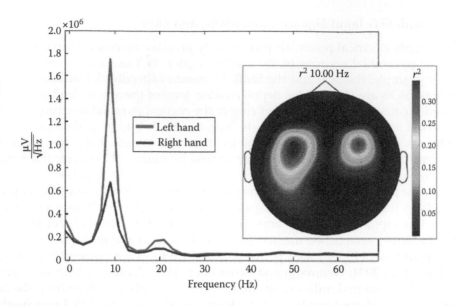

FIGURE 9.2

Exemplary spectral representation (SR) of the sensorimotor rhythm at electrode FC3 (left) and its associated brain topography (BT, right). The black line in the SR indicates motor imagery of the right hand, which leads to greater event-related desynchronization than motor imagery of the left hand (gray line). In this case a binary choice would be possible by moving a cursor on a computer screen downward by imagining right-hand movement and upward by imagining left-hand movement (see Figure 9.1). In the BT, brain activation in the sensorimotor areas of a healthy participant when imagining right- versus left-hand movement at a frequency of 10 Hertz is displayed.

of 83% on average in 9 naïve healthy subjects when contrasting motor imagery of the left hand with that of the foot or motor imagery of the left hand with that of the foot. Reports of high accuracies were also found in larger participant groups (Blankertz et al. 2010; Guger et al. 2003). Blankertz et al. (2010) most recently found an average online accuracy of above 75% in a sample of 80 healthy BCI novices. Also, ALS patients were able to achieve SMR BCI control with an average accuracy of 78% by contrasting imagery of left-hand, right-hand, or feet movements with a resting state (Kübler et al. 2005).

The P300 ERP is a positive electrical deflection occurring in the time window between 200 and 700 ms following provocation of stimuli (see Figure 9.3). Large P300 ERPs are elicited upon the perception of rare target stimuli presented within a stream of frequently occurring standard, nontarget stimuli, in the so called "oddball" paradigm (Donchin 1981; Sutton et al. 1965). The P300 is usually largest over centroparietal regions, at electrode positions Cz and Pz. The P300 ERP is autonomously elicited by visual, auditory, or tactile stimulation with an oddball (Farwell and Donchin 1988; Pritchard 1981) which allows for significant BCI control within the first session in most subjects, healthy and impaired alike (Section 9.2).

Stepwise linear discriminant analysis (SWLDA) is commonly used as P300 signal classification algorithm because of its reliability (Donchin, Spencer, and Wijesinghe 2000; Furdea et al. 2009; Krusienski et al. 2008; Sellers and Donchin 2006) and low computational requirements (Lotte et al. 2007). SWLDA separates the segmented epochs into target and nontarget classes and both obtain equal covariance matrices. In a series of stepwise regression, features that increase the distinction between the two classes are included in the model whereas those with less predictive validity are excluded. This process is repeated

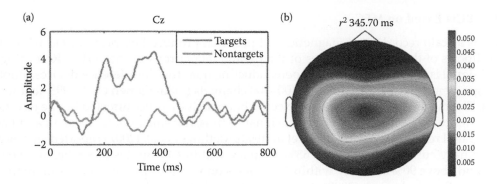

FIGURE 9.3

Exemplary P300 event-related potential epoch and brain topography in a healthy subject. (a) The P300 is elicited by the target stimuli and depicted in red whereas the activity associated with the nontarget stimuli is displayed in green. (b) Topography: The P300 is most prominent at the centroparietal region of the cortex.

until a most suitable model for the distinction between targets and nontargets is detected or when a predefined number of features are tested and no further improvement of the model is possible (Krusienski et al. 2008).

A feasibility test of the P300 Speller, originally designed by Farwell and Donchin (1988), with 100 healthy volunteers, showed its immediate usability in naïve subjects. After a 5-minute introduction, more than 85% of the volunteers were able to operate the BCI at 80%–100% accuracy in a text entry task (Guger et al. 2009). Kleih et al. (2010) even found 100% accuracy in 29 of 33 healthy volunteers. The minimum introductory period and ease-of-use has a high clinical relevance. At present, the P300-based BCI appears to be the most feasible communication approach in patients with major impairment or LIS (Kübler and Birbaumer 2008; Nijboer, Birbaumer, and Kübler 2010). Numerous clinical studies have shown the efficacy of the P300 BCI in paralyzed patients with four choice responses, for example, "YES/NO/PASS/END" or "UP/DOWN/LEFT/RIGHT" for cursor movement (Piccione et al. 2006; Sellers and Donchin 2006; Silvoni et al. 2009), six choices (Hoffmann et al. 2008), and more than 25 choices using the P300 Speller (Kübler et al. 2009).

Motivation of the BCI users and habituation (Ravden and Polich 1999) has been mentioned as possible factors that can influence the P300 ERP in long-term BCI use (Kübler, Neumann, et al. 2001). Working with a group of ALS patients that used the P300 BCI for 40 weeks, Nijboer, Sellers, et al. (2008) addressed the issue of habituation and found no significant changes over time in the P300 amplitude and latencies. Most recently, we studied the effect of motivation and emotion on performance with the P300 BCI and found moderate effects of motivation in healthy subjects (Kleih et al. 2010) and only minor effects of emotion (Lukito et al., under revision). Taken together, the minimal time needed for adapting the BCI to the individual user, the high possible accuracy, and easiness-of-use render the P300 BCI the most promising candidate for daily use at the patients' home.

We only briefly mention here SSVEPs that have been used for BCI applications such as orthoses and neuroprostheses (Müller-Putz and Pfurtscheller 2008; Müller-Putz et al. 2006). The SSVEP is evoked at the occipital cortical area as a response to stimulation with flickering light-emitting diodes (LEDs). The SSVEP oscillations are of the same frequency as the stimulation; thus, the LED toward which the user fixates their gaze can be detected (Müller-Putz et al. 2006). The successful use of the SSVEP BCI, with accuracies of up to 100%, was achieved in a study by Martinez, Bakardjian, and Cichocki (2007). The SSVEP BCIs await testing with target patient groups.

9.3.2 BCIs Based on MEG

MEG is a scalp recording of magnetic field potential produced by primary electrical current dipoles of the apical dendrites of the pyramidal neurons in the cortex. Recording of MEG signal is accomplished with superconducting quantum interference devices coupled with gradiometers at approximately 100–300 channels (Hämäläinen et al. 1993; Ioannides 2006). The magnetic field induced by electric brain activity is not affected by the electrical conductance of the head volume. MEG signal is, thus, not smeared by the skull and has a high spatial resolution (Hämäläinen et al. 1993). Mellinger et al. (2007) reported significant SMR binary cursor control above 63% accuracy within 64 minutes in six healthy volunteers and above 90% accuracy within 32 minutes only in four participants. A more recent report by Battapady et al. (2009) stated 86% cross-validation classification accuracy of the MEG BCI in predicting movement intention in four directions on a single trial basis. The ultra sensitivity to micro-scale signal and obligatory operationalization in magnetically shielded enclosure renders the MEG unlikely to become a cheap, practical, and portable communication device. Nonetheless, the MEG may evolve as a clinical tool for rehabilitation in the future (Buch et al. 2008; Daly et al. 2009; Wang et al. 2010; see Section 9.4.2.2).

9.3.3 BCIs with Hemodynamic Input Signals

Both fMRI- and fNIRS-based BCIs are dependent on local changes of deoxygenated hemoglobin owing to fluctuating cerebral blood flow and cerebral metabolic rate of oxygen (Uludağ, Dubowitz, and Buxton 2005). The fMRI detects the blood oxygen level-dependent (BOLD) signal and measures neural activity in cortical and subcortical brain regions with high spatial resolution. The recently applied parallel computation of fMRI data with BOLD signal acquisition and analysis resulted in a novel rtfMRI feedback technique that supports near-real-time correspondence between physiological signal and behavior (Bagarinao, Nakai, and Tanaka 2006; Sitaram et al. 2007). This technological advance has been applied in a neurofeedback rtfMRI BCI involving modulation of BOLD signal using motor imagery and affective state imagery (Caria et al. 2007; Sitaram et al. 2007; Weiskopf et al. 2003) and was also tested as a neurorehabilitation strategy for chronic pain and emotional dysregulation (deCharms et al. 2005; Ruiz et al. 2008; Section 9.4.2.3). An alternative rtfMRI BCI paradigm involves spatial pattern recognition of cortical responses during a mental task. Yoo et al. (2004) detected distinct cortical activation patterns associated with left/right-hand motor imagery, mental speech, and mental arithmetic that were then translated into four-direction cursor control. Accuracy beyond 90% was recorded for three subjects in a spatial navigation task to direct a ball out of a two-dimensional maze (Yoo et al. 2004). In principle, this rtfMRI BCI cursor control could become a clinic-based communication facilitator, for example, such as proposed by Sorger et al. (2009), to serve as a diagnostic tool and reduce the number of misdiagnoses between locked-in state and other disorders of consciousness, for example, the minimally conscious state.

fNIRS posits another possibility for noninvasive hemodynamic brain response measurement with better portability than the fMRI. The method is based on passing coherent light sources of two or more wavelengths through layers of brain tissue. The light intensity changes as it is scattered and absorbed in the brain and blood vessels, allowing detection of metabolic changes of deoxygenated and oxygenated blood as a result. The fNIRS signal has only been recently exploited for BCI control (Sitaram, Caria, and Birbaumer 2009; Wriessnegger, Kurzmann, and Neuper 2008). In a study by Luu and Chau (2009) nine healthy volunteers were presented with images of two types of drinks and asked to mentally decide on their preference. Hemodynamic response to this question was classified correctly at an accuracy level within 75%–84% (Luu and Chau 2009). Investigation in 40 ALS patients (17 in the locked-in state) by Naito et al. (2007) showed that 40% of LIS patients and 70% of early-stage ALS patients displayed fNIRS BCI control. These patients were presented with a binary choice question with a "YES" answer elicited by mental calculations and a "NO" answer by a relaxed state. Those who succeeded achieved a performance with up to 80% accuracy, thereby indicating the feasibility of fNIRS BCI for meaningful communication in patients. Significant challenges for future optimization of fNIRS BCI technology include the influence of human hair on signal strength and optode (light detector) and motion artifacts that affect the signal quality. On the other hand, near-infrared spectroscopy (NIRS) is portable and can, thus, be brought to the patients' bedside and fNIRS offers high spatial resolution. The present high costs of an NIRS system may also be reduced when fNIRS gains popularity as a measurement tool for the blood oxygen level in the brain.

9.3.4 NOVEL BCIs: Investigating Input Modalities and Input Signal Combinations

A growing number of studies have attempted to establish BCIs that do not rely on vision for operation by patients, specifically for locked-in and nonresponsive patients (see Section 9.2). For example, auditory neurofeedback of SCP (Hinterberger et al. 2005; Pham et al. 2005) and SMR (Nijboer, Furdea, et al. 2008) or auditory ERPs (Halder et al. 2010; Hong et al. 2009; Höhne et al. 2011; Schreuder et al. 2011; Hill and Schölkopf 2012) were explored. Likewise, vibrotactile presentation of feedback was investigated for SMR (Cincotti et al. 2007; Müller-Putz et al. 2006) and the P300 (Brouwer and van Erp 2010; Nijboer, Birbaumer, and Kübler 2010). The new methods usually comprise a limited number of possible responses, for example, binary "YES" or "NO" (Halder et al. 2010) or four choices (Sellers and Donchin 2006), but the proof of principle has also been shown for a 5×5 matrix in healthy subjects (Furdea et al. 2009) and ALS patients in the locked-in state (Kübler et al. 2009). Performance with accuracy above 70% has been reported.

To obtain a greater variety for controlling assistive devices, recent studies have investigated the feasibility of hybrid BCIs for integration of different, most preferably ALL available, input signals for BCI control (Leeb et al. 2011). The hybrid BCIs allow for multiple input signals to potentially accommodate a wider range of users because they are not restricted to brain activity as input and allow the user to switch to brain-based control in case of muscular fatigue. A recent offline study showed that simultaneous classification of data from SSVEP and SMR tasks was indeed feasible and a trend toward improvement of offline performance using the hybrid approach was seen in comparison to SSVEP and SMR alone (Allison et al. 2010; Brunner et al. 2010). A follow-up study by Pfurtscheller et al. (2010) successfully demonstrated the compatibility of an SSVEP device (an orthosis; see Section 9.4.1.2) and a motor imagery-based "brain switch" (Pfurtscheller and Solis-Escalante 2009) that utilized SMR input. The switch enabled switching the orthosis ON/OFF to prevent unintended movement by inadvertently gazing in the direction of the LEDs. This method significantly reduced false response by 50% in four of six healthy volunteers.

9.3.5 Intracortical BCIs

Intracortical BCIs are based on neurophysiological recording techniques and directly modulated by neuronal activity through changes of single- or multi-unit action potential

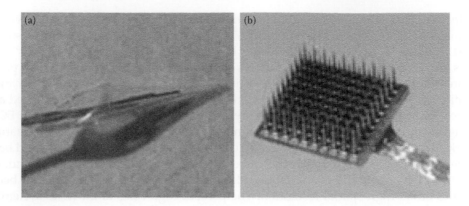

FIGURE 9.4
Intracortical electrodes. (a) Neurotrophic electrode. The electrode is approximately 1.5 mm long and has a diameter of 0.1–0.4 mm. (From Bartels, J. et al. 2008. *Journal of Neuroscience Methods* 174 (2): 168–76. With permission.) (b) Microelectrode BrainGate™ Sensor. The electrode tips are spaced by 400 μm. (From Donoghue, J. P. et al. 2007. *Journal of Physiology* 579 (Pt 3): 603–11. With permission.)

or local field potential. The signal has the highest temporal and spatial resolution and thus potentially provides the best control for the BCI* (Leuthardt et al. 2009). Targeted cortical area for intracortical implant is the primary motor cortex M1, where neuronal tuning of property toward movement kinematics has been observed in non-human primates, thus significant for the development of BCI neuroprostheses and orthoses (Carmena et al. 2003; Lebedev et al. 2005).

To date, two intracortical BCI sensors have been established and tested in patients (Hochberg et al. 2006; Kennedy and Bakay 1998). A first trial by Kennedy et al. (2000; see also Kennedy and Bakay 1998) made used of the individually implanted neurotrophic electrode (see Figure 9.4). On the basis of the findings from the animal studies, the sensor was implanted in the hand area of the M1 cortical layers 4 and 5 in an ALS patient (Kennedy and Bakay 1998), who, within a few months, controlled her neuronal signal and turned it "ON" and "OFF" without failing, aided by visual and audio feedback. Subsequently, operation of a computer cursor, a visual keyboard, and a virtual hand by a brainstem stroke patient was reported (Kennedy et al. 2000; Kennedy et al. 2004). Using a distinctive approach and sensor, Hochberg et al. (2006) implanted BrainGate™ microelectrode sensor in the arm area of M1 of a patient with high SCI. Accuracy of controlling a computer cursor was reported to be 73%–95% in the "center-out task" that consisted of moving the cursor from the center of the screen toward targets at the periphery, and with this movement thus bringing a robot arm under volitional control.

9.3.6 Electrocorticography BCI

The ECoG relies on surface potential recording of neural activity on the epidural or subdural surface of the brain achieved by a flat electrode array that detects higher spatial resolution, higher amplitude, and wider frequency bandwidth than the EEG (Hinterberger et al. 2008; Leuthardt et al. 2004; Schalk et al. 2007). Accordingly, ECoG has a high signal-to-noise ratio and the wide bandwidth of ECoG enables utilization of μ, β, and higher-frequency γ

---

* For an alternative discussion, see Wolpaw and McFarland (2004) who achieved comparable cursor control with noninvasive approach.

oscillations for BCI input signal. Owing to ethical considerations almost all ECoG-based BCI trials were conducted in patients with intractable epilepsy who received implantation for subsequent surgery (Huggins et al. 2007; Leuthardt et al. 2009).

Trials of ECoG-based BCI in epileptic patients typically showed remarkable performance. Online cursor control above 70% accuracy for binary choice has been seen in 12 patients across three studies (Felton et al. 2007; Leuthardt et al. 2004; Leuthardt et al. 2006). Remarkably, the ECoG implants were located at a variety of cortical sites, including the auditory cortex, and patients used different strategies, for example, motor and speech imagery, actual movement,* and speech, for SMR control. One exceptional performance was displayed by a patient who was able to direct the cursor toward eight targets with more than 80% accuracy (Felton et al. 2007). In response to these findings, Hinterberger et al. (2008) investigated five patients with epilepsy in a spelling task with an SMR-based TTD (see Section 9.4.1.1), and observed that most patients were able to operate the TTD for communication. Taking into consideration the robust results from animal studies and the relatively short learning period for control of ECoG signal in past human studies, Hill et al. (2006) implanted an ALS patient with ECoG BCI. Informed consent was taken by the method of salivary pH-controlled BCI that was tested in this patient previously at 100% accuracy (Wilhelm, Jordan, and Birbaumer 2006). However, no BCI control could be established which was attributed to the diminishing ability to carry out motor imagery. In a recent study by Brunner and colleagues (2011), an incredibly high performance of 17 characters per minute with the ECoG-based BCI was reported. This result seems very promising; however, the reported result is based on a single case so far.

9.4 Applications of BCI for Neuroadaptation and Neurorehabilitation

Majorly impaired patients with ALS, SCI, and stroke need suitable assistive devices to compensate for loss of motor functions. In the first part of this section, we discuss a variety of technological advances, for example, communication devices, Internet browsers, "Brainpainter," orthosis, and mobility solutions, which are proposed by the BCI research community. The second part of this section presents evidence for neuroadaptation in the context of BCI devices. Details of most recent findings from animal and human studies are presented followed by the discussion on the projected use of BCI as a tool for neurorehabilitation strategy in SCI and stroke patients. We conclude this section with a series of recent findings in the field of neurofeedback. Specifically, we describe briefly the possible usage of BCIs for rehabilitation of epilepsy, ADHD, chronic pain, and emotion dysregulation.

9.4.1 BCIs as Assistive-Technological Answer for Motor-Disabled Users

9.4.1.1 Communication Devices

Communication has been cited as an important index of well-being in LIS patients (Bach 1993). It is thus highly desirable to satisfy the need for communication in these patients. The SCP-based TTD was the first BCI device that was tested successfully for communication in LIS patients diagnosed with ALS (Birbaumer et al. 1999). In TTD, the alphabet

---

* A BCI control using actual movement cannot be considered as a true BCI control.

was split into two groups to select with binary decision. After the first selection, the selected letter group (e.g., letters A to D) was halved again and a group consisting of half the letters of the first one was selected. The procedure was repeated until the target letter was singled out for selection. In a subsequent trial, the longest ever published message was written using the TTD (Neumann et al. 2003) in which patient HPS, who had used the BCI with and without experimenters for 11 years, described his strategy to control the cursor with SCP. Despite the low speed of communication with a maximum of three letters per minute, patient HPS wrote letters to his friends and directives for his caregivers using the BCI.

But also the P300 Speller (see Section 9.3.1) was shown to be a promising communication device for ALS patients (Kübler et al. 2009; Nijboer, Sellers, et al. 2008; Sellers and Donchin 2006). In the study by Nijboer, Sellers et al. (2008), four ALS patients used the P300 Speller for free communication and spelled sentences with up to 79 characters. Therefore, the usefulness and effectiveness of the application of BCI for complex communication in severely disabled users are clearly shown.

9.4.1.2 Development of BCI Orthoses and Neuroprostheses

The loss of hand function such as grasping ability is a significant impairment in stroke or tetraplegic SCI patients. This loss is perceived as most devastating among SCI patients because of the limitations it imposes for independent living and gainful employment (Peckham et al. 2001). It was, thus, a major breakthrough when Keith et al. (1989) introduced the Freehand® (NeuroControl, Cleveland, Ohio) system that subsequently proved to be highly successful in tetraplegic patients. The Freehand® system works by the principle of functional electrical stimulation (FES). It sends electrical stimulation through electrodes implanted in muscle groups in the disabled hand and forearm to initiate grasping movement activated by contralateral shoulder movement, which is detected by a shoulder position sensor and transmitted by radio signal to an implanted coil receiver on the ipsilateral chest (Peckham et al. 2001).

The fact that the Freehand® system relies on the presence of residual shoulder movement and first and foremost, the fact that it is no longer produced limits the assistive device options for SCI patients with injury at C4 level. However, Pfurtscheller, Guger, et al. (2000) discovered that noninvasive BCI orthosis control is feasible and compatible with the Freehand® system (Müller-Putz et al. 2005). This was a promising finding with regard to the future of noninvasive neuroprostheses. Müller-Putz and Pfurtscheller (2008) also showed the successful use of an SSVEP BCI-based asynchronous control, that is, self-paced hand prosthesis. Interestingly, the LEDs that evoked the SSVEP were attached directly to the prosthesis so that the movement triggered by the LED the user fixated on was intuitive. The successful use of a SSVEP based orthosis was also demonstrated by Ortner and colleagues in 2011. The average positive predictive value for six out of seven subjects was 78% which reveals good control without prior feedback (Ortner et al. 2011). Finally, Krusienski, Cox, and Shih (2010) recently reported a robotic interface for manipulating arbitrary objects on the basis of commands delivered from a modified P300 Speller application. The system is still in the development phase and tests with ECoG signals are planned (D. J. Krusienski, personal communication). Taken together, the use of BCI controlled prostheses and orthoses have achieved significant results such that BCI-controlled neuroprosthetic devices can be realized in the near and intermediate future.

9.4.1.3 Mobility Solution and "Smart Homes"

Majorly impaired individuals such as LIS patients continue to engage in meaningful social contact with significant others and the community despite their disability (Laureys et al. 2005). Social contact, of course, implies some degree of mobility. A survey among 77 experienced users of assistive technology revealed increased mobility as an important aspect of well-being that they would like to improve (Zickler et al. 2009). Indeed, among physically impaired individuals manual wheelchairs can be a source of social barriers because of the great difficulty in maneuvering (Chaves et al. 2004). Therefore, various studies have attempted to provide a mobility solution for patients by developing a BCI-controlled wheelchair that can assist users who can no longer rely on residual motor movement for mobility control. Research to date has shown that a wheelchair can be successfully directed using BCI with the P300 input signal (Iturrate et al. 2009; Pires and Nunes 2002) and the SMR as input signal (Galán et al. 2008). Leeb et al. (2007) tested the wheelchair steering of one SCI patient in a virtual environment with up to 100% directional accuracy. For patients, a mobility solution does not mean to approach a destination only; it can also mean to bring objects closer within reach. Millàn et al. (2004) equipped a Khepera (K-team Corporation, Switzerland) mobile robot with BCI control and trained two healthy volunteers to drive the robot using signals derived from motor imagery of hands, relaxed state, and mental cube rotation. Control over the mobile robot was achieved after a few days of learning. Although this research was originally motivated by the idea of providing better wheelchair control, the research has thrown some light on the possibility of automatization for other mobile appliances.

In its broadest sense, the concept of "smart home" refers to all technology that supports various home-based activities (Gentry 2009). Technologies that allow remote controlling and automatization of devices are, by today's standard, commonplace, and such technologies hold the potential for supporting physically impaired individuals and their caregivers alike. Babiloni et al. (2007) presented a promising study that showed that wheelchair-bound patients with Duchenne muscular dystrophy could use an SMR-based BCI to control several domotic-adapted appliances such as a door opener or BCI-controlled television ("ON/ OFF " switch and change of channel). All patients controlled the system successfully at the end of the training and reported increased confidence in their ability to interact with their environment (Babiloni et al. 2007). In comparison to BCI-controlled domotic devices the residual muscle-controlled domotic devices still yield higher control accuracies (Cincotti et al. 2008). This is by no means unexpected as BCI operation relies on input signals with far fewer degrees of freedom. It has been suggested that more mental states should be recognized to achieve fine control of BCI-actuated devices (Millàn et al. 2004). Invention of assistive technology that gives a higher degree of autonomy for disabled patients in their home environment is an attainable challenge for the BCI research community.

9.4.1.4 BCI and Entertainment: A Nonconventional Aspect of the BCI

Conventional assistive technologies for enabling communication and movement are not the only types of applications that the BCI community has developed. Addressing the LIS patients' wish to participate in social life (Laureys et al. 2005; Leon-Carrion et al. 2002), various BCIs have been developed to satisfy users' needs for entertainment and creative expression (Kübler et al. 2008; Moore 2003). Elaborating on the real-world application of BCI, Moore (2003) reported a system that translated EEG activity into musical output, thus allowing people musical expression and self-determined composition. Kübler et al. (2008) modified the P300 6 × 6 letter matrix to create a "Brainpainting" application that contains options for color, shape, zoom, and other supporting painting functions. This application has recently been tested successfully in three ALS patients (Münßinger et al. 2010) and all stated that they enjoy having an output channel for creative expression. The paintings produced by these patients and some artists were exhibited in Rostock, Germany in 2012 (http://www.kunst-hallerostock.de/pingoergosum.html) in an exhibition called "Pingo ergo sum."

More BCI applications have been created for ALS patients such as the BCI Internet browser (Bensch et al. 2007; Karim et al. 2006; Mugler et al. 2008). The P300 BCI-based web browser, in particular, has been tested with three ALS patients (Mugler et al. 2010). All patients successfully navigated through the Internet and mastered the task to order a book through an online vendor. Attempts to develop various BCI-based gaming applications have also been undertaken (Finke, Lenhardt, and Ritter 2009; Tangermann et al. 2008). Playing complex games, such as pinball, was also found to be feasible using noninvasive BCI. Healthy volunteers controlled the pinball machine by imagining two different movements to operate the left and right paddles (Tangermann et al. 2008). In the Finke et al. (2009) computer game, figures could be moved in illusional worlds using the P300 BCI. The authors pointed out that, in the future, gaming applications could possibly be played by two or three players in a competitive setting that offers more challenges for both the physically impaired and the non-impaired users. All BCI applications presented here can support disabled people to engage in more social activities and interactions with their environment, and also aim at enabling them to share the electronic world (e-inclusion, www.tobi-project.org).

9.4.2 The Potential of BCIs for Neurorehabilitation

BCI control requires co-adaptation from both the human and the computer side of the interface. Nonetheless, different BCI groups put their own emphasis on one of the two adaptive directions. The BCI approach founded on the neurofeedback principle (Birbaumer et al. 1999; Miner, McFarland, and Wolpaw 1998; Pfurtscheller, Neuper, et al. 2000) predominantly relies on the learning of voluntary regulation of EEG parameters. In this approach, positive reinforcement (operant conditioning) for every successful attempt is given to encourage users who cannot produce required responses at the beginning of their training. Other approaches of BCI broadly utilize the machine-learning capacity for classification of neural states, for example, tuning curve of neurons (Donoghue et al. 2007; Hochberg et al. 2006), or EEG pattern into a discernible BCI input signal (Krauledat et al. 2008; Müller et al. 2008; Vidaurre and Blankertz 2009), which decreases the amount of operant training necessary for reliable control.

The term neuroadaptation described in this section refers to the feedback training and operant learning part of the interaction, that is, the neural learning contribution within the brain–machine co-adaptation. The following sections present the most recent evidence of neuroadaptation in the context of animal and human studies. We also discuss the recently conjectured possible usage of BCI as an addition to the current physical rehabilitation in stroke and SCI patients and the role of motor imagery in promoting neuroplasticity. Finally, most recent findings in neurofeedback rehabilitation are described.

9.4.2.1 BCI Learning and Neuroadaptation: Studies in Primates and Findings in Humans

Studies of intracortical BCI in macaque monkeys have revealed long-term neurophysiological changes in the cortex after BCI operation (Carmena et al. 2003; Jarosiewicz et al. 2008;

Lebedev et al. 2005). In these studies, the monkeys are typically trained to operate a cursor (e.g., in the center-out task; see Section 9.3.5), initially using a hand-controlled joystick, while recording of neural tuning and machine learning are taking place. Subsequently, the joystick is disconnected from cursor operation, or taken away entirely, such that the monkey operates the cursor by brain control only. Learning-associated increase of a single neuron contribution to task performance was observed in cortical areas M1, S1, dorsal premotor cortex (PMd), and supplementary motor area (SMA), and the contribution of dominant control was distributed from M1 to other cortical areas at the end of the training period, which distinctly showed the development of cortical reorganization associated with learning (Carmena et al. 2003). Most recent findings show that long-term use of neuroprosthesis in the macaque monkeys results in a stable cortical map that is readily recalled and robust against interference (Ganguly and Carmena 2009).

Despite extensive findings from studies on non-human primates, no comparable report of neuroadaptation in human BCI studies has been made. Early clinical studies of the SCP-based BCI (Birbaumer et al. 1999; Neumann et al. 2004) provided some insights on the mechanism of neuroadaptation in BCI learning. Neumann et al. (2004) showed that ALS patients can increasingly self-regulate their SCP at a specific EEG channel. The patient first controlled BCI using widespread frontal, central, and parietal cortical areas. In the course of more than 150 training runs, a task-related change in polarity of SCP (positive vs. negative) occurred below the Cz electrode in central cortical areas only, indicating response automatization or focalization (Neumann et al. 2004). No similar observations have been reported in the context of P300 BCI. In fact, a patient study by Nijboer, Sellers, et al. (2008) showed no changes in the P300 ERP amplitude over 10 and more BCI training sessions (see Section 9.3.1).

Although our knowledge of BCI-induced neuroplasticity in the human brain is presently limited, it is very likely that plastic changes occur in the brain during the use of BCI devices. This is evident from the numerous results from non-human primate studies cited above (Carmena et al. 2003; Lebedev et al. 2005; Zacksenhouse et al. 2007). Indeed, BCI-induced neuroplasticity and neuroadaptation is important in the attainment of successful and finer control of BCI devices. Most notably, BCI-guided neuroplasticity can potentially play an important role in the development of a new neurorehabilitation strategy to support current physiotherapeutic regimes for patients with injuries of the central nervous system, such as stroke and SCI (Wang et al. 2010; see below).

9.4.2.2 Motor Imagery and the Augmentation of Plasticity

Cortical reorganization (Elbert and Rockstroh 2004) can facilitate regaining muscle control by manifesting in the expansion of cortical somatotopy due to increased synaptic activity, for example, through repeated practice of skills or functions. In the case of cerebral injury, adjacent cortical areas frequently replace the functions previously sustained by the lesioned areas and this provides a basis for post-injury rehabilitation. Traditional rehabilitation strategy for stroke-induced paralysis either focuses on repeated forced use of the afflicted body parts, or, in the case of hemiparesis stroke, involves constraint-induced movement therapy, that is, by restraining the unaffected limb and suppressing a patient's "learned non-use" of the semi-paralyzed limb (Taub and Uswatte 2003). Naturally, both strategies require reasonable amount of residual motor function in the affected limb.

In recent years, motor imagery training has emerged as a potential strategy for neurorehabilitation. Imagined movement is closely related to planning of movement and it is a component of broad motor representation which, in ordinary circumstances, is unconscious to us all (Jeannerod 1995). Research has established that motor imagery activates cortical areas similar to those activated by voluntary movement in healthy subjects (Pfurtscheller and Neuper 1997). Its proposed clinical utility for neurological disorders such as stroke and SCI, however, requires evidence of preserved motor cortical areas that respond to motor imagery training despite motor impairment. Indeed, it has been shown that stroke and SCI patients also retain cortical neuroplasticity in their motor cortex (Buch et al. 2008; Cramer et al. 2007). Even in patients with neurodegenerative disorders such as ALS, motor imagery can elicit significantly stronger BOLD response than in healthy controls (Lulé et al. 2007; see Figure 9.5a) in a number of cortical areas. It is, thus, plausible that motor imagery training can have a significant impact on the cortical reorganization and plasticity. In support to this argument, a systematic review comprising 10 different studies and 121 patients (Braun et al. 2006) concluded that additional motor imagery training in conjunction with the primary therapy did have an effect on recovery after stroke.

The observations of cortical reorganization and neuroplasticity in stroke and SCI patients while imagining movement suggest the readiness of the cortical areas to adapt motor imagery training. Nevertheless, current rehabilitation strategy offers little to patients with slight or absent residual motor function in the affected limb. After a year of intensive rehabilitation, a third of such patients regain poor residual movement only or none at all (Lai et al. 2002), which renders further intervention using current treatment of choice impossible. To find an alternative solution, Buch et al. (2008) investigated an MEG BCI hand orthosis control in eight chronic stroke patients with a plegic hand. MEG was used here because of the minimal effect a lesion has on the MEG signal. By relying on the motor imagery-evoked SMR signals from the ipsilesional or contralesional side of the cortex, the patients were able to control the orthosis at a success rate above 70% over the training period. Variability in performance was noticed, with one patient showing chance-level performance despite training (Buch et al. 2008).

Preserved cortical and subcortical areas have also been reported during motor imagery study in chronic complete SCI patients (Alkadhi et al. 2005). However, a later study published in the same year reported abnormalities of motor imagery-induced activation resulting in increased disturbance of brain activation pattern, poor modulation of function, and substantial reduction of activation volume in precentral and postcentral gyri (Cramer et al. 2005). Most interestingly, Cramer et al. (2007) subsequently observed improvement of tongue motor task performance in complete SCI patients and healthy controls after a week of motor imagery training without feedback. Improvement of feet motor performance was also evident in the healthy controls, although not in SCI patients. From such studies, one can conjecture the positive influence a long-term SMR-based BCI has on the motor cortex of impaired patients. To test this hypothesis, Enzinger et al. (2008) compared the BOLD signal between an SCI patient (who has been a long-term user of BCI devices since 1999) and five healthy age-matched volunteers during motor imagery of the limbs (left vs. right hand, left vs. right foot) and, for the healthy participants, during the active limb movement task. Overall, participants displayed significant activation of the SMC, SMA, and pre-SMA areas contralateral to the moved or imagined limb. The patient showed greater activation of the SMC area during motor imagery than healthy volunteers during real movement (see Figure 9.5b).

These results demonstrate that long-term usage of BCI based on neurofeedback at the very least preserves or, perhaps, promotes recovery. Such findings prompted Daly et al. (2009) to do a case study of neurorehabilitation by using BCI and FES (see Section 9.4.1.2). The stroke patient in this study regained volitional control of an isolated index finger movement after the ninth BCI and FES session (see also Section 9.4.1.2). Control of relaxed muscle

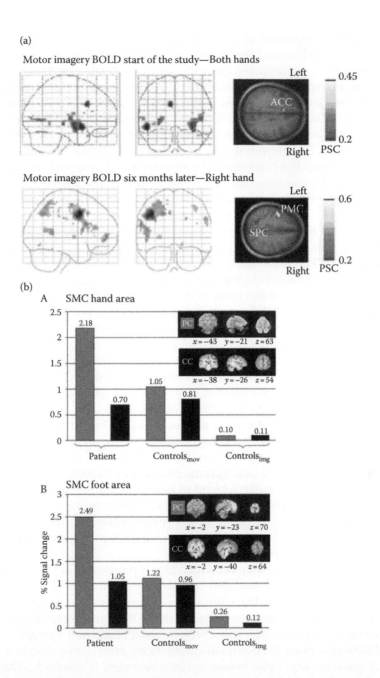

FIGURE 9.5

Motor imagery, cortical plasticity, and brain–computer interface. (a) Statistical parametric map of the motor imagery of right- and left-hand movements of healthy controls minus patients with amyotrophic lateral sclerosis (ALS) shows significant reduction for ALS patients (top). After 6 months, signal from around the same area was increased in ALS patients compared to that in controls. Blood oxygen level-dependent (BOLD) signal from the motor imagery of the right hand was increased to 60% in ALS patients compared to that in controls (bottom). PSC, percentage signal change. (From Lulé, D. et al. 2007. *Neurorehabilitation and Neural Repair* 21 (6): 518–26.) (b) BOLD signals from the sensorimotor cortex of the hand and foot area of SCI patients during motor imagery are stronger than that of real movements in healthy controls. PC, patient cluster; CC, control cluster. (From Enzinger, C. et al. 2008. *Experimental Brain Research* 190 (2): 215–23.)

state was considerably improved by more than 80%, which was a significant achievement because impaired neural control for relaxed muscle state could obstruct recovery (Daly et al. 2009). Partial recovery occurred after BCI feedback trials based on attempted movement of the same extremity, FES treatment, and whole-arm practice. Taking into account the accumulating evidence of improved motor imagery performance with action observation (Conson et al. 2009; Neuper et al. 2009; Sakamoto et al. 2009), Wang et al. (2010) proposed a neurorehabilitation paradigm that coupled MEG BCI motor imagery training with observation of action. This proposal was intended to optimize the amount of information transmitted through the corticospinal pathways and to support recovery in patients. Preliminary comparison between an SCI patient (incomplete major impairment) and a healthy control displayed a shorter period of SMR power reduction and an earlier SMR power "rebound" in the SCI patient during motor imagery and action observation, which in turn suggested that the temporal and spatial characteristics of SMR power modulation could be used as a training parameter during action imitation and a visually cued movement task. Recently, Picchiori et al. (2011) discovered that motor cortical excitability as measured with the transcranial magnetic stimulation in 10 healthy volunteers was modulated during motor imagery of the hand and was enhanced after six to eight sessions of BCI training. Taken together, all these studies demonstrated not only that motor imagery BCI training enhances motor cortex functioning but also that optimal paradigms for BCI-induced neurorehabilitation in patients are unquestionably emerging.

It must be noted that the development of a neurorehabilitation paradigm with BCI-induced neuroplasticity is still at its infancy. However promising, the few studies cited here are yet to show more concrete evidence of functional change of the chronically impaired limb owing to BCI training. Daly et al. (2009) conceded in their report that the regained volitional index finger movement in their patient could not be attributed specifically to the BCI and FES training alone. It has been suggested that successive motor imagery training in a "stepwise fashion," for example, in graduated steps from the premotor cortex to the cerebellum, can facilitate guided neuroplastic changes in the brain (Dobkin 2003; Sitaram et al. 2007). Given the current research trend in neurorehabilitation and BCI, there is, thus, an urgent need for careful design of optimum BCI-based neurorehabilitation protocols. Daly et al. (2009) and Wang et al. (2010) have already indicated that additional strategies such as electrostimulation and action observation are important factors that may influence the success of a rehabilitative outcome.

Also a central issue is the decision on which target patients could benefit from BCI in a neurorehabilitation protocol, for example, complete or incomplete SCI patients, chronic or acute stroke patients. With regard to acute stroke, it is imperative to clarify what contribution the BCI neurorehabilitation strategy can make to the current treatment of choice, that is, forced movement and constraint-induced treatment (Taub and Uswatte 2003). Murphy and Corbett (2009) described the diminishing plasticity after stroke akin to a "closing time window" that must be kept open before optimal recovery is reached. Whether BCI can assume the role as the "window keeper" to keep it open is an interesting conjecture that is worth exploring. In principle, an investigation of this idea from the perspective of BCI is technologically possible with the assistance of rtfMRI technology. Sitaram et al.'s (2007) idea of stepwise guided neuroplastic changes (see above) could be realized both cortically and subcortically by utilizing the rtfMRI technique, and this in turn would support investigations in patients with stroke lesion at various brain regions. It must be noted, however, that there are presently limited numbers of repertoires of guided training (e.g., motor imagery and attempted movement) that patients can use to locally control their neural activation. These repertoires need expanding such that patients are able to promote neuroplasticity optimally not only at the motor cortex but also upstream and downstream neural projections.

As a last note on this topic, there are instances when the steps taken for "enabling" and "curing"* a patient are at odds with one another. For example, in the interest of enabling stroke patients, readily acquired SMR signals from ipsilesional sites have been used as a BCI control input in some patients (Buch et al. 2008; Wisneski et al. 2008). By gaining proficient control of the SMR at the ipsilesional sites and thus promoting plasticity in these regions, patients can operate orthoses (and other types of BCI devices) that can help in their day-to-day assisted living. From the point of view of neuroplasticity-based rehabilitation, however, promotion of plasticity from the contralateral motor cortex is most desirable for "curing," or restoring, the function of the impaired limb (Murphy and Corbett 2009). The decision on which path to take for an individual patient using the BCI (i.e., neuroadaptation to enable function or neurorehabilitation to restore function) is a complex matter both practically and ethically. In this regard, significant amounts of research and expert guidance are needed.

9.4.2.3 Neurofeedback in Neurological and Psychological Disorders

Several neurofeedback applications, which have been formally developed within the BCI framework or otherwise, are presently undergoing further research or clinical trials. Most notably, SCP and SMR neurofeedback therapy has been used in epilepsy (Lubar and Bahler 1976; Sterman and Egner 2006; Sterman, Macdonald, and Stone 1974; Strehl et al. 2005). A meta-analysis about the effectiveness of neurofeedback training on seizure control in epilepsy patients by Tan et al. (2009) revealed that out of 10 studies comprising 87 patients altogether, 74% of patients reported fewer seizures per week after neurofeedback training, thus supporting neurofeedback training as a feasible intervention in these patients.

Neurofeedback training can also be given to children with ADHD (Lubar and Lubar 1984; Monastra et al. 2005). A study by Strehl et al. (2005) demonstrated that 23 children diagnosed with ADHD displayed significant improvement in attention and behavior after neurofeedback training. This effect was stable even in the 6-month (Strehl et al. 2007) and 2-year follow-up studies (Arns et al. 2009). A meta-analysis of 15 neurofeedback studies on ADHD (Arns et al. 2009) has shown large effect size for the intervention on impulsivity and inattention. A medium effect size was also observed for hyperactivity.

Concerning neurorehabilitation in chronic pain, the usage of rtfMRI coupled BCIs is a relatively novel strategy (deCharms et al. 2005). In a single-day study, it was shown that healthy participants receiving noxious thermal stimuli and most importantly patients with chronic pain could be trained to control activation of the rostral anterior cingulate cortex brain area using BOLD feedback. Several strategies such as attention toward painful stimuli and perception about nature and intensity of the stimuli were used as a means to control BOLD neurofeedback signals. At the end of the study, all participants experienced corresponding changes in their subjective perception of pain whereas patients rated more than 50% decrease in subjective experience of pain (deCharms et al. 2005). No similar observation was derived from control studies using cognitive or behavioral practice of pain control without rtfMRI feedback, with feedback from a different brain region or with sham feedback from a different subject's rtfMRI response. The neurofeedback intervention was also more than twice as effective as autonomic biofeedback strategies (monitoring

---

* Here we use the term "cure" to describe a restoration of functions through exploitation of the neuroplastic nature of the brain. The term "enabling" refers to help regaining of functions using assistive devices instead.

of skin conductance, heart rate, and respiration) to induce relaxation. Therefore, the subjective rating of the experience of pain after training was specific to the rtfMRI BCI feedback. It would be interesting to see whether the result of this study can be applied to other types of chronic pain such as the phantom limb pain.

Emotion regulation is another area in which BCI can potentially be useful for. Phan et al. (2004) have previously identified the insula and medial frontal cortex as brain regions activated by aversive images during rtfMRI. Through a case study, Weiskopf et al. (2003) reported that a healthy volunteer was able to gain control on a local BOLD response at the anterior cingulate cortex. Following this result, Caria et al. (2007) tested the ability of healthy subjects to control specifically the activity of their right anterior insula using rtfMRI. In this study, participants used affective mental imagery to activate the region of interest and to return it to baseline level and hence control a continuous visual feedback in the form of a "thermometer bar" (Caria et al. 2007). Further investigation showed that subjects who had learnt to increase anterior insula activation rated the valence of fear-evoking images of the International Affective Picture System (IAPS, Lang, Bradley, and Cuthbert 2008) more negatively than did subjects who received noncontingent feedback (unpublished result). Undoubtedly, this is an important finding because emotional dysregulation is a common feature in various psychological disorders including schizophrenia (Williams et al. 2004). Recent findings from two stable schizophrenia patients showed that control of BOLD signal at the right and left insula was possible after 16 training sessions (Ruiz et al. 2008). A subsequent report on these patients stated that there was an increase in the percentage of BOLD signal in comparison to that at the start of the study (Sitaram, Caria, and Birbaumer 2009). From these findings, it can be expected that BCI-coupled neurofeedback research will offer a plethora of possible clinical applications in the future.

9.5 Clinical, Practical, and Ethical Considerations Surrounding BCI

Throughout its development, the BCI encountered a number of challenges and issues. The following section presents the current clinical and practical issues that were often discussed within the BCI community. We also outline past and recent findings in BCI research that can provide solutions for these issues. As a closing commentary, we discuss the ethical concerns with regard to the promotion of communication in locked-in patients and those who are majorly impaired.

9.5.1 Clinical and Practical Issues

Several publications have identified a variety of clinical and practical issues related to current and future use of BCIs (Cincotti et al. 2006; Kübler et al. 2006). As described elsewhere in this chapter, clinical studies involving patients have predominantly been carried out in ALS, SCI, and stroke patients and in ECoG BCI patients receiving treatment for intractable epilepsy. In addition, many BCI studies were carried out with healthy volunteers. However, as a communication channel the BCI should ideally match its users' distinct requirement. The current research still needs to address deeper the differential indication of which patients or which patient group is most suitably assisted by BCIs in the future. For instance, Piccione et al. (2006) suggested that some diseases, for example, such as multiple sclerosis may impact BCI performance more than others; cognitive impairment as found in some ALS patients can also lead to poor BCI performance. At any rate, after approximately two decades of intense research robust findings from BCI research can be used as a guide to formulate the target patient inclusion/exclusion criteria.

The first international meeting of BCI technology outlined the primary objective of the BCI community: to provide an alternative communication technology for paralyzed individuals (Wolpaw et al. 2000). It is, thus, an encouraging finding that many majorly disabled and LIS patients are able to use the BCI at the criterion level, that is, equal or above 70% accuracy, for effective communication (Kübler and Birbaumer 2008; Silvoni et al. 2009). On the other hand, results of BCI trials in completely locked-in patients have largely been negative (Kübler and Birbaumer 2008). Arguably, these are the patients with the highest need for communication among the patient groups. Indeed, residual motor functions such as eye blink that could serve as a means of communication in LIS no longer exist in completely locked-in patients. The primary cause of the negative results of the BCI trial in these patients is the absence of classifiable neural signal. It has been suggested that neural signal deterioration is related to the extinction of goal-directed thinking due to loss of contingency between intention and consequences (Kübler and Birbaumer 2008; Kübler, Nijboer, and Birbaumer 2007). Detected awareness in completely locked-in patients in vegetative state (Owen et al. 2006) posits a new challenge to this hypothesis. Willful modulation of BOLD response in patients who diagnosed with the vegetative state or minimally conscious state (Monti et al. 2010), although few, suggests that the deteriorating link between intention and consequence cannot be the sole explanation for the loss of classifiable neural signal in the completely locked-in state. Further, BCI research with completely locked-in patients is necessary before concrete conclusions can be drawn.

It is generally acknowledged that a BCI should be ready to wear and easy to handle (Kaufmann et al. 2012) by caregivers or significant others caring for the patient (Kübler et al. 2006). A survey conducted in Germany, Austria, and Italy among 77 users of assistive technology who were severely impaired with neurological/neuromuscular diseases (47%), SCI (37%), and cerebrovascular disorders (16%), identified functionality, possibility of independent use, and ease of use as most important for BCI use in daily life (Zickler et al. 2009). Naturally, the diversity of the user group to which a BCI has to be adapted constitutes a challenge for BCI. For instance, involuntary muscle spasm in a patient could disturb electrode placement as reported in one study (Kübler, Kotchoubey et al. 2001). Such issues may lead to alteration in the design of the BCI itself and the application of more conservative methods of muscle artifact removal. BCI training often depends on the presence of experts such as BCI research scientists or engineers in the patients' home, though the presence of BCI experts in the patients' proximity may cause discomfort and intrusion of privacy. Furthermore, the current cumbersome treatment of electrode cap, gel, and lengthy training may deter potential users from using the BCI (Nijboer, Sellers et al. 2008). Despite these downsides, exemplary patients have used a BCI for communication and interaction at home without the presence of experts from the supervising BCI laboratory (Neumann et al. 2003; Vaughan et al. 2006). With regard to the "ease of use" and "functionality," invasive ECoG BCI may present a further solution because of its high signal-to-noise ratio, permanent electrode placement, and resistance to muscle artifacts (Huggins et al. 2007). However, invasive BCIs may need closer and costlier experts' supervision in practice and surgery that may reduce its acceptance by the patients.

Several technological developments can potentially remedy some of the practical issues mentioned above. Firstly, it has been shown that a BCI telemonitoring system supported by an Internet connection can be used effectively by a patient for research purposes (Müller, Neuper, and Pfurtscheller 2003). Telemonitoring systems can easily bridge a connection between users and experts in instances where long geographical distance may present logistic difficulty. This in turn will ensure the availability of support and care for patients at wider clinical catchment areas while simultaneously maintaining the patients' much-needed privacy. Secondly, the currently developed dry EEG electrode and wireless system presents an attractive prospect for a BCI prototype. The dry electrodes offer vast improvement in the BCI application in patients and eliminate the need for constant cleaning of the electrode gel from the hair at the end of BCI use. Studies have shown that minimum application of six dry electrodes has an information transfer rate comparable to that of other mainstream BCI. A high correlation of SMR recording using dry electrodes to customary EEG has also been reported (Gargiulo et al. 2008; Popescu et al. 2007). A wireless BCI system enhances the cosmetic appearance of invasive BCI and the users' safety by reducing health risks related to transcutaneous implants. This system also supports general minimization of the BCI that can be battery-powered and easily attached to the patient's bed or wheelchair (Edlinger and Guger 2005). It must also be noted that the NIRS BCI is one of the forward solutions for wearability issues in BCI. More research on the reliability of the NIRS BCI in patient population is thus necessary. Thirdly, an independent initiation of BCI can enhance the quality of life of patients who are otherwise completely dependent on caregivers and significant others. A study of the self-initiation of BCI by brisk inspiration-triggered changes of heart rate showed high prediction rate in most healthy volunteers (Scherer, Müller-Putz, and Pfurtscheller 2007). Although this method requires relatively less training than another known method of BCI self-initiation (Kaiser et al. 2001), its application for patients with artificial ventilation is limited. Self-initiation controlled by brain activity, as demonstrated with SCP, overcomes the need of muscular activity even if it requires more operationalization time. Last but not least, the hybrid BCI (Brunner et al. 2010) can potentially be useful in providing better control and switching of BCI input signals, which protects users against fatigue, boredom, and probable signal detection failure.

9.5.2 Ethical Considerations

Is it ethically justified to use the BCI to facilitate communication with LIS patients? We answer this question with a resounding "YES." Phillips (2006) argued that reasonable quality of life in LIS is a prior requirement to BCI implementation. In fact, plenty of evidence shows that LIS patients do have a meaningful life (see Figure 9.6). Numerous studies have confirmed low levels of major depression and functional coping strategy in ALS patients (Houpt, Gould, and Norris 1977; Lulé et al. 2008; Rabkin et al. 2005). LIS patients, in general, have intact linguistic and cognitive faculties and retain the capacity to enjoy social life by going out and meeting friends (Laureys et al. 2005). Unsurprisingly, the presence of communication has been reported as a determinant for well-being in these patients (Bach 1993; Lulé et al. 2008), which raises the significance of BCI's contribution in facilitating patients' interaction with their immediate surroundings and the larger social community, for example, through the Internet and e-mails (Mugler et al. 2008; Mugler et al. 2010). By facilitating communication, the BCI can also assist the therapy process in LIS patients diagnosed with depression. Therefore, though the capacity for well-being must be taken as an ethical justification for BCI use, evidence of the opposite (e.g., the presence of depression) should not be taken hastily as a reason to reject BCI use in LIS patients.

Notwithstanding the offers of modern technology manifesting through the BCI, we have to take into account its possible contribution to an unrealistic expectation of cure

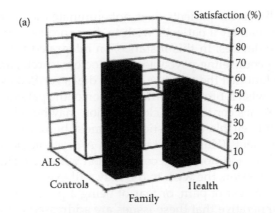

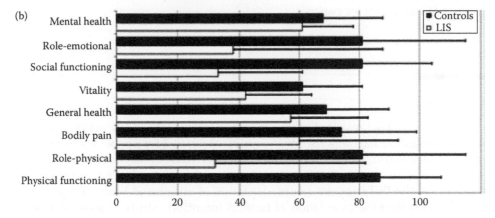

FIGURE 9.6
Quality of life and patients with locked-in syndrome. (a) Patients with amyotrophic lateral scelrosis rated more life satisfaction with regard to their family than controls. Understandably the satisfaction rating of their health condition is lower than that of controls. (b) General health status subjective rating (Short Form-36) of 17 patients in chronic locked-in state owing to brainstem lesion. (From Lulé, D. et al. 2009. *Progress in Brain Research* 177: 339–51.)

that is influential in a LIS patient's life decision. Undue optimism and the expectation of imminent cure are known to predict ALS patients' commitment to elective long-term mechanical ventilation that prolongs their life expectancy (Rabkin et al. 2006). The unwarranted hope in gaining benefit from scientific development places patients in the position of "special vulnerability" for consenting to BCI clinical trials (Clausen 2008). In this context, researchers and clinicians share the responsibility of taking the necessary precautions to prevent any misunderstanding in patients caused by their own personal expectation or by the over-enthused media portrayal of BCI. This responsibility entails an extensive researcher–patient dialogue prior to taking informed consent in clinical trials and a responsible engagement of public interest in the field of BCI (Haselager et al. 2009). The BCI community is aware of these circumstances and an ethically sound protocol for initiating BCI training in patients was written in 2003 (Neumann and Kübler 2003; IEEE special issue on BCI). The awareness of ethical issues in the BCI community is also reflected by the inclusion of an Ethics group in the current large-scale integrating project TOBI funded by the European Union (www.tobi-project.org).

Evidence of good quality of life in LIS patients does not eliminate the most challenging ethical issue in BCI application, namely a patient's wish to die expressed through competent use of BCI communication devices. In this instance, an integrated psychosocial and medical intervention involving counseling psychologists, doctors, carers, and significant others is a necessity. It is important that the patient's wish to die is verified over the course of several sessions and that this wish is brought to the attention of the patients' doctors and significant others (with the patient's consent). Suicide ideation may be related to depression in patients; thus, valid and reliable diagnostic tools must be used to estimate the degree of depression in these patients (Hammer et al. 2008). A psychological intervention for major depressive disorder and, additionally, a consultation with a psychiatrist will be necessary. In the absence of depression, the wish to die may still exist in patients because of anticipated poor quality of life, fear of pain, or fear of being a psychosocial burden on others (Kurt et al. 2007). It is imperative that these issues are addressed exhaustively as a part of the palliative care for patients.

9.6 Conclusion

To summarize, we have presented in this chapter current state-of-the-art BCIs and various cutting-edge research that demonstrate the utility of the BCI for people with motor impairment. BCIs play a significant role in establishing alternative means of environmental control, most notably in the form of a communication device for locked-in patients. As an assistive device, the BCI supports neuroadaptation of an injured brain and provides new channels for enabling the translation of human intention into functions. This has been facilitated by the extraction of a variety of neural signals such as SCP, SMR, and evoked potential from the EEG signal. In addition, BCIs can potentially play a larger role for guiding neuroadaptation processes in stroke and SCI patients toward functional recovery. This unprecedented role of BCIs was made possible by the advent of modern brain imaging technology such as NIRS, MEG, and rtfMRI that allow control of neural activation locally. We acknowledge that, presently, several issues must be addressed in the practical and clinical aspects of the BCI. Specifically, with regard to the projected role of the BCI as a rehabilitation tool to augment plasticity, some questions on the role of BCI in relation to the current treatment of choice, specifications of target patients, and the optimum paradigm for efficacy investigations of this BCI-assisted neurorehabilitation strategy call for significant clarification. However, the few studies conducted in this field have shown promising results, which in themselves are incentives toward more extensive research in the future. We have also presented other practical and clinical issues often discussed in past publications and, by reviewing possible solutions that are currently still being developed, it is hoped that these issues will soon be a problem of the past. Last but not least, there have been ethical concerns surrounding the applications and the development of the BCI for individuals with LIS. In the last section, we attempted to clarify these issues; specifically, we submitted evidence of the continuously meaningful life in LIS patients and the BCI community's commitment to provide choices and an even better quality of life for these individuals. Within the last two decades, the field of BCI has flourished and we sincerely believe that it is still capable of making more contributions.

Acknowledgments

This work is supported by the European ICT Programme Project FP7-224631 (TOBI). S. C. K. and S. L. contributed equally to the manuscript. This chapter only reflects the authors' views and funding agencies are not liable for any use that may be made of the information contained herein. We also thank Sebastian Halder, Carolin Ruf, and Claudia Zickler for their contributions to the manuscript.

References

Alkadhi, H., P. Brugger, S. H. Boendermaker, G. Crelier, A. Curt, M. C. Hepp-Reymond, and S. S. Kollias. 2005. What disconnection tells about motor imagery: Evidence from paraplegic patients. *Cerebral Cortex* 15 (2): 131–40.

Allison, B. Z., C. Brunner, V. Kaiser, G. R. Müller-Putz, C. Neuper, and G. Pfurtscheller. 2010. Toward a hybrid brain-computer interface based on imagined movement and visual attention. *Journal of Neural Engineering* 7 (2): 026007. doi:10.1088/1741-2560/7/2/026007.

American Psychiatric Association. 2000. *Diagnostic and Statistical Manual of Mental Disorders (DSM-IV-TR)*. Washington, DC: American Psychiatric Association.

Arns, M., S. de Ridder, U. Strehl, M. Breteler, and A. Coenen. 2009. Efficacy of neurofeedback treatment in ADHD: The effects on inattention, impulsivity and hyperactivity—A meta-analysis. *Clinical EEG & Neuroscience* 40 (3): 180–9.

Babiloni, F., F. Cincotti, M. Marciani, S. Salinari, L. Astolfi, A. Tocci, F. Aloise, F. De Vico Fallani, S. Bufalari, and D. Mattia. 2007. The estimation of cortical activity for brain-computer interface: Applications in a domotic context. *Computational Intelligence and Neuroscience* 2007: 91651. doi:10.1155/2007/91651.

Bach, J. R. 1993. Amyotrophic lateral sclerosis. Communication status and survival with ventilatory support. *American Journal of Physical Medicine and Rehabilitation* 72 (6): 343–9.

Bagarinao, E., T. Nakai, and Y. Tanaka. 2006. Real-time functional MRI: Development and emerging applications. *Magnetic Resonance in Medical Sciences* 5 (3): 157–65.

Bamford, J. 1992. Clinical examination in diagnosis and subclassification of stroke. *Lancet* 339 (8790): 400–2.

Bartels, J., D. Andreasen, P. Ehirim, H. Mao, S. Seibert, E. J. Wright, and P. Kennedy. 2008. Neurotrophic electrode: Method of assembly and implantation into human motor speech cortex. *Journal of Neuroscience Methods* 174 (2): 168–76.

Battapady, H., P. Lin, T. Holroyd, M. Hallett, X. Chen, D. Y. Fei, and O. Bai. 2009. Spatial detection of multiple movement intentions from SAM-filtered single-trial MEG signals. *Clinical Neurophysiology* 120 (11): 1978–87.

Bauer, G., F. Gerstenbrand, and E. Rumpl. 1979. Varieties of the locked-in syndrome. *Journal of Neurology* 221 (2): 77–91.

Bensch, M., A. A. Karim, J. Mellinger, T. Hinterberger, M. Tangermann, M. Bogdan, W. Rosenstiel, and N. Birbaumer. 2007. Nessi: An EEG-controlled web browser for severely paralyzed patients. *Computational Intelligence and Neuroscience* 2007: 71863. doi:10.1155/2007/71863.

Birbaumer, N. and L. G. Cohen. 2007. Brain-computer interfaces: Communication and restoration of movement in paralysis. *Journal of Physiology* 579 (Pt 3): 621–36.

Birbaumer, N., N. Ghanayim, T. Hinterberger, I. Iversen, B. Kotchoubey, A. Kübler, J. Perelmouter, E. Taub, and H. Flor. 1999. A spelling device for the paralysed. *Nature* 398 (6725): 297–8.

Blankertz, B., F. Losch, M. Krauledat, G. Dornhege, G. Curio, and K. R. Müller. 2008. The Berlin brain-computer interface: Accurate performance from first-session in BCI-naive subjects. *IEEE Transactions on Biomedical Engineering* 55 (10): 2452–62.

Blankertz, B., C. Sannelli, S. Halder, E. M. Hammer, A. Kübler, K. R. Müller, G. Curio, and T. Dickhaus. 2010. Neurophysiological predictor of SMR-based BCI performance. *NeuroImage* 51 (4): 1303–9.

Bononati, A., P. Cicinelli, F. Pichiorri, F. Cincotti, F. Babiloni, and D. Mattia. 2010. Motor imagery-based brain computer interface: Contribution of TMS to the understanding of training-induced effects on motor cortical excitability. Paper presented at the *TOBI—Tools for Brain-Computer Interaction Workshop 2010: Integrating Brain–Computer Interfaces with Conventional Assistive Technology*, Graz, Austria, February 3–4, 2010.

Braun, S. M., A. J. Beurskens, P. J. Borm, T. Schack, and D. T. Wade. 2006. The effects of mental practice in stroke rehabilitation: A systematic review. *Archives of Physical Medicine and Rehabilitation* 87 (6): 842–52.

Brouwer, A.-M. and J. B. F. van Erp. 2010. A tactile P300 brain-computer interface. *Frontiers in Neuroprosthetics* 4: 19. doi:10.3389/fnins.2010.00019.

Brunner, C., B. Z. Allison, D. J. Krusienski, V. Kaiser, G. R. Müller-Putz, G. Pfurtscheller, and C. Neuper. 2010. Improved signal processing approaches in an offline simulation of a hybrid brain-computer interface. *Journal of Neuroscience Methods* 188 (1): 165–73.

Brunner, P., A. L. Ritaccio, J. F. Emrich, H. Bischof, and G. Schalk. 2011. Rapid communication with a "P300" matrix speller using electrocorticographic signals (ECoG). *Frontiers in Neuroscience* 5: 5. doi: 10.3389/fnins.2011.00005.

Buch, E., C. Weber, L. G. Cohen, C. Braun, M. A. Dimyan, T. Ard, J. Mellinger et al. 2008. Think to move: A neuromagnetic brain-computer interface (BCI) system for chronic stroke. *Stroke* 39 (3): 910–7.

Caria, A., R. Veit, R. Sitaram, M. Lotze, N. Weiskopf, W. Grodd, and N. Birbaumer. 2007. Regulation of anterior insular cortex activity using real-time fMRI. *NeuroImage* 35 (3): 1238–46.

Carmena, J. M., M. A. Lebedev, R. E. Crist, J. E. O'Doherty, D. M. Santucci, D. F. Dimitrov, P. G. Patil, C. S. Henriquez, and M. A. L. Nicolelis. 2003. Learning to control a brain-machine interface for reaching and grasping by primates. *PLoS Biology* 1 (2): e42. doi:10.1371/journal.pbio.0000042.

Chaves, E. S., M. L. Boninger, R. Cooper, S. G. Fitzgerald, D. B. Gray, and R. A. Cooper. 2004. Assessing the influence of wheelchair technology on perception of participation in spinal cord injury. *Archives of Physical Medicine and Rehabilitation* 85 (11): 1854–8.

Cincotti, F., L. Bianchi, G. Birch, C. Guger, J. Mellinger, R. Scherer, R. N. Schmidt, O. Y. Suarez, and G. Schalk. 2006. BCI meeting 2005—workshop on technology: Hardware and software. *IEEE Transactions on Neural Systems and Rehabilitation Engineering* 14 (2): 128–31.

Cincotti, F., L. Kauhanen, F. Aloise, T. Palomaki, N. Caporusso, P. Jylänki, D. Mattia et al. 2007. Vibrotactile feedback for brain-computer interface operation. *Computational Intelligence and Neuroscience* 2007: 48937. doi:10.1155/2007/48937.

Cincotti, F., D. Mattia, F. Aloise, S. Bufalari, G. Schalk, G. Oriolo, A. Cherubini, M. G. Marciani, and F. Babiloni. 2008. Non-invasive brain-computer interface system: Towards its application as assistive technology. *Brain Research Bulletin* 75 (6): 796–803.

Clausen, J. 2008. Moving minds: Ethical aspects of neural motor prostheses. *Biotechnology Journal* 3 (12): 1493–501.

Conson, M., M. Sara, F. Pistoia, and L. Trojano. 2009. Action observation improves motor imagery: Specific interactions between simulative processes. *Experimental Brain Research* 199 (1): 71–81.

Cramer, S. C., L. Lastra, M. G. Lacourse, and M. J. Cohen. 2005. Brain motor system function after chronic, complete spinal cord injury. *Brain* 128 (Pt 12): 2941–50.

Cramer, S. C., E. L. Orr, M. J. Cohen, and M. G. Lacourse. 2007. Effects of motor imagery training after chronic, complete spinal cord injury. *Experimental Brain Research* 177 (2): 233–42.

Daly, J. J., R. Cheng, J. Rogers, K. Litinas, K. Hrovat, and M. Dohring. 2009. Feasibility of a new application of noninvasive Brain Computer Interface (BCI): A case study of training for recovery of volitional motor control after stroke. *Journal of Neurologic Physical Therapy* 33 (4): 203–11.

Daly, J. J. and J. R. Wolpaw. 2008. Brain-computer interfaces in neurological rehabilitation. *Lancet Neurology* 7 (11): 1032–43.

deCharms, R. C., F. Maeda, G. H. Glover, D. Ludlow, J. M. Pauly, D. Soneji, J. D. E. Gabrieli, and S. C. Mackey. 2005. Control over brain activation and pain learned by using real-time functional MRI. *Proceedings of the National Academy of Sciences of the United States of America* 102 (51): 18626–31.

DeVivo, M., F. Biering-Sorensen, S. Charlifue, V. Noonan, M. Post, T. Stripling, and P. Wing. 2006. International spinal cord injury core data set. *Spinal Cord* 44 (9): 535–40.

Dobkin, B. H. 2003. Functional MRI: A potential physiologic indicator for stroke rehabilitation interventions. *Stroke* 34 (5): e23–8.

Dobkin, B. H. 2007. Brain-computer interface technology as a tool to augment plasticity and outcomes for neurological rehabilitation. *Journal of Physiology* 579 (Pt 3): 637–42.

Donchin, E. 1981. Presidential address, 1980. Surprise! . . . Surprise? *Psychophysiology* 18 (5): 493–513.

Donchin, E., K. M. Spencer, and R. Wijesinghe. 2000. The mental prosthesis: Assessing the speed of a P300-based brain-computer interface. *IEEE Transactions on Rehabilitation Engineering* 8 (2), 174–9.

Donoghue, J. P., A. Nurmikko, M. Black, and L. R. Hochberg. 2007. Assistive technology and robotic control using motor cortex ensemble-based neural interface systems in humans with tetraplegia. *Journal of Physiology* 579 (Pt 3): 603–11.

Edlinger, G. and C. Guger. 2005. Laboratory PC and mobile pocket PC brain-computer interface architectures. *Conference Proceedings IEEE Engineering in Medicine and Biology Society* 5, 5347–50.

Elbert, T. and B. Rockstroh. 2004. Reorganization of human cerebral cortex: The range of changes following use and injury. *Neuroscientist* 10 (2): 129–41.

Enzinger, C., S. Ropele, F. Fazekas, M. Loitfelder, F. Gorani, T. Seifert, G. Reiter, C. Neuper, G. Pfurtscheller, and G. Müller-Putz. 2008. Brain motor system function in a patient with complete spinal cord injury following extensive brain-computer interface training. *Experimental Brain Research* 190 (2): 215–23.

Farwell, L. A. and E. Donchin. 1988. Talking off the top of your head: Toward a mental prosthesis utilizing event-related brain potentials. *Electroencephalography and Clinical Neurophysiology* 70 (6): 510–23.

Felton, E. A., J. A. Wilson, J. C. Williams, and P. C. Garell. 2007. Electrocorticographically controlled brain-computer interfaces using motor and sensory imagery in patients with temporary subdural electrode implants. Report of four cases. *Journal of Neurosurgery* 106 (3): 495–500.

Finke, A., A. Lenhardt, and H. Ritter. 2009. The MindGame: A P300-based brain-computer interface game. *Neural Networks* 22 (9): 1329–33.

Furdea, A., S. Halder, D. J. Krusienski, D. Bross, F. Nijboer, N. Birbaumer, and A. Kübler. 2009. An auditory oddball (P300) spelling system for brain-computer interfaces. *Psychophysiology*, 46 (3): 617–25.

Galán, F., M. Nuttin, E. Lew, P. W. Ferrez, G. Vanacker, J. Philips, and J. d. R. Millán. 2008. A brain-actuated wheelchair: Asynchronous and non-invasive brain-computer interfaces for continuous control of robots. *Clinical Neurophysiology* 119 (9): 2159–69.

Ganguly, K. and J. M. Carmena. 2009. Emergence of a stable cortical map for neuroprosthetic control. *PLoS Biology* 7 (7): e1000153. doi:10.1371/journal.pbio.1000153.

Gargiulo, G., P. Bifulco, R. A. Calvo, M. Cesarelli, and C. v. S. A. Jin. 2008. A mobile EEG system with dry electrodes. Paper presented at the *IEEE Biomedical Circuits and Systems Conference: Intelligent Biomedical Systems* (BioCAS), Baltimore, MD, November 20–22, 2008.

Gentry, T. 2009. Smart homes for people with neurological disability: State of the art. *NeuroRehabilitation* 25 (3): 209–217.

Graimann, B., J. E. Huggins, S. P. Levine, and G. Pfurtscheller. 2002. Visualization of significant ERD/ERS patterns in multichannel EEG and ECoG data. *Clinical Neurophysiology* 113 (1): 43–7.

Guger, C., S. Daban, E. Sellers, C. Holzner, G. Krausz, R. Carabalona, F. Gramatica, and G. Edlinger. 2009. How many people are able to control a P300-based brain-computer interface (BCI)? *Neuroscience Letters* 462 (1): 94–8.

Guger, C., G. Edlinger, W. Harkam, I. Niedermayer, and G. Pfurtscheller. 2003. How many people are able to operate an EEG-based brain-computer interface (BCI)? *IEEE Transactions on Neural Systems and Rehabilitation Engineering* 11 (2): 145–7.

Halder, S., M. Rea, R. Andreoni, F. Nijboer, E. M. Hammer, S. C. Kleih, N. Birbaumer, and A. Kübler. 2010. An auditory oddball brain-computer interface for binary choices. *Clinical Neurophysiology* 121 (4): 516–23.

Hämäläinen, M., R. Hari, R. Ilmoniemi, J. Knuutila, and O. V. Lounasmaa. 1993. Magnetoencephalography: Theory, instrumentation, and applications to noninvasive studies of the working human brain. *Reviews of Modern Physics* 65 (2): 413–97.

Hammer, E. M., S. Häcker, M. Hautzinger, T. D. Meyer, and Kübler. 2008. Validity of the ALS-Depression-Inventory (ADI-12)—A new screening instrument for depressive disorders in patients with amyotrophic lateral sclerosis. *Journal of Affective Disorders* 109 (1–2): 213–9.

Haselager, P., R. Vlek, J. Hill, and F. Nijboer. 2009. A note on ethical aspects of BCI. *Neural Networks* 22 (9): 1352–7.

Hill, N. J. T. N. Lal, M. Schroder, T. Hinterberger, B. Wilhelm, F. Nijboer, U. Mochty et al. 2006. Classifying EEG and ECoG signals without subject training for fast BCI implementation: Comparison of nonparalyzed and completely paralyzed subjects. *IEEE Transactions on Neural Systems and Rehabilitation Engineering* 14 (2): 183–6.

Hill, N. J. and B. Schölkopf. 2012. An online brain-computer interface based on shifting attention to concurrent streams of auditory stimuli. *Journal of Neural Engineering* 9 (2): 026011.

Hinterberger, T., G. Widman, T. N. Lal, J. Hill, M. Tangermann, W. Rosenstiel, B. Schölkopf, C. Elger, and N. Birbaumer. 2008. Voluntary brain regulation and communication with electrocortico-gram signals. *Epilepsy & Behavior* 13 (2): 300–6.

Hinterberger, T., B. Wilhelm, J. Mellinger, B. Kotchoubey, and N. Birbaumer. 2005. A device for the detection of cognitive brain functions in completely paralyzed or unresponsive patients. *IEEE Transactions on Biomedical Engineering* 52 (2): 211–20.

Hochberg, L. R., M. D. Serruya, G. M. Friehs, J. A. Mukand, M. Saleh, A. H. Caplan, A. Branner, D. Chen, R. D. Penn, and J. P. Donoghue. 2006. Neuronal ensemble control of prosthetic devices by a human with tetraplegia. *Nature* 442 (7099): 164–71.

Hoffmann, M., R. Sacco, J. P. Mohr, and T. K. Tatemichi. 1997. Higher cortical function deficits among acute stroke patients: The stroke data bank experience. *Journal of Stroke and Cerebrovascular Diseases* 6 (3): 114–20.

Hoffmann, U., J. M. Vesin, T. Ebrahimi, and K. Diserens. 2008. An efficient P300-based brain-computer interface for disabled subjects. *Journal of Neuroscience Methods* 167 (1): 115–25.

Höhne, J., M. Schreuder, B. Blankertz, and M. Tangermann. 2011. A novel 9-class auditory ERP paradigm driving a predictive text entry system. *Frontiers in Neuroscience* 5: 99.

Hong, B., B. Lou, J. Guo, and S. Gao. 2009. Adaptive active auditory brain computer interface. *Conference Proceedings IEEE Engineering in Medicine and Biology Society* 2009: 4531–4.

Houpt, J. L., B. S. Gould, and F. H. Norris. 1977. Psychological characteristics of patients with amyotrophic lateral sclerosis (ALS). *Psychosomatic Medicine* 39 (5): 299–303.

Huggins, J., S. P. Levine, B. Graimann, S. Y. Chun, and J. A. Fessler. 2007. Electrocorticogram as a brain-computer interface signal source. In *Toward Brain-Computer Interfacing*, edited by G. Dornhege, J. d. R. Millán, T. Hinterberger, D. J. McFarland, and K. R. Müller, 129–46. Cambridge, MA: The MIT Press.

Ioannides, A. A. 2006. Magnetoencephalography as a research tool in neuroscience: State of the art. *Neuroscientist* 12 (6) : 524–44.

Iturrate, I., J. M. Antelis, A. Kübler, and J. Minguez. 2009. A noninvasive brain-actuated wheelchair based on a P300 neurophysiological protocol and automated navigation. *IEEE Transactions on Robotics* 25 (3): 614–27.

Jarosiewicz, B., S. M. Chase, G. W. Fraser, M. Velliste, R. E. Kass, and A. B. Schwartz. 2008. Functional network reorganization during learning in a brain-computer interface paradigm. *Proceedings of the National Academy of Sciences of the United States of America* 105 (49): 19486–91.

Jeannerod, M. 1995. Mental imagery in the motor context. *Neuropsychologia* 33 (11): 1419–32.

Kaiser, J., J. Perelmouter, I. H. Iversen, N. Neumann, N. Ghanayim, T. Hinterberger, A. Kübler, B. Kotchoubey, and N. Birbaumer. 2001. Self-initiation of EEG-based communication in paralyzed patients. *Clinical Neurophysiology* 112 (3): 551–4.

Karim, A. A., T. Hinterberger, J. Richter, J. Mellinger, N. Neumann, H. Flor, A. Kübler, and N. Birbaumer. 2006. Neural Internet: Web surfing with brain potentials for the completely paralyzed. *Neurorehabilitation and Neural Repair* 20 (4): 508–15.

Katz, R. T., A. J. Haig, B. B. Clark, and R. J. DiPaola. 1992. Long-term survival, prognosis, and life-care planning for 29 patients with chronic locked-in syndrome. *Archives of Physical Medicine and Rehabilitation* 73 (5): 403–8.

Kaufmann, T., S. Völker, L. Gunesch, and A. Kübler. 2012. Spelling is just a click away—a user-centered brain-computer interface including auto-calibration and predictive text entry. *Frontiers in Neuroscience* 6: 72.

Keith, M. W., P. H. Peckham, G. B. Thrope, K. C. Stroh, B. Smith, J. R. Buckett, K. L. Kilgore, and J. W. Jatich. 1989. Implantable functional neuromuscular stimulation in the tetraplegic hand. *Journal of Hand Surgery* 14 (3): 524–30.

Kennedy, P. R. and R. A. Bakay. 1998. Restoration of neural output from a paralyzed patient by a direct brain connection. *NeuroReport* 9 (8): 1707–11.

Kennedy, P. R., R. A. Bakay, M. M. Moore, K. Adams, and J. Goldwaithe. 2000. Direct control of a computer from the human central nervous system. *IEEE Transactions on Rehabilitation Engineering* 8 (2): 198–202.

Kennedy, P. R., M. T. Kirby, M. M. Moore, B. King, and A. Mallory. 2004. Computer control using human intracortical local field potentials. *IEEE Transactions on Neural Systems and Rehabilitation Engineering* 12 (3): 339–44.

Kleih, S. C., F. Nijboer, S. Halder, and A. Kübler. 2010. Motivation modulates the P300 amplitude during brain-computer interface use. *Clinical Neurophysiology* 121 (7): 1023–31.

Kleih, S. C., T. Kaufmann, C. Zickler, S. Halder, F. Leotta, F. Cincotti, F. Aloise et al. 2011. Out of the frying pan into the fire—the P300-based BCI faces real-world challenges. *Progress in Brain Research* 194: 27–46. Review.

Krauledat, M., M. Tangermann, B. Blankertz, and K. R. Muller. 2008. Towards zero training for brain-computer interfacing. *PLoS One* 3 (8): e2967. doi:10.1371/journal.pone.0002967.

Krusienski, D. J., D. Cox, and J. Shih. 2010. Control of a robotic manipulator using EEG and ECoG signals. Paper presented at the *TOBI: Tools for Brain-Computer Interaction Workshop 2010: Integrating Brain–Computer Interfaces with Conventional Assistive Technology*, Graz, Austria, February 3–4, 2010.

Krusienski, D. J., E. W. Sellers, D. J. McFarland, T. M. Vaughan, and J. R. Wolpaw. 2008. Toward enhanced P300 speller performance. *Journal of Neuroscience Methods* 167 (1): 15–21.

Kübler, A. and N. Birbaumer. 2008. Brain-computer interfaces and communication in paralysis: Extinction of goal directed thinking in completely paralysed patients? *Clinical Neurophysiology* 119 (11): 2658–66.

Kübler, A., A. Furdea, S. Halder, E. M. Hammer, F. Nijboer, and B. Kotchoubey. 2009. A brain-computer interface controlled auditory event-related potential (p300) spelling system for locked-in patients. *Annals of the New York Academy of Sciences* 1157:90–100.

Kübler, A., Halder, S., Furdea, A., and Hösle, A. 2008. Brain painting—BCI meets art. Paper presented at the *4th International Brain-Computer Interface Workshop and Training Course*, Graz University of Technology, Austria.

Kübler, A., B. Kotchoubey, J. Kaiser, J. R. Wolpaw, and N. Birbaumer. 2001. Brain-computer communication: Unlocking the locked in. *Psychological Bulletin* 127 (3): 358–75.

Kübler, A., V. K. Mushahwar, L. R. Hochberg, and J. P. Donoghue. 2006. BCI meeting 2005—workshop on clinical issues and applications. *IEEE Transactions on Neural Systems and Rehabilitation Engineering* 14 (2): 131–4.

Kübler, A., N. Neumann, J. Kaiser, B. Kotchoubey, T. Hinterberger, and N. Birbaumer. 2001. Brain-computer communication: Self-regulation of slow cortical potentials for verbal communication. *Archives of Physical Medicine and Rehabilitation* 82 (11): 1533–9.

Kübler, A., N. Neumann, B. Wilhelm, T. Hinterberger, and N. Birbaumer. 2004. Brain-computer predictability of brain-computer communication. *Journal of Psychophysiology* 18 (2–3): 121–9.

Kübler, A., F. Nijboer, and N. Birbaumer. 2007. Brain-computer interfaces for communication and motor control - Perspectives on clinical applications. In *Toward Brain-Computer Interfacing*, edited by G. Dornhege, J. d. R. Millán, T. Hinterberger, D. J. McFarland, and K. R. Müller, 373–91. Cambridge, MA: The MIT Press.

Kübler, A., F. Nijboer, J. Mellinger, T. M. Vaughan, H. Pawelzik, G. Schalk, D. J. McFarland, N. Birbaumer, and J. R. Wolpaw. 2005. Patients with ALS can use sensorimotor rhythms to operate a brain-computer interface. *Neurology* 64 (10): 1775–7.

Kurt, A., F. Nijboer, Matuz, and A. Kübler. 2007. Depression and anxiety in individuals with amyotrophic lateral sclerosis: Epidemiology and management. *CNS Drugs* 21 (4): 279–91.

Lai, S. M., S. Studenski, P. W. Duncan, and S. Perera. 2002. Persisting consequences of stroke measured by the Stroke Impact Scale. *Stroke* 33 (7): 1840–4.

Lang, P. J., M. M. Bradley, and B. N. Cuthbert. 2008. International affective picture system (IAPS): Affective ratings of pictures and instruction manual. *Technical Report A-8*, University of Florida, Gainesville, FL.

Laureys, S., F. Pellas, P. Van Eeckhout, S. Ghorbel, C. Schnakers, F. Perrin, J. Berré et al. 2005. The locked-in syndrome : What is it like to be conscious but paralyzed and voiceless? *Progress in Brain Research* 150: 495–511.

Lebedev, M. A., J. M. Carmena, J. E. O'Doherty, M. Zacksenhouse, C. S. Henriquez, J. C. Principe, and M. A. L. Nicolelis. 2005. Cortical ensemble adaptation to represent velocity of an artificial actuator controlled by a brain-machine interface. *Journal of Neuroscience* 25 (19): 4681–93.

Leeb, R., D. Friedman, G. R. Müller-Putz, R. Scherer, M. Slater, and G. Pfurtscheller. 2007. Self-paced (asynchronous) BCI control of a wheelchair in virtual environments: A case study with a tetraplegic. *Computational Intelligence and Neuroscience* 2007: 79642. doi:10.1155/2007/79642.

Leeb, R., H. Sagha, R. Chavarriaga, and J. del R. Millan. 2010. Multimodal fusion of muscle and brain signals for a hybrid-BCI. *Engineering in Medicine and Biology Society (EMBC), 2010 Annual International Conference of the IEEE Center for Neuroprosthetics*, Ecole Polytech. Fed. de Lausanne, Lausanne, Switzerland.

Leon-Carrion, J., P. van Eeckhout, R. Dominguez-Morales Mdel, and F. J. Perez-Santamaria. 2002. The locked-in syndrome: A syndrome looking for a therapy. *Brain Injury* 16 (7): 571–82.

Leuthardt, E. C., K. J. Miller, G. Schalk, R. P. Rao, and J. G. Ojemann. 2006. Electrocorticography-based brain computer interface—The Seattle experience. *IEEE Transactions on Neural Systems and Rehabilitation Engineering* 14 (2): 194–8.

Leuthardt, E. C., G. Schalk, J. Roland, A. Rouse, and D. W. Moran. 2009. Evolution of brain-computer interfaces: Going beyond classic motor physiology. *Neurosurgical Focus* 27 (1): e4. doi:10.3171/2009.4.FOCUS0979.

Leuthardt, E. C., G. Schalk, J. R. Wolpaw, J. G. Ojemann, and D. W. Moran. 2004. A brain-computer interface using electrocorticographic signals in humans. *Journal of Neural Engineering* 1 (2): 63–71.

Lotte, F., M. Congedo, A. Lecuyer, F. Lamarche, and B. Arnaldi. 2007. A review of classification algorithms for EEG-based brain-computer interfaces. *Journal of Neural Engineering* 4 (2): R1–13.

Lubar, J. F. 1998. Electroencephalographic biofeedback methodology and the management of epilepsy. *Integrative Physiological and Behavioral Science* 33 (2): 176–207.

Lubar, J. F. and W. W. Bahler. 1976. Behavioral management of epileptic seizures following EEG biofeedback training of the sensorimotor rhythm. *Biofeedback and Self Regulation* 1 (1): 77–104.

Lubar, J. O. and Lubar, J. F. 1984. Electroencephalographic biofeedback of SMR and beta for treatment of attention deficit disorders in a clinical setting. *Biofeedback and Self-Regulation* 9 (1): 1–23.

Lukito, S., S. Halder, P. Bretherton, B. Kotchoubey, C. Vögele, and A. Kübler. Under revision. Depressed mood, emotion, and communication using an oddball (P300) brain-computer interface (BCI).

Lulé, D., V. Diekmann, J. Kassubek, A. Kurt, N. Birbaumer, A. C. Ludolph, and Eduard Kraft. 2007. Cortical plasticity in amyotrophic lateral sclerosis: Motor imagery and function. *Neurorehabilitation and Neural Repair* 21 (6): 518–26.

Lulé, D., S. Häcker, A. Ludolph, N. Birbaumer, and A. Kübler. 2008. Depression and quality of life in patients with amyotrophic lateral sclerosis. *Deutsches Ärzteblatt International* 105 (23): 397–403.

Lulé, D., C. Zickler, S. Häcker, M. A. Bruno, A. Demertzi, F. Pellas, S. Laureys, and A. Kübler. 2009. Life can be worth living in locked-in syndrome. *Progress in Brain Research* 177: 339–51.

Lutzenberger, W., T. Elbert, B. Rockstroh, and N. Birbaumer. 1979. The effects of self-regulation of slow cortical potentials on performance in a signal detection task. *International Journal of Neuroscience* 9 (3): 175–83.

Lutzenberger, W., T. Elbert, B. Rockstroh, and N. Birbaumer. 1982. Biofeedback produced slow brain potentials and task performance. *Biological Psychology* 14 (1–2): 99–111.

Luu, S. and T. Chau. 2009. Decoding subjective preference from single-trial near-infrared spectroscopy signals. *Journal of Neural Engineering* 6 (1): 016003. doi:10.1088/1741-2560/6/1/016003.

Martinez, P., H. Bakardjian, and A. Cichocki. 2007. Fully online multicommand brain-computer interface with visual neurofeedback using SSVEP paradigm. *Computational Intelligence and Neuroscience* 2007: 94561. doi:10.1155/2007/94561.

Mayes, R., C. Bagwell, and J. Erkulwater. 2008. ADHD and the rise in stimulant use among children. *Harvard Review of Psychiatry* 16 (3): 151–66.

McDonald, J. W. and C. Sadowsky. 2002. Spinal-cord injury. *Lancet* 359 (9304): 417–25.

McFarland, D.J. and J. R. Wolpaw. 2008. Sensorimotor rhythm-based brain-computer interface (BCI): model order selection for autoregressive spectral analysis. *Journal of Neural Engineering* 5 (2): 155–62.

McFarland, D. J., L. A. Miner, T. M. Vaughan, and J. R. Wolpaw. 2000. Mu and beta rhythm topographies during motor imagery and actual movements. *Brain Topography* 12 (3): 177–86.

Mellinger, J., G. Schalk, C. Braun, H. Preissl, W. Rosenstiel, N. Birbaumer, and A. Kübler. 2007. An MEG-based brain-computer interface (BCI). *NeuroImage* 36 (3): 581–93.

Millàn, J. D., F. Renkens, J. Mourino, and W. Gerstner. 2004. Noninvasive brain-actuated control of a mobile robot by human EEG. *IEEE Transactions on Biomedical Engineering* 51 (6): 1026–33.

Millán, J. d. R., R. Rupp, G. R. Müller-Putz, R. Murray-Smith, C. Giugliemma, M. Tangermann, C. Vidaurre et al. 2010. Combining brain–computer interfaces and assistive technologies: State-of-the-art and challenges. *Frontiers in Neuroscience* 4: 161.

Miner, L. A., D. J. McFarland, and J. R. Wolpaw. 1998. Answering questions with an electroencephalogram-based brain-computer interface. *Archives of Physical Medicine and Rehabilitation* 79 (9): 1029–33.

Monastra, V. J., S. Lynn, M. Linden, J. F. Lubar, J. Gruzelier, and T. J. LaVaque. 2005. Electroencephalographic biofeedback in the treatment of attention-deficit/hyperactivity disorder. *Applied Psychophysiology and Biofeedback* 30 (2): 95–114.

Monti, M. M., A. Vanhaudenhuyse, M. R. Coleman, M. Boly, J. D. Pickard, L. Tshibanda, A. M. Owen, and S. Laureys. 2010. Willful modulation of brain activity in disorders of consciousness. *The New England Journal of Medicine* 362 (7): 579–89.

Moore, M. M. 2003. Real-world applications for brain-computer interface technology. *IEEE Transactions on Neural Systems and Rehabilitation Engineering* 11 (2): 162–5.

Mugler, E., M. Bensch, S. Halder, W. Rosenstiel, M. Bogdan, N. Birbaumer, and A. Kübler. 2008. Control of an Internet browser using the P300 event-related potential. *International Journal of Bioelectromagnetism* 10 (1): 56–63.

Mugler, E., C. Ruf, S. Halder, M. Bensch, and A. Kübler. 2010. Design and implementation of a P300-based brain-computer interface for controlling an Internet browser. *IEEE Transactions on Neural Systems and Rehabilitation Engineering* 18 (6): 599–609.

Müller, G. R., C. Neuper, and G. Pfurtscheller. 2003. Implementation of a telemonitoring system for the control of an EEG-based brain-computer interface. *IEEE Transactions on Neural Systems and Rehabilitation Engineering* 11 (1): 54–9.

Müller, K. R., M. Tangermann, G. Dornhege, M. Krauledat, G. Curio, and B. Blankertz. 2008. Machine learning for real-time single-trial EEG-analysis: From brain-computer interfacing to mental state monitoring. *Journal of Neuroscience Methods* 167 (1): 82–90.

Müller-Putz, G. R. and G. Pfurtscheller. 2008. Control of an electrical prosthesis with an SSVEP-based BCI. *IEEE Transactions on Biomedical Engineering* 55 (1): 361–4.

Müller-Putz, G. R., R. Scherer, C. Neuper, and G. Pfurtscheller. 2006. Steady-state somatosensory evoked potentials: Suitable brain signals for brain-computer interfaces? *IEEE Transactions on Neural Systems and Rehabilitation Engineering* 14 (1): 30–7.

Müller-Putz, G. R., R. Scherer, G. Pfurtscheller, and R. Rupp. 2005. EEG-based neuroprosthesis control: A step towards clinical practice. *Neuroscience Letters* 382 (1–2): 169–74.

Münßinger, J., S. Halder, S. C. Kleih, A. Furdea, V. Raco, A. Hösle, and A. Kübler. 2010. Brain painting: First evaluation of a new braincomputer interface application with ALS-patients and healthy volunteers. *Frontiers in Neuroscience* 4: 182.

Murphy, T. H. and D. Corbett. 2009. Plasticity during stroke recovery: From synapse to behaviour. *Nature Reviews Neuroscience* 10 (12): 861–72.

Naito, M., Y. Michioka, K. Ozawa, Y. Ito, M. Kiguchi, and T. Kanazawa. 2007. A communication means for totally locked-in ALS patients based on changes in cerebral blood volume measured with near-infrared light. *IEICE Transactions on Information and Systems* 90: 1028–37.

Neumann, N. and N. Birbaumer. 2003. Predictors of successful self control during brain-computer communication. *Journal of Neurology, Neurosurgery & Psychiatry* 74 (8): 1117–21.

Neumann, N., T. Hinterberger, J. Kaiser, U. Leins, N. Birbaumer, and A. Kübler. 2004. Automatic processing of self-regulation of slow cortical potentials: Evidence from brain-computer communication in paralysed patients. *Clinical Neurophysiology* 115 (3): 628–35.

Neumann, N. and A. Kübler. 2003. Training locked-in patients: A challenge for the use of brain-computer interfaces. *IEEE Transactions on Neural Systems and Rehabilitation Engineering* 11 (2): 169–72.

Neumann, N., A. Kübler, J. Kaiser, T. Hinterberger, and N. Birbaumer. 2003. Conscious perception of brain states: Mental strategies for brain-computer communication. *Neuropsychologia* 41 (8): 1028–36.

Neuper, C., R. Scherer, S. Wriessnegger, and G. Pfurtscheller. 2009. Motor imagery and action observation: Modulation of sensorimotor brain rhythms during mental control of a brain-computer interface. *Clinical Neurophysiology* 120 (2): 239–47.

Nijboer, F., N. Birbaumer, and A. Kübler. 2010. The influence of psychological state and motivation on Brain-Computer Interface performance in patients with amyothropic lateral sclerosis—A longitudinal study. *Frontiers in Neuroscience* 4: 55. doi:10.3389/fnins.2010.00055.

Nijboer, F., A. Furdea, I. Gunst, J. Mellinger, D. J. McFarland, N. Birbaumer, and A. Kübler. 2008. An auditory brain-computer interface (BCI). *Journal of Neuroscience Methods* 167 (1): 43–50.

Nijboer, F., E. W. Sellers, J. Mellinger, M. A. Jordan, T. Matuz, A. Furdea, S. Halder et al. 2008. A P300-based brain-computer interface for people with amyotrophic lateral sclerosis. *Clinical Neurophysiology* 119 (8): 1909–16.

Ortner, R., B. Z. Allison, G. Korisek, H. Gaggl, and G. Pfurtscheller. 2011. An SSVEP BCI to control a hand orthosis for persons with tetraplegia. *Neural Systems and Rehabilitation Engineering, IEEE Transactions on* 19 (1): 1–5.

Owen, A. M., M. R. Coleman, M. Boly, M. H. Davis, S. Laureys, and J. D. Pickard. 2006. Detecting awareness in the vegetative state. *Science* 313 (5792): 1402.

Patterson, J. R. and M. Grabois. 1986. Locked-in syndrome: A review of 139 cases. *Stroke* 17 (4): 758–64.

Peckham, P. H., M. W. Keith, K. L. Kilgore, J. H. Grill, K. S. Wuolle, G. B. Thrope, P. Gorman et al. for the Implantable Neuroprothesis Research Group. 2001. Efficacy of an implanted neuroprosthesis for restoring hand grasp in tetraplegia: A multicenter study. *Archives of Physical Medicine and Rehabilitation* 82 (10): 1380–8.

Pfurtscheller, G. 1992. Event-related synchronization (ERS): An electrophysiological correlate of cortical areas at rest. *Electroencephalography and Clinical Neurophysiology* 83 (1): 62–9.

Pfurtscheller, G., C. Brunner, A. Schlögl, and F. H. Lopes da Silva. 2006. Mu rhythm (de)synchronization and EEG single-trial classification of different motor imagery tasks. *NeuroImage* 31 (1): 153–9, doi: 10.1016/j.neuroimage.2005.12.003.

Pfurtscheller, G., C. Guger, G. Müller, G. Krausz, and C. Neuper. 2000. Brain oscillations control hand orthosis in a tetraplegic. *Neuroscience Letters* 292 (3): 211–4.

Pfurtscheller, G. and F. H. Lopes da Silva, eds. 2005. *Event-Related Desynchronization (ERD) and Event-Related Synchronization (ERS)*, 5th ed. Philadelphia, PA: Lippincott, Williams & Wilkins.

Pfurtscheller, G., G. Müller, and G. Korisek. 2002. [Mental activity hand orthosis control using the EEG: A case study]. *Rehabilitation (Stuttgart)* 41 (1): 48–52.

Pfurtscheller, G. and C. Neuper. 1997. Motor imagery activates primary sensorimotor area in humans. *Neuroscience Letters* 239 (2–3): 65–8.

Pfurtscheller, G. and C. Neuper. 2005. EEG-based brain-computer interfaces. In *Electroencephalography: Basic Principles, Clinical Applications, and Related Fields*, 5th ed., edited by E. Niedermeyer and F. da Silva, 1265–71. Philadelphia, PA: Lippincott, Williams & Wilkins.

Pfurtscheller, G., C. Neuper, C. Guger, W. Harkam, H. Ramoser, A. Schlogl, B. Obermaier, and M. Pregenzer. 2000. Current trends in Graz brain-computer interface (BCI) research. *IEEE Transactions on Rehabilitation Engineering* 8 (2): 216–9.

Pfurtscheller, G. and T. Solis-Escalante. 2009. Could the beta rebound in the EEG be suitable to realize a "brain switch"? *Clinical Neurophysiology* 120 (1): 24–9.

Pfurtscheller, G., R. Scherer, G. R. Müller-Putz, and F. H. Lopes da Silva. 2008. Short-lived brain state after cued motor imagery in naive subjects. *European Journal of Neuroscience* 28(7): 1419–26.

Pfurtscheller, G., T. Solis-Escalante, R. Ortner, P. Linortner, and G. R. Müller-Putz. 2010. Self-paced operation of an SSVEP-based orthosis with and without an imagery-based "brain switch": A feasibility study towards a hybrid BCI. *IEEE Transactions on Neural Systems and Rehabilitation Engineering* 18 (4): 409–14.

Pham, M., T. Hinterberger, N. Neumann, A. Kübler, N. Hofmayer, A. Grether, B. Wilhelm, J.-J. Vatine, and N. Birbaumer. 2005. An auditory brain-computer interface based on the self-regulation of slow cortical potentials. *Neurorehabilitation & Neural Repair* 19 (3): 206–18.

Phan, K. L., D. A. Fitzgerald, K. Gao, G. J. Moore, M. E. Tancer, and S. Posse. 2004. Real-time fMRI of cortico-limbic brain activity during emotional processing. *NeuroReport* 15 (3): 527–32.

Phillips, L. H., II. 2006. Communicating with the "locked-in" patient: Because you can do it, should you? *Neurology* 67 (3): 380–1.

Piccione, F., F. Giorgi, P. Tonin, K. Priftis, S. Giove, S. Silvoni, G. Palmas, and F. Beverina. 2006. P300-based brain computer interface: Reliability and performance in healthy and paralysed participants. *Clinical Neurophysiology* 117 (3): 531–7.

Pichiorri, F., F. De Vico Fallani, F. Cincotti, F. Babiloni, M. Molinari, S. C. Kleih, C. Neuper, A. Kübler, and D. Mattia. 2011. Sensorimotor rhythm-based brain–computer interface training: The impact on motor cortical responsiveness. *Journal of Neural Engineering* 8: 1–9.

Pires, G. and U. Nunes. 2002. A wheelchair steered through voice commands and assisted by a reactive fuzzy-logic controller. *Journal of Intelligent & Robotic Systems* 34 (3): 301–14.

Popescu, F., S. Fazli, Y. Badower, B. Blankertz, and K. R. Muller. 2007. Single trial classification of motor imagination using 6 dry EEG electrodes. *PLoS One* 2 (7): e637. doi:10.1371/journal.pone.0000637.

Pritchard, W. S. 1981. Psychophysiology of P300. *Psychological Bulletin* 89 (3): 506–40.

Rabkin, J. G., S. M. Albert, M. L. Del Bene, I. O'Sullivan, T. Tider, L. P. Rowland, and H. Mitsumoto. 2005. Prevalence of depressive disorders and change over time in late-stage ALS. *Neurology* 65 (1): 62–7.

Rabkin, J. G., S. M. Albert, T. Tider, M. L. Del Bene, I. O'Sullivan, L. P. Rowland, and H. Mitsumoto. 2006. Predictors and course of elective long-term mechanical ventilation: A prospective study of ALS patients. *Amyotrophic Lateral Sclerosis* 7 (2): 86–95.

Ravden, D. and J. Polich. 1999. On P300 measurement stability: Habituation, intra-trial block variation, and ultradian rhythms. *Biological Psychology* 51 (1): 59–76.

Rowland, L. P. and N. A. Shneider. 2001. Medical progress: Amyotrophic lateral sclerosis. *The New England Journal of Medicine* 344 (22): 1688–700.

Ruiz, S., R. Sitaram, B. Várkuti, S. Lee, A. Caria, C. Plewnia, S. Soekadar, R. Veit, V. Singh, and N. Birbaumer. 2008. Learned control of insular activity and functional connectivity changes using fMRI brain computer interface in schizophrenia. *Schizophrenia Research* 102 (1–2, Suppl. 2): 92.

Sakamoto, M., T. Muraoka, N. Mizuguchi, and K. Kanosue. 2009. Combining observation and imagery of an action enhances human corticospinal excitability. *Neuroscience Research* 65 (1): 23–7.

Schalk, G., J. Kubanek, K. J. Miller, N. R. Anderson, E. C. Leuthardt, J. G. Ojemann, D. Limbrick, D. Moran, L. A. Gerhardt, and J. R. Wolpaw. 2007. Decoding two-dimensional movement trajectories using electrocorticographic signals in humans. *Journal of Neural Engineering* 4 (3): 264–75.

Scherer, R., G. R. Müller-Putz, and G. Pfurtscheller. 2007. Self-initiation of EEG-based brain-computer communication using the heart rate response. *Journal of Neural Engineering* 4 (4): L23–9.

Schreuder, M., J. Höhne, M. Treder, B. Blankertz, and M. Tangermann. 2011. Performance optimization of ERP-based BCIs using dynamic stopping. *Conference Proceedings IEEE Engineering in Medicine and Biology Society*.

Sellers, E. W. and E. Donchin. 2006. A P300-based brain-computer interface: Initial tests by ALS patients. *Clinical Neurophysiology* 117 (3) : 538–48.

Silvoni, S., C. Volpato, M. Cavinato, M. Marchetti, K. Priftis, A. Merico, P. Tonin, K. Koutsikos, F. Beverina, and F. Piccione. 2009. P300-based brain–computer interface communication: Evaluation and follow-up in amyotrophic lateral sclerosis. *Frontiers in Neuroprosthetics* 3: 60. doi:10.3389/neuro.20.001.2009.

Sitaram, R., A. Caria, and N. Birbaumer. 2009. Hemodynamic brain-computer interfaces for communication and rehabilitation. *Neural Networks* 22 (9): 1320–8.

Sitaram, R., A. Caria, R. Veit, T. Gaber, G. Rota, A. Kübler, and N. Birbaumer. 2007. fMRI Brain-Computer Interface: A tool for neuroscientific research and treatment. *Computational Intelligence and Neuroscience* 2007: 25487. doi:10.1155/2007/25487.

Smith, E. and M. Delargy. 2005. Locked-in syndrome. *British Medical Journal* 330 (7488): 406–9.

Sorger, B., B. Dahmen, J. Reithler, O. Gosseries, A. Maudoux, S. Laureys, and R. Goebel. 2009. Another kind of 'BOLD Response': Answering multiple-choice questions via online decoded single-trial brain signals. *Progress in Brain Research* 177: 275–92.

Sterman, M. B., and T. Egner. 2006. Foundation and practice of neurofeedback for the treatment of epilepsy. *Applied Psychophysiology and Biofeedback* 31 (1): 21–35.

Sterman, M. B., L. R. Macdonald, and R. K. Stone. 1974. Biofeedback training of the sensorimotor electroencephalogram rhythm in man: Effects on epilepsy. *Epilepsia* 15 (3): 395–416.

Strehl, U., C. Gani, S. Kaller, and N. Birbaumer. 2007. Long term stability of neurofeedback in children with ADHD. *Journal of Neural Transmission* 114 (7): LIX.

Strehl, U., B. Kotchoubey, T. Trevorrow, and N. Birbaumer. 2005. Predictors of seizure reduction after self-regulation of slow cortical potentials as a treatment of drug-resistant epilepsy. *Epilepsy & Behavior* 6 (2): 156–66.

Sutton, S., M. Braren, J. Zubin, and E. R. John. 1965. Evoked-potential correlates of stimulus uncertainty. *Science* 150 (700): 1187–8.

Tan, G., J. Thornby, D. C. Hammond, U. Strehl, B. Canady, K. Arnemann, and D. A. Kaiser. 2009. Meta-analysis of EEG biofeedback in treating epilepsy. *Clinical EEG and Neuroscience* 40 (3): 173–9.

Tangermann, M., M. Krauledat, K. Grzeska, M. Sagebaum, B. Blankertz, C. Vidaurre, and K. R. Müller. 2008. *Playing pinball with non-invasive BCI*. Paper presented at the *Advances in Neural Information Processing Systems (NIPS) 21: Proceedings of the 2008 Conference*, Vancouver, British Columbia, Canada, December 8–10, 2008, pp. 1641–8.

Taub, E. and G. Uswatte. 2003. Constraint-induced movement therapy: Bridging from the primate laboratory to the stroke rehabilitation laboratory. *Journal of Rehabilitation Medicine* 41(Suppl): 34–40.

Uludağ, K., D. J. Dubowitz, and R. B. Buxton. 2005. Basic principles of functional MRI. In *Clinical MRI*, edited by R. Edelman, J. Hesselink, and M. Zlatkin, 249–87. San Diego: Elsevier.

Vaughan, T. M., D. J. McFarland, G. Schalk, W. A. Sarnacki, D. J. Krusienski, E. W. Sellers, and J. R. Wolpaw. 2006. The Wadsworth BCI research and development program: At home with BCI. *IEEE Transactions on Neural Systems and Rehabilitation Engineering* 14 (2): 229–33.

Vidaurre, C. and B. Blankertz. 2009. Towards a cure for BCI illiteracy. *Brain Topography* 23 (2): 194–8.

Wang, W., J. L. Collinger, M. A. Perez, E. C. Tyler-Kabara, L. G. Cohen, N. Birbaumer, S. W. Brose, A. B. Schwartz, M. L. Boninger, and D. J. Weber. 2010. Neural interface technology for rehabilitation: Exploiting and promoting neuroplasticity. *Physical Medicine and Rehabilitation Clinics of North America* 21 (1): 157–78.

Weiskopf, N., R. Veit, M. Erb, K. Mathiak, W. Grodd, R. Goebel, and N. Birbaumer. 2003. Physiological self-regulation of regional brain activity using real-time functional magnetic resonance imaging (fMRI): Methodology and exemplary data. *NeuroImage* 19 (3): 577–86.

Wilhelm, B., M. Jordan, and N. Birbaumer. 2006. Communication in locked-in syndrome: Effects of imagery on salivary pH. *Neurology* 67 (3): 534–5.

Williams, L. M., P. Das, A. W. Harris, B. B. Liddell, M. J. Brammer, G. Olivieri, D. Skerrett et al. 2004. Dysregulation of arousal and amygdala-prefrontal systems in paranoid schizophrenia. *American Journal of Psychiatry* 161 (3): 480–9.

Wisneski, K. J., N. Anderson, G. Schalk, M. Smyth, D. Moran, and E. C. Leuthardt. 2008. Unique cortical physiology associated with ipsilateral hand movements and neuroprosthetic implications. *Stroke* 39 (12): 3351–9.

Wolpaw, J. R. N. Birbaumer, W. J. Heetderks, D. J. McFarland, P. H. Peckham, G. Schalk, E. Donchin, L. A. Quatrano, C. J. Robinson, and T. M. Vaughan. 2000. Brain-computer interface technology: A review of the first international meeting. *IEEE Transactions on Rehabilitation Engineering* 8 (2): 164–73.

Wolpaw, J. R. and D. J. McFarland. 2004. Control of a two-dimensional movement signal by a noninvasive brain-computer interface in humans. *Proceedings of the National Academy of Sciences of the United States of America* 101 (51): 17849–54.

World Health Organization. 2004. *ICD-10: International Statistical Classification of Diseases and Related Health Problems Tenth Revision*. Geneva: World Health Organization.

Wriessnegger, S. C., J. Kurzmann, and C. Neuper. 2008. Spatio-temporal differences in brain oxygenation between movement execution and imagery: A multichannel near-infrared spectroscopy study. *International Journal of Psychophysiology* 67 (1): 54–63.

Yoo, S. S., T. Fairneny, N. K. Chen, S. E. Choo, L. P. Panych, H. Park, S. Y. Lee, and F. A. Jolesz. 2004. Brain-computer interface using fMRI: Spatial navigation by thoughts. *NeuroReport* 15 (10): 1591–5.

Zacksenhouse, M., M. A. Lebedev, J. M. Carmena, J. E. O'Doherty, C. Henriquez, and M. A. Nicolelis. 2007. Cortical modulations increase in early sessions with brain-machine interface. *PLoS One* 2 (7): e619. doi:10.1371/journal.pone.0000619.

Zickler, C., V. Di Donna, V. Kaiser, A. Al-Khodairy, S. C. Kleih, A. Kübler, M. Malavasi et al. 2009. BCI applications for people with disabilities: Defining user needs and user requirements. Paper presented at the *AAATE 25th Conference*, Florence, Italy, August 31–September 2, 2009.

10

Neuroadaptive Systems: Challenges and Opportunities in Creating Symbiotic Relationships between Humans and the Machines They Use

Joseph V. Cohn and Tracey L. Wheeler

CONTENTS

10.1 Introduction

Recently, there has been a profound resurgence of interest in expanding the effectiveness of human machine symbiotic systems. This renaissance has been fueled in no small part by advances in two diverse and broad fields—neuroscience and engineering. Advances in neuroscience have contributed to a strong growth in understanding how the human brain effectively processes information leading to behavior. Theoretically, this understanding should provide the insights necessary for enabling machines to better adapt to their users. At the same time advances in engineering have enabled significant reductions in the size, weight, and power requirements of modern computers, as well as increasing overall computational capabilities. These advances have removed many of the limitations commonly associated with building practical and easy-to-use human–machine symbiotic systems.

Traditional approaches to creating human–machine symbiotic systems have focused on engineering or machine learning techniques to establish couplings between humans and their machines (Cooley 2007). For example, many of the cognitive architectures that are intended to allow the machine to infer human intention are based on computer processing metaphors, not on actual brain dynamics. This is a direct result of the levels of technology available to understand and represent the processes through which the human brain transforms information into action. Until very recently, neither the imaging technologies nor the analytic capabilities were available to truly link actual brain activity to behavior. As a result, when one wished to create human–machine systems one was forced to do so by basing this integration on observed behaviors, and building predictive models of human behavior on these observed behaviors.

Of course, the ideal is to directly link high fidelity representations of human behavior with machine operating systems. These representations may be found in the neural processes leading to the actual observed behavior. Just as understanding the equations of motion provides a much broader set of capabilities than inferring these equations from a limited set of observations (Kelso 1995), so too understanding and modeling the dynamics of neural activity as it leads to behavior should provide a much richer and more robust set of models than those based on the actual observed behavior alone. Today, advances in neuroscience and engineering provide the basis for building these "equations of motion" for the brain and for using brain-based techniques to create and maintain very robust human–machine interactions.

Collectively, systems that incorporate elements of the brain's activity to enable human–machine interactions are known as neuroadaptive systems. This chapter explores the underlying rationale for using these systems compared to other kinds of human–machine systems and the impact that recent advances in areas such as neuroimaging, neural decoding, and neural modeling have had and will continue to have on the development and extension of neuroadaptive systems. Several example applications that are ideally suited to neuroadaptive systems are also provided.

10.2 Defining Neuroadaptation and Neuroadaptive Systems

In the strictest sense, neuroadaptation is the process through which neural communication is altered after repeated exposure to a stimulus. This alteration could involve changes to the type, quantity, or distribution of proteins in a nerve cell's membrane (Even et al. 2008), changes in the dynamics of neurotransmitter release (Xiao et al. 2009), changes in gene expression (Polesskaya et al. 2007), and even alterations to nerve cell morphology (McDonald et al. 2005; McDonald et al. 2007; Bergstrom et al. 2008). Traditionally, neuroadaptation research has focused on understanding the mechanisms through which drug addiction develops (Kalivas 2007). However, the basic principles of neuroadaptation—changes in the dynamics between neural connections—also serve to explain how learning occurs, how memories form, and how brain plasticity arises.

Neuroadaptive systems use the detailed output of their human users' neural activity in order to effectively adapt their behavior to the behavior of their users. This requires more than simply taking a snapshot of brain action. As the term neuroadaptive suggests, the brain is not a static organ. It changes with experience (Cohn, Stripling, and Kruse 2005), creating new connections and optimizing older ones; it varies with emotional and physiological state, impacting and influencing higher-order processes (Glimcher and Rustichini 2004); and it is primed by changes in environmental context (Aamodt and Wang 2008). The end result of the brain's inherent dynamicity is often changes in observed behavior (Cohn, Stripling, and Kruse 2005). Consequently, while it should be possible to create a closed-loop human–machine symbiotic system that can adapt its overall performance on the basis of representations of brain activity, care must be taken to understand precisely how to transform neural activity into representations of the behavior they encode.

10.3 Why Neuroadaptive Systems

The notion of creating dynamically adaptive closed-loop human–machine systems is not new. As early as the 1940s, researchers were concerned with the question of how to represent the human element in human–machine systems. Using the terminology of the time, Bates (1947), Craik (1947, 1948), and others attempted to explain human performance in terms of control theory with the goal of developing engineering representations of the human that could be used to improve human–machine systems (Birmingham and Taylor 1954). Others, like Chapanais (1951), applied a similar approach for analyzing human error in human–machine systems. In all cases, the properties of the human being modeled were only at the observed behavior level. For example, Fitts' speed-accuracy tradeoff (Fitts 1954; Fitts and Peterson 1964) emphasizes the development of basic relationships guiding human motor planning. Stevens' power law describes the relationship between the magnitude of a physical stimulus and its perceived intensity (Stevens 1957), and the Hick–Hyman law relates decision response time to the number of possible choices (Hick 1952; Hyman 1953). One of the primary applications for this line of research was to develop more effective and responsive aviation systems (Adams 1957; McRuer and Jex 1967; Young 1969). More broadly, fully automated systems that could perform tasks in the absence of actual human controller inputs were also envisioned as resulting from this line of research, as were human assistive systems (i.e., symbiotic systems; Licklider 1960).

In a classic sense, automation may be thought of as a means of substituting human actions with those of a machine (Parsons 1985; Parasuraman and Riley 1997). The reasons for automating certain tasks range from safety considerations to cost and efficiency considerations (Weiner and Curry 1980; Weiner 1989). Inherent to the notion of automation is the idea that of an overall pool of tasks, some may be allocated to a system or machine, whereas others may be allocated to a human. In the most conservative sense (e.g., Licklider 1960), automation requires a strict parsing of tasks—those at which a machine may excel and those at which a human may excel. Along those lines, Parasuraman, Sheridan, and Wickens (2000) proposed a set of discrete levels of automation to be implemented on the basis of overall task context. Yet, as Rouse (1977) and Woods (1996) suggest, these kinds of approaches to automation are brittle. Situations change, information changes, and people change, often as a consequence of using automation (Woods 1996) and the allocation of tasks between humans and machines should be able to change, dynamically and in real time to provide the most effective assistance.

Adaptive automation—automation that allows for control of tasks to be passed in real time, between human and machine—represents one attempt to bridge the human–machine gap of classic automation (Scerbo 1996). This kind of automation seeks to optimize human–machine interactions by changing task demands in response to user performance. A direct result of this kind of automation is that the task environment is restructured, dynamically, in terms of *what* tasks are automated, *how* they are automated, and *when* they are automated (Rouse, Geddes, and Curry 1988). A key consideration in adaptive automation is the means through which the adaptation is triggered. Early attempts at creating adaptive techniques focused on a purely artificial intelligence approach (Rouse 1977), merging expert systems with knowledge-based representations of human performance (or, loosely, cognition) to detect and assess task context, and develop adaptive strategies (e.g., Hammer and Small 1995). A significant disadvantage with this approach is that although representations of the human operator may be gleaned from psychometric measures (speed and accuracy types of measures), the level of fidelity of these representations is typically orders of magnitude less than that of representations of the system and task environment. Furthermore, the rate at which this information may be accumulated is similarly challenged. Human behavior typically evolves over a timescale measured in seconds, whereas machine action may occur over a millisecond to second timescale. In other words, currently available measures of the human are rate limiting in human–machine systems, even those that are adaptive.

Recent attempts to get around the human representation challenge have focused on adding another dimension of measurement, based on neurophysiologically detected processes (Morrison and Gluckman 1994). The basic premise is that by including neurophysiological measures, it should be possible to gain higher levels of fidelity, over a shorter time course, for the kinds of human representation needed to make adaptive automation effective, beyond simple observationally behavior-based ones. These richer metrics would, therefore, serve as a more effective input into a dynamic and adaptive automation system (Scerbo 1996). Such measures include (Scerbo et al. 2001; Cohn, Stripling, and Kruse 2005):

- Heart rate variability
- Eye-based responses (e.g., eye blinks, pupil diameter)
- Galvanic skin response
- Neural-based signals (electroencephalography, functional magnetic resonance imaging, functional near-infrared imaging)

These measurements provide a vast improvement over traditional measures that feed into adaptive automation developed to make use of them (e.g., Schmorrow 2005; Schmorrow, Stanney, and Reeves 2007) and, collectively, have pushed the field of adaptive automation far ahead of where it might otherwise be. At the same time, while these measures provide a more effective diagnostic metric indicating when automation might be useful, they don't provide deeper descriptions of *what* tasks should be automated, *how* they should be automated, and *when* they must be automated. These determinations, in the current approach, are left to predefined strategies that are implemented on the basis of the triggering of these measures (Rouse, Geddes, and Curry 1988).

Neuroadaptive systems seek to address this gap by enabling adaptive interactions between humans and their machines, using deeper and more representative measures of human neural action underlying behavior than those used in traditional adaptive automation technologies. With these representations, high-fidelity individualized models of human performance can be crafted, which can be expected to behave in a manner analogous to that in which the human brain on which they are based will behave. Although still in their infancy, neuroadaptive systems are beginning to be realized as a direct result of recent advances in neuroscience and engineering.

10.4 Foundations of Neuroadaptive Systems

10.4.1 Basis of Neuroadaptive Systems

Neuroadaptive systems are based on the idea that understanding human cognition is key to understanding human behavior, because cognition is how the human brain transforms sensed information into behavior. Wickens and Hollands (2000) and others have proposed a four-stage model of human information processing, including sensing information, perceiving information (through working memory), decision making, and response selection. It is possible to reduce this model to a three-stage one that treats perceiving and decision making as two ends of a cognitive process continuum, in order to highlight the important role that cognition plays in driving human action. This model includes sensing (detecting information through different sensory organs), cognition (transforming information through neurocognitive processes), and acting (as a result of) on that transformation.

Figure 10.1 illustrates this information processing flow and highlights how, today, information from the human operator may be captured and used to drive adaptive automation systems. On the one hand, adaptive automation technologies may work at the "sensing" stage—using psychophysiological measurement techniques to detect when sensory processes are active—or very early into the "cognition" stage—detecting the onset of certain cognitive processes or ensemble measures of cognitive state, like workload. In this control scheme, the neural signals serve as little more than a response selection trigger. Measures indicating that information has been sensed may be sent to a model, which, in turn, selects an output from the adaptive technology on the basis of a predetermined set of criteria, usually context- and task-specific. On the other hand, adaptive automation technologies may work at the "acting" stage, using observed behaviors as a means of inferring how the brain's cognitive processes may work. These inferences are captured in a cognitive architecture or cognitive model, which is then used to select an output from the adaptive technology, again, on the basis of a predetermined set of criteria. In this control scheme, the behavior signals serve as the only indicator that cognition has occurred. Because models based on inferred cognition are context-, task-, and user-specific, predictions of the type of automation, timing of automation, and extent of automation based on these models are often unable to adapt to new contexts, tasks, and users without significant ad hoc modifications (for an in-depth discussion, see Gluck and Pew 2005). Solving modeling challenge is core to enabling neuroadaptive systems.

Figure 10.2 provides two different ways of illustrating this challenge (Newell 1994; Schmorrow, Cohn, and Nicholson 2009). First, this challenge can be represented in terms

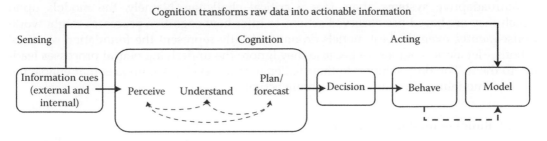

FIGURE 10.1
Information processing flow.

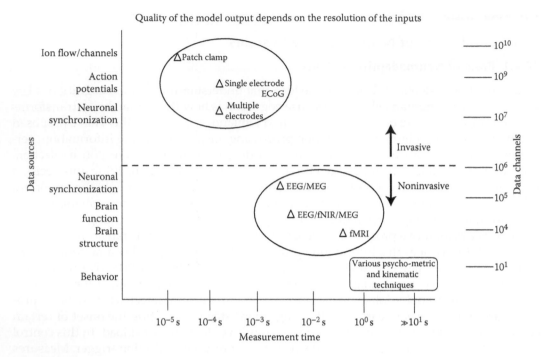

FIGURE 10.2
The resolution challenge.

of the amount of information or the channels of information available to populate a model. Neural data clearly provides a significant amount of information, over a very rapid time course, leaving open the possibility of creating high-fidelity real-time models of user performance that can intelligently drive adaptive automation. In contrast, behavior data provides comparatively little information, leading to the development of basic models of performance that are highly constrained. Second, this challenge can be represented in terms of the time required to capture the required information to populate a model. Neural activity takes place on the millisecond timescale, opening up the possibility for near-real-time development and updating of models based on that type of information. In contrast, behavior takes place on the second or seconds timescale, even though the actual intent to act may have been formed within hundreds of milliseconds of sensing relevant information (Luu et al. 2010). Models based on behavior data simply cannot keep pace with the actions of the adaptive systems that they are meant to inform.

Neuroadaptive systems, then, face a critical challenge. Namely, the models upon which they are based use observed actions to infer how cognitive processes might work. Consequently, even the best models do not faithfully represent the foundation of users' actions—let alone, cognition—because they ignore the underlying neural processes leading to them. The only solution to this challenge is to develop techniques that enable the accurate modeling of cognition using brain activity.

10.4.2 Building on Recent Advances

On the surface, addressing this challenge may appear to be a tall order. Interpreting actual meaning from neural activity has been a long-sought dream of the neuroscience community. The reliance of cognitive models on observed behavior is in many ways a tacit admission that, while there is a great need to "go to the brain," in the past available technologies and theories simply precluded doing this, making observed actions the most readily accessible feature of human behavior that could be accessed to provide critical data to populate models.

Recently, though, there has been a shift in theories of the brain, made possible by advances in neuroimaging technologies and data analysis techniques. The notion that the brain is made of discrete centers, each responsible for a portion of the information processing chain, has given way to a more dynamic and integrative conception. Under this framework, different areas of the brain each contribute, in different ways depending on the task environment and user state, to ensemble brain processes leading ultimately to behavior (Singer 1999; Philiastides and Sajda 2007). Cognition, in this view, is the interaction and integration of "building blocks" like perception, attention, and memory, which, in turn, results from activity across multiple brain regions. These regions form "ad hoc" networks across the physical substrate of the brain via synchronization signals that bind different neural centers together, for brief periods of time (Palva, Palva, and Kaila 2005; Kahana 2006; Osipova et al. 2006; Singer 1999).

These advances have been made possible as direct result of developments in three core domains (see Table 10.1):

- Detection technologies
- Decoding methodologies
- Modeling frameworks

10.4.3 Detection Technologies

The notion that human behavior is the result of coordinated activity across the brain is not new (Kelso 1995). However, access to the brain has been one of the key limiting steps in demonstrating coordinated activity across the brain as behavior develops. As new technologies, such as functional magnetic resonance imaging, (Logothetis 2001), dense-array electroencephalography (Junghöfer et al. 2000), and other types of tools, become increasingly refined, simplified, and incorporated into the researcher's toolkit, the ability to capture neural action simultaneously across multiple regions will continue to grow. As one example, Philiastides and Sajda (2007) used an electroencephalography-based paradigm to illustrate the integration of different neural regions over time, as participants formed and acted upon a rapid decision-making task. As a second example, Luu et al. (2010)

TABLE 10.1

Challenges in Neuroadaptive Systems

Challenge	Outcome	Enablers
Detect: Neural processes underlying cognition	Record neural activity occurring in multiple structures across the brain as cognition develops	Brain imaging technologies
Decode: Neural data into representations of cognition	Establish rule sets for translating neural activity into cognitive behavior	Brain imaging technologies; advances in neuroscience theory
Model: Brain activity to predict behavior	Develop approaches to modeling behavior that incorporate activity/response of the brain	Advances in neuroscience theory; development of neurocognitive modeling

demonstrated that it was possible to use dense-array electroencephalography to detect neural activity occurring in multiple structures across the brain as a cognitive process known as intuition develops. Furthermore, they also report signals that indicate ad hoc network formation.

10.4.4 Decoding Methodologies

Access to integrated neural data is necessary but not sufficient for interpreting it in terms of cognitive processes. New processes for analyzing these multivariate data sets must also be established and refined, and efforts to do so have led to the development, refinement, and application of these multivariate analytical techniques to data captured as participants perform a range of cognitive tasks. Briefly, multivariate decoding takes into account the full spatial pattern of brain activity, measured simultaneously across many regions, and enables the decoding of the current "cognitive state" from measured brain activity (Haynes and Rees 2006). Using this approach, it is possible to build classifiers that can distinguish between various cognitive behaviors, provided an adequate training set can be identified. Decoding routines have recently been applied to accurately decode meaning (i.e., simple thoughts) from neural activity (Mitchell et al. 2004; Mitchell et al. 2008). What is most exciting is that these algorithms not only can decode on the basis of the training they were built from but also can, in fact, predict patterns of brain activity for thousands of other concepts with relatively high accuracies within and between participants (Kay et al. 2008; Shinkareva et al. 2008).

10.4.5 Modeling Frameworks

Perhaps, the greatest challenges still remain in the domain of modeling—developing cognitive models based on how information flows, and is processed, across the brain, to simulate what the content of cognition will look like, based on neural activity. One approach that continues to gain momentum is to take existing cognitive models and link them to neural data. For example, one of the better-known cognitive modeling approaches is ACT-R (Anderson 1996). ACT-R is an implementable theory of how human cognition works, based on the underlying assumption that knowledge is encoded from the environment and synthesized into "cognition," leading to behavior. Within the ACT-R framework, modules and buffers represent knowledge and processing of that knowledge, with cognition emerging through their activation. In its executable form, the timing and sequencing of model components is based on observed behaviors, and the output is typically timing and accuracy predictions.

Because a key output of ACT-R is timing, one important hypothesis about the accuracy with which ACT-R reflects underlying, coordinated, neural activity could be stated as follows:

H_0: If ACT-R represents how the brain produces cognition, then the timing of module and buffer activity should predict/reflect timing of corresponding brain region activity. (Anderson et al. 2008)

For example, ACT-R incorporates a visual buffer (Anderson et al. 2008). Imaging studies suggest that the functional action of such a visual buffer is contained in a region of the brain known as the fusiform area. Therefore, one test of how well ACT-R's visual buffer represents activity in the fusiform area is to determine how closely the timing of the visual buffer's activity predicts the timing in the corresponding fusiform area during a cognitive task (Anderson et al. 2008). Studies currently being conducted suggest that there is strong correspondence (Anderson et al. 2008), indicating that ACT-R may be one modeling framework suitable for representing activity captured at the neural level.

10.5 Application Areas

When considering areas to which neuroadaptive technologies may be applied, it is important to make an assessment from the "to what end" perspective. All too often, neuroscience-based technologies are presented as solutions because of their "wow" factor, when significantly less complex solutions may work just as well. Nevertheless, there are at least three general application domains where neuroadaptive technologies could make a significant impact (see Table 10.2):

- Decision support
- Human–robot teams
- Learning and memory

10.5.1 Decision Support

Computers can process super-ordinate amounts of data in a short time, but programming them to detect patterns is extremely difficult. Humans, on the other hand, are adept at pulling out patterns from large amounts of data; yet are limited in the rate at which they can apply these cognitive abilities to new problems (Hodgkinson, Langan-Fox, and Sadler-Smith 2008). Currently, there is no simple way to combine the strengths of human pattern recognition ability with the strengths of computer processing speed to enable better decision support tools. Potential solutions to building decision support tools that take advantage of these strengths would enable the human decision maker to guide the computer in its data analysis efforts, and allow the computer to present the results of this analysis in a format that is quickly understandable by the human, who would then provide additional feedback as needed to hone in on effective decisions and courses of action. The main challenge with this type of solution is that traditional decision aids rely on overt feedback from human decision makers, which occurs on a timescale of seconds and minutes, much

TABLE 10.2

Three Application Areas for Neuroadaptive Systems

Decision Support	Human–Robot Teams	Learning and Memory
Challenge: Decision making under stress, with incomplete information	Challenge: Human team members can anticipate each others' actions—robots can only do so for limited contexts/tasks	Challenge: Ability to store and recall information is limited
Neuroadaptive systems: Anticipate decision-making bottlenecks; present alternate solutions including partial or full automation	Neuroadaptive systems: Represent cognitive processes leading to actions, enabling robots to understand and anticipate human actions	Neuroadaptive systems: Understand neural basis of these limits to mitigate/exploit them

greater than the typical speeds at which today's software-based decision support systems operate. Yet, it is becoming increasingly clear that humans make decisions far earlier in the decision-making process than once thought (Ambady and Rosenthal 1993; Rensink 2004; Winerman 2005) and that these early-onset decisions may be detected in neural imaging data as early as a few hundred milliseconds after data cues are presented (Luu et al. 2010).

Neuroadaptive technologies could be developed that detect and decode human thoughts and intention on the basis of brain activity, and combine these data with adaptive data analysis techniques like genetic algorithmic modeling to build an adaptive, symbiotic human–computer decision support system. Such a system would monitor neural markers of early decision making and combine this with bio-inspired modeling techniques for analyzing supra-ordinate amounts of information to develop symbiotic human–machine decision–aiding strategies that increase decision–making accuracy, while decreasing decision–making time.

10.5.2 Human–Robot Teams

Human–robot teams will be an important component of future workspace, creating complex but potentially more effective teams. This complexity stems from the almost infinite number of possible human behaviors and collective team outcomes. Human team members, practicing together over time, develop "mental models" of their team members' performance (Lim and Klein 2006). With these mental models, team members are able to predict and anticipate each other's potential responses to a given challenge, and compensate for those if needed (Wilson et al. 2007). Robots, however, are not able to develop such anticipatory and predictive models—today, the best that can be done is to encode a series of stimulus–response rules. Yet, hard coding the wide range of potential stimulus–response sets for informing robot team members is impractical. Consequently, current approaches to using robots to support specific actions as part of a team—for example, within the Army, supporting Urban Area Operations—emphasize tele-operation, requiring one or more designated soldiers to serve as an Operator/Controller. This creates an artificial barrier between the human and the robot, imposes additional personnel requirements, introduces significant performance lags in time-critical scenarios, and reduces the effective support robots can bring to their teammates. To make this interaction more effective, intuitive communication, collaboration, and problem solving between humans and their robot teammates must be supported. This requires technology solutions, grounded in both neuroscientific and cybernetic approaches, which provide robots with the basic abilities to interact with people using human-like representations, strategies, and knowledge—solutions that may be provided by neuroadaptive systems.

10.5.3 Learning and Memory

Learning is the neurocognitive process through which information is encoded into memory (Cohn and Forsythe 2008). Quick and accurate information recall, therefore, critically depends on effectively consolidating relevant information into memories. With the growing trends in developing information systems that display increasingly greater amounts of data, new technologies are needed to optimize the neurocognitive processes underlying the storage of information into memory. The traditional memory theory divides this process into two stages: (1) acquiring information into working memory; and (2) encoding this information into long-term memory (Wickens and Hollands 2000). Recent findings indicate that memorization and subsequent recall are optimized when these two processes are coordinated in time (Lisman and Idiart 1995). To do this effectively, however, requires identifying the basic neural markers of these memory processes and using the timing of these markers to correctly phase the presentation of the to-be-remembered information to ensure coordination.

At the neural scale, memory formation depends on interactions between different patterns of nerve cell activity (Sederberg et al. 2003) that appear as waves of synchronization across the brain (Singer 1999; Axmacher et al. 2006). Two of the most important frequencies are gamma and theta (Kahana, Seelig, and Madsen 2001; Kahana 2006), both of which are essential for acquiring, encoding, and recalling memories (Mormann et al. 2005; Osipova et al. 2006). Computational models (Lisman and Idiart 1995) suggest that gamma waves enable the acquisition of information into working memory, whereas theta waves facilitate the subsequent encoding of this information into long-term memory (Jensen and Lisman 2005). These findings are supported by recent demonstrations that link these frequency signals with cognitive performance on memory tasks (Logar et al. 2008). Consequently, neuroadaptive technologies that can detect gamma and theta patterns should provide the timing cues necessary to correctly stage information presentation to optimize the acquisition and encoding of information into memories, leading to more effective and accurate recall.

10.6 Conclusion

The field of neuroadaptation lies at the intersection of neuroscience and engineering. Collectively, advances in these areas continue to enable the development of a comprehensive theory, and associated technologies, that will ultimately allow humans and their machines to cooperatively achieve a shared set of goals. Although past attempts at developing truly neuroadaptive systems have not completely achieved the vision of closed-loop symbiosis, they have paved the way for increasingly more sophisticated theories and technologies that will enable the attainment of this vision. Most recently, advances on several fronts have significantly advanced the state of the art in human–machine interactions. It remains to be seen to what extent researchers will be able to integrate these advances in new and exciting ways to support human performance.

Conflicts of Interest

Views, opinions, and/or findings contained in this chapter are those of the authors and should not be interpreted as representing official views or policies, either expressed or implied, of the Defense Advanced Research Projects Agency or the Department of Defense. Distribution Statement "A" (Approved for Public Release, Distribution Unlimited).

References

Aamodt, S. and S. Wang. 2008. *Welcome to Your Brain. Why You Lose Your Car Keys but Never Forget How to Drive and Other Puzzles of Everyday Life*. New York: Bloomsbury.
Adams, J. A. 1957. *Some Considerations in the Design and Use of Dynamic Flight Simulators*. Air Force Research Report AFPTRC-TN-57-51. Texas: Lackland Air Force Base.

Ambady, N. and R. Rosenthal. 1993. Half a minute: Predicting teacher evaluations from thin slices of behavior and physical attractiveness. *Journal of Personality and Social Psychology* 64: 431–41.

Anderson, J. R. 1996. ACT: A simple theory of complex cognition. *American Psychologist* 51: 355–65.

Anderson, J. R., C. S. Carter, J. M. Fincham, Y. Qin, S. M. Ravizza, and M. Rosenberg-Lee. 2008. Using fMRI to test models of complex cognition. *Cognitive Science* 32: 1323–48.

Axmacher, N., F. Mormann, G. Fernandez, C. Elger, and J. Fell. 2006. Memory formation by neuronal synchronization. *Brain Research Reviews* 52: 170–82.

Bates, J. A. V. 1947. Some characteristics of a human operator. *Journal of the Institute of Electrical Engineering* 94: 298–304.

Bergstrom, H. C., C. G. McDonald, H. T. French, and R. F. Smith. 2008. Continuous nicotine administration produces selective, age-dependent structural alteration of pyramidal neurons from prelimbic cortex. *Synapse* 62 (1): 31–9.

Birmingham, H. P. and F. V. Taylor. 1954. A design philosophy for man-machine control systems. *Proceedings of the I.R.E.* 42 (12): 1748–58.

Chapanais, A. 1951. Theory and methods for analyzing errors in man-machine systems. *Annals of the New York Academy of Sciences* 51: 1179–203.

Cooley, M. 2007. Cognition, communication and interaction: Transdisciplinary perspectives on interactive technology. In *On Human-Machine Symbiosis. Human-Computer Interaction Series*, edited by S. P. Gill, 457–85. London: Springer.

Cohn, J. V. and C. J. Forsythe. 2008. The effective use of performance enhancing technologies: Mechanisms, applications and policies. *Technology* 11: 107–26.

Cohn, J. V., R. Stripling, and A. Kruse. 2005. Investigating the transition from novice to expert. In *Foundations of Augmented Cognition*, edited by D. Schmorrow, 946–53. Mahwah, NJ: Lawrence Erlbaum Associates.

Craik, K. J. W. 1947. Theory of the human operator in control systems I: The operation of the human operator in control systems. *British Journal of Psychology* 38 (2): 56–61.

Craik, K. J. W. 1948. Theory of the human operator in control systems II: Man as an element in a control system. *British Journal of Psychology* 38 (3): 142–8.

Even, N., A. Cardona, M. Soudant, P. J. Corringer, J. P. Changeux, and I. Cloëz-Tayarani. 2008. Regional differential effects of chronic nicotine on brain alpha 4-containing and alpha 6-containing receptors. *Neuroreport* 19 (15): 1545–50.

Fitts, P. M. 1954. The information capacity of the human motor system in controlling the amplitude of movement. *Journal of Experimental Psychology* 47 (6): 381–91.

Fitts, P. M. and J. R. Peterson. 1964. Information capacity of discrete motor responses. *Journal of Experimental Psychology* 67 (2): 103–12.

Glimcher, P. W. and A. Rustichini. 2004. Neuroeconomics: The consilience of brain and decision. *Science* 306 (5695): 447–52.

Gluck, K. A. and R. W. Pew. 2005. *Modeling Human Behavior with Integrated Cognitive Architectures: Comparison, Evaluation and Validation*. Mahwah, NJ: Lawrence Erlbaum Associates.

Hammer, J. M. and R. L. Small. 1995. An intelligent interface in an associate system. In *Human/Technology Interaction in Complex Systems*, Vol. 7, edited by W. B. Rouse, 1–44. Greenwich, CT: JAI Press.

Haynes, J.-D. and G. Rees. 2006. Decoding mental states from brain activity in humans. *Nature Reviews Neuroscience* 7 (7): 523–34.

Hick, W. E. 1952. On the rate of gain of information. *Quarterly Journal of Experimental Psychology* 4: 11–26.

Hodgkinson, G. P., J. Langan-Fox, and E. Sadler-Smith. Intuition: A fundamental bridging construct in the behavioral sciences. *British Journal of Psychology* 99 (1): 1–27.

Hyman, R. 1953. Stimulus information as a determinant of reaction time. *Journal of Experimental Psychology* 45: 188–96.

Jensen, O. and J. E. Lisman. 2005. Hippocampal sequence-encoding driven by a cortical multi-item working memory buffer. *Trends in Neuroscience* 28 (2): 67–72.

Junghöfer, M., T. Elbert, D. M. Tucker, and B. Rockstroh. 2000. Statistical control of artifacts in dense array EEG/MEG studies. *Psychophysiology* 37 (4): 523–32.

Kahana, M. J. 2006. The cognitive correlates of human brain oscillations. *The Journal of Neuroscience* 26 (6): 1669–72.

Kahana, M. J., D. Seelig, and J. R. Madsen. 2001. Theta returns. *Current Opinion in Neurobiology* 11: 739–44.

Kalivas, P. W. 2007. Neurobiology of cocaine addiction: Implications for new pharmacotherapy. *American Journal on Addictions* 16 (2): 71–8.

Kay, K. N., T. Naselaris, R. J. Prenger, and J. L. Gallant. 2008. Identifying natural images from human brain activity. *Nature* 452: 352–5.

Kelso, J. A. S. 1995. *Dynamic Patterns: The Self-Organization of Brain and Behavior*. Cambridge, MA: MIT Press.

Licklider, J. C. R. 1960. Man-computer symbiosis. *IEEE Transactions on Human Factors in Electronics* 1: 4–11.

Lim, B. C. and K. J. Klein. 2006. Team mental models and team performance: A field study of the effects of team mental model similarity and accuracy. *Journal of Organizational Behaviour* 27: 403–18.

Lisman, J. E. and M. A. P. Idiart. 1995. Short-term memories in oscillatory subcycles. *Science* 267 (5203): 1512–5.

Logar, V., A. Belič, B. Koritnik, J. Brežan, J. Zidar, R. Karba, and D. Matko. 2008. Using ANNs to predict a subject's response based on EEG traces. *Neural Networks* 21: 881–7.

Logothetis, N. K. 2001. Neurophysiological investigation of the basis of the fMRI signal. *Nature* 412: 150.

Luu, P., A. Geyer, C. Fidopiastis, G. Campbell, T. Wheeler et al. 2010. Reentrant processing in intuitive perception. *PLoS One* 5 (3): e9523.

McDonald, C. G., V. K. Dailey, H. C. Bergstrom, T. L. Wheeler, A. K. Eppolito, L. N. Smith, and R. F. Smith. 2005. Periadolescent nicotine administration produces enduring changes in dendritic morphology of medium spiny neurons from nucleus accumbens. *Neuroscience Letters* 385 (2): 163–7.

McDonald, C. G., A. K. Eppolito, J. M. Brielmaier, L. N. Smith, H. C. Bergstrom, M. R. Lawhead, and R. F. Smith. 2007. Evidence for elevated nicotine-induced structural plasticity in nucleus accumbens of adolescent rats. *Brain Research* 1151: 211–8.

McRuer, D. T. and H. R. Jex. 1967. A review of quasi linear pilot models. *IEEE Transactions on Human Factors in Electronics* 3: 231–49.

Mitchell, T. M., R. Hutchinson, R. S. Niculescu, F. Pereira, X. Wang, M. A. Just, and S. D. Newman. 2004. Learning to decode cognitive states from brain images. *Machine Learning* 57: 145–75.

Mitchell, T. M., S. V. Shinkareva, A. Carlson, K.-M. Chang, V. L. Malave, R. A. Mason, and M. A. Just. 2008. Predicting human brain activity associated with the meanings of nouns. *Science* 320: 1191–5.

Mormann, F., J. Fell, N. Axmacher, B. Weber, K. Lehnertz, C. E. Elger, and G. Fernandez. 2005. Phase/amplitude reset and theta-gamma interaction in the human medial temporal lobe during a continuous word recognition memory task. *Hippocampus* 15: 890–900.

Morrison, J. G. and J. P. Gluckman. 1994. Definitions and prospective guidelines for the application of adaptive automation. In *Human Performance in Automated Systems: Current Research and Trends*, edited by M. Mouloua and R. Parasuraman, 256–63. Hillsdale, NJ: Lawrence Erlbaum Associates.

Newell, A. 1994. *Unified Theories of Cognition*. Cambridge, MA: Harvard University Press.

Osipova, D., A. Takashima, R. Oostenveld, G. Fernandez, E. Maris, and O. Jensen. 2006. Theta and gamma oscillations predict encoding and retrieval of declarative memory. *The Journal of Neuroscience* 26 (28): 7523–31.

Palva, J. M., S. Palva, and K. Kaila. 2005. Phase synchrony among neuronal oscillations in the human cortex. *The Journal of Neuroscience* 25 (15): 3962–72.

Parasuraman, R. and V. Riley. 1997. Humans and automation: Use, misuse, disuse, abuse. *Human Factors* 39: 230–53.

Parasuraman, R., T. B. Sheridan, and C. D. Wickens. 2000. A model for types and levels of human interaction with automation. *IEEE Transactions on Systems, Man, and Cybernetics—Part A: Systems and Humans* 30: 286–97.

Parsons, H. M. 1985. Automation and the individual: Comprehensive and comparative views. *Human Factors* 27: 99–112.

Philiastides, M. G. and P. Sajda. 2007. EEG-informed fMRI reveals spatiotemporal characteristics of perceptual decision making. *The Journal of Neuroscience* 27 (48): 13082–91.

Polesskaya, O. O., K. J. Fryxell, A. D. Merchant, L. L. Locklear, K. F. Ker, C. G. McDonald, A. K. Eppolito, L. N. Smith, T. L. Wheeler, and R. F. Smith. 2007. Nicotine causes age-dependent changes in gene expression in the adolescent female rat brain. *Neurotoxicology and Teratology* 29 (1): 126–40.

Rensink, R. A. 2004. Visual sensing without seeing. *Psychological Science* 15: 27–32.

Rouse, W. B. 1977. Human-computer interaction in multitask situations. *IEEE Transactions Systems, Man, and Cybernetics* 7: 293–300.

Rouse, W. B., N. D. Geddes, and R. E. Curry. 1988. An architecture for intelligent interfaces: Outline of an approach to supporting operators of complex systems. *Human-Computer Interaction* 3: 87–122.

Scerbo, M. W. 1996. Theoretical perspectives on adaptive automation. In *Automation and Human Performance: Theory and Applications*, edited by R. Parasuraman and M. Mouloua, 37–63. Mahwah, NJ: Lawrence Erlbaum Associates.

Scerbo, M. W., F. G. Freeman, P. J. Mikulka, R. Parasuraman, R., F. Di Nocero, and J. P. Lawrence, III. 2001. The efficacy of physiological measures for implementing adaptive technology. NASA TP-2001-211018. Hampton, VA: NASA Langley Research Center.

Schmorrow, D., J. Cohn, and D. Nicholson, eds. 2009. *PSI Handbook of Virtual Environments for Training and Education: Developments for the Military and Beyond—Volume 1, Learning Requirements and Metrics*. Santa Barbara, CA: Praeger Security International.

Schmorrow, D. D. 2005. *Foundations of Augmented Cognition*. Mahwah, NJ: Lawrence Erlbaum Associates.

Schmorrow, D. D., K. Stanney, and L. Reeves. 2007. *Foundations of Augmented Cognition: Past, Present and Future*. Arlington, VA: Strategic Analysis.

Sederberg, P. B., M. J. Kahana, M. W. Howard, E. J. Donner, and J. R. Madsen. 2003. Theta and gamma oscillations during encoding predict subsequent recall. *The Journal of Neuroscience* 23 (34): 10809–14.

Shinkareva, S. V., R. A. Mason, V. L. Malave, W. Wang, T. M. Mitchell, and M. A. Just. 2008. Using fMRI brain activation to identify cognitive states associated with perception of tools and dwellings. *PLoS ONE* 3: e1394.

Singer, W. 1999. Neuronal synchrony: A versatile code for the definition of relations? *Neuron* 24: 49–65.

Stevens, S. S. 1957. On the psychophysical law. *Psychological Review* 64 (3): 153–81.

Weiner, E. L. 1989. *Human Factors of Advanced Technology ("Glass Cockpit") Transport Aircraft*. NASA Technical Report 117528. Moffett Field, CA: NASA—Ames Research Center.

Weiner, E. L. and R. E. Curry. 1980. Flight deck automation: Promises and problems. *Ergonomics* 23: 995–1011.

Wickens, C. D. and J. G. Hollands. 2000. *Engineering Psychology and Human Performance*, 3rd ed. Upper Saddle River, NJ: Prentice Hall.

Wilson, K. A., E. Salas, H. A. Priest, and D. Andrews. 2007. Errors in the heat of battle: Taking a closer look at shared cognition breakdowns through teamwork. *Human Factors* 49: 243–56.

Winerman, L. 2005. A "sixth sense?" Or merely mindful caution? *Monitor on Psychology* 36 (3): 62.

Woods, D. D. 1996. Decomposing automation: Apparent simplicity, real complexity. In *Automation and Human Performance: Theory and Applications*, edited by R. Parasuraman and M. Mouloua 3–18. Mahwah, NJ: Lawrence Erlbaum Associates.

Xiao, C., R. Nashmi, S. McKinney, H. Cai, J. M. McIntosh, and H. A. Lester. 2009. Chronic nicotine selectively enhances alpha4beta2* nicotinic acetylcholine receptors in the nigrostriatal dopamine pathway. *The Journal of Neuroscience* 29 (40): 12428–39.

Young, L. R. 1969. On adaptive manual control. *IEEE Transactions on Man-Machine Systems* 10: 292–331.

11

Eye-Tracking Data Analysis and Neuroergonomics

Heiner Bubb and Martin Wohlfarter

CONTENTS

11.1 Neuroergonomics and Information Processing

In 1945, the physicist Felix Bloch of Stanford University, along with Edward Purcell of Harvard University, succeeded in measuring the so-called nuclear spin resonance of liquids. Both researchers received the Nobel Prize in physics for this detection. The effect is based on the fact that the nucleons of atoms have their own rotation; this rotation is the spin that generates a magnetic field. If (a probe of) a material is brought in a strong homogeneous magnetic field, the single spins of the nucleons perform a precession movement around the direction of the magnetic field of the electromagnet (they behave like a spinning top influenced by a force, in this case that of the magnetic field). Simultaneously, another electric inductor generates another weaker altering magnetic field perpendicular to the measuring field (the frequency of which is changed slowly). If the frequency of the measuring field matches the precession movement of the respective nuclear spins, its direction tilts as a result of this resonance process. The energy necessary for this tilting is measured by the measuring coil as increased current consumption. Because atoms have different resonance frequencies, depending on their number of protons and neutrons, the type of the atoms can be detected. This method of nuclear spin resonance is used for magnetic resonance tomography and magnetic resonance imaging (MRI), which are especially prominent in the medical field. Using the MRI technique generally involves having the test person or patient rest in a lying position, back down, on a sliding bed which is then slid into an electric inductor, which generates a high-frequency magnetic field. In an adjacent room, a computer that is connected to the magnetic resonance tomography machine receives the data output. The received data are typically sectional images of the body that can be combined into a spatial picture containing coordinates not only of the body surface but also of internal organs and the skeleton. In 1992, Seiji Ogawa and coworkers discovered that with this nuclear spin tomography the oxygenation of the hemoglobin in blood cells was being detected. Consequently, it was possible to indirectly track the blood flow of the brain to a nearly exact measurement in space and time. Assumedly, the brain areas that show a large blood supply are also those areas that are especially active, which means that this technology permits the measurement of a fully conscious person lying in the scanner tube. In addition to medical uses, this sort of technology is used in basic and applied research settings, where, for example, participants solve different types of problems or perform various types of tasks while in the scanner. This form of MRI coupled with tasks is called functional magnetic resonance imaging (fMRI).

In the 1990s, Parasuraman took fMRI methodology and applied it to the field of ergonomics, creating a new branch of ergonomics called "neuroergonomics." He described neuroergonomics as ". . . studies [that] involve an examination of the neural bases of such perceptual and cognitive functions as seeing, hearing, attending, remembering, deciding and planning in relation to technologies and settings in the real world" (Parasuraman 2003). In this description, an essential ergonomic research direction is touched upon, addressing in particular increasingly intelligent machines. Indeed, it has to be asked whether ergonomic knowledge can be gained from MRI experiments. At least under the current technical conditions MRI experiments are still more experimental than applicative; this is primarily because such experiments require a person to lie in the machine. Additionally, owing to the spatial restrictions of the machine, experiments are typically oriented around presenting visual (e.g., pictures) or acoustical stimuli to a test person. As a result, experiments are also limited to more a simplistic scheme, where button presses can communicate task responses. A more detailed investigation of fMRI shows that this methodology does not directly measure neural processes but rather correlates a certain task with activated brain areas.

This procedure has a methodological problem in terms of its application. Grau (2003) states that the fascinating contrast sharpness of the published pictures is the product of an idealization, as the actual values measured by the detectors hardly differ; that is why the measured signals are optimized by means of statistical procedures. Subcomponents of the brain do not work in isolation of each other, but rather the whole brain operates constantly and some regions are more required than others according to different tasks. This background activity of the brain is the focus of the research in particular nowadays.

The research team of Marcus E. Raichle, when dealing with slow cortical potentials, recognized that certain neuron groups fire about every tenth of a second. The problem is that slow to very slow potential fluctuations or waves on the surface of the brain are normally not recorded by an electroencephalogram. These very slow waves have a large influence on remaining events. The higher-frequency electric activity synchronizes itself with the phases of the slow fluctuations. According to Raichle (2010), a comparison to a symphony orchestra fits to a certain extent. As all the different instruments play to the same rhythm, they generate specific sound scenery. This image applied to the brain reveals that the extremely slow oscillations correspond to the beat of the conductor. Indeed, the performers—the single brain system—are not given a common beat, but rather they are given access to a vast archive in the brain, full of memories and other information. Without this access, life would not be possible in this complicated and constantly changing world. The very slow waves allow right calculations to take place at the right time. Additionally, this sophisticated system of internal brain self-adjustment has to occasionally follow surrounding conditions; new or unexpected sensations or specific actions come to the foreground. As soon as these systems "switch off" again, because the order is finished, the internal communication traffic of very slow potential fluctuations revives again.

The well-known neurophysiologist Wolf Singer claimed that perception is the reality reconstructed by our brain. Today, perception is considered to be based on the coordinated activity of many cortical areas. During an interview with Epping (2009), Singer said, "you must fancy this so: The system is constantly active, everybody talks all the time with all, and they generate constantly incredibly complicated patterns. Then, an incoming message enters via the ears or eyes and this message spreads out like a brush fire. While doing so, it changes everywhere a little the state. But only some of it penetrates till the consciousness."

To optimally design informatory tasks there has to be an idea of how a user sees, for example, technical equipment, the so-called internal picture of the outside world of the user and, in particular, how this picture possibly changes during use. To get an idea of these processes, already established neuroscientific knowledge needs to be accessed. For ergonomic application, illustrated in Figure 11.1, a sort of shell model appears suitable. In the most central shell, processes occurring in the neuron cells are considered. Their changes occur in synaptic connections during information transfers. In the next higher shell, the different effects of the different connection possibilities of the neuron cells are taken into account. It is known that the receptor cells connect with the following cells to complex and hyper-complex cells. Many special aspects of perception can be understood, as described in the following paragraphs.

The next higher located shell refers to the functional aerials of the brain, that is, the knowledge that can assign specific mental activities to certain local areas in the brain (much of this knowledge has been acquired by MRI studies on patients with cerebral lesions).

The external shell contains internal representations of the outside world, which are also referred to as "internal models," which are represented by specific connections of the neuron cells. Such internal models often cover locally several areas of the brain. According to Singer, their contents can be conscious or unconscious depending on the external condition (see Epping 2009). However, even in the last case, they can be a cause for actions observable from the outside.

The idea of human information processing using the mentioned shells has to be confirmed in their fundamental structure by specific fMRI experiments, in addition to complementary psychological and physiological experiments. All in all, these experiments

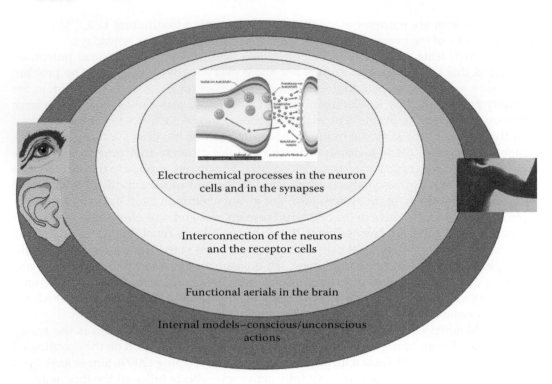

Electrochemical processes in the neuron
cells and in the synapses

Interconnection of the neurons
and the receptor cells

Functional aerials in the brain

Internal models—conscious/unconscious
actions

FIGURE 11.1
(See color insert.) Shell model of human information processing.

give a better idea of how human data processing is structured. However, to derive conclusions about the design of technical devices, it is necessary to achieve a realistic experimental scenario that allows us to also monitor brain activity. At the moment, this is only achieved by observing several visible reactions of the brain as far as possible, from the outside, in a strict temporal order. An excellent "peer tube" into the brain is the study of eye movements. This is primarily because gazes directed to an object (so-called areas of interest, AOI) are normally unconscious. Also, the movement of the corporeal extremities is controlled only partly consciously. The observation of these movements as well as the capturing of external information that influences the organism (noise, acceleration, thermal stimulus, smell) is an essential means of exploring what happens in the brain, along with the basic knowledge of neurophysiology and psychology.

Still, in principle, only certain activities can be ascertained at one time. Examining traffic and the interaction between driver–vehicle is worthwhile and important because it concerns the human himself and the material costs of the consequences of an accident. Actually, the car is mostly a prime example for ergonomically designing the human–machine interaction for the following reasons:

- The vehicle demands almost all ergonomic design areas (design of the environment, anthropometric and information technical design).
- The "unqualified" driver makes the highest demands on the ergonomic design.
- The driving task is easy and clear to describe: the vehicle has to be moved in such a way that no objects standing or moving on the street are touched. However, in

different traffic situations this task can become quite complicated and, therefore, very demanding.

- In the vehicle, basic interactions occur between the human and machine, namely "tracking" (i.e., following the course given by the street and other road users), "selecting," and "deciding" (i.e., making a decision on the basis of the traffic situation; for instance, with the change of traffic light from "green" to "red," deciding to "stop" or "still drive through," or deciding whether some control elements have to be operated in the vehicle to accomplish "tertiary tasks" (see below)).

The following sections are concerned with car driving in connection with human information processing. First, a theoretical model will be presented regarding ideas based on the knowledge gained from neurological findings as well as accompanying physiological and psychological experiments. The ideas of this model will be specified and verified by experimental findings.

11.2 Car Driving from the Viewpoint of Information Processing

Traffic safety research focuses on two important issues: how task information gets into the brain of the driver and how it is processed. A model of human information processing is considered to understand driver behavior more comprehensively. Figure 11.2 shows a general model that is drawn as a rectangle, in agreement with the system technique rules. The left side represents the information put in, characterized by the sense organs. The right side represents the information put out, characterized by speech and posture or movement of the upper and lower extremities. Both input and output sides are connected by the

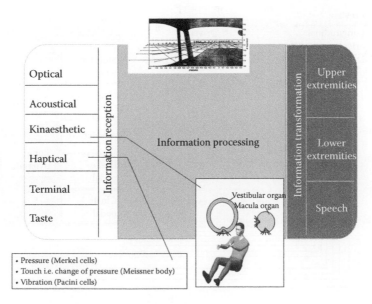

FIGURE 11.2
(See color insert.) General model of human information processing.

central information processing unit—the brain. A specific property of human information processing is convergence–divergence behavior. This means that from the immense amount of information coming in (more than 10^6 bits per second), only a portion of it can actively be processed (about 3 to 4 bits per second). However, on the output side, much more information can be observed by unconscious, autonomously initiated behavior, causing many muscles to become innerved.

In 1971, Rockwell reported that when driving a car about 90% of the information relevant to decision making is absorbed by the visual canal. This sensory canal, therefore, is of special importance for leading a car in traffic. Nevertheless, it has to be taken into consideration that, besides the visual canal, information perceived from the kinesthetic as well as the acoustic sensory canals are also important for correct car driving (Bubb 1977; Timpe 2001). Particularly, acceleration and the feeling of speed are supported by both these senses.

In explaining the interaction between the driver and the vehicle through scientific means, the human driver has to be described in technical terminology. The goal is to simulate this interaction in order to improve it by appropriate design. For this description, the closed-loop paradigm is suitable. The closed loop generally serves as a basic scheme of ergonomics (see Helander 1988; Bubb 1993; Schmidtke 1993; and Figure 11.3). In the 1940s and 1950s, modeling of the human operator by methods of the control theory, having their origin in the cybernetics of Wiener (1948) and Shannon and Weaver (1949), expected human information processing to be treated as a natural science, similar to that of physics (Jürgensohn 1997).

Driving a car can be seen under this closed-loop paradigm like any control system of a machine. The driving task is thus determined by the course of the road, vehicles, and other

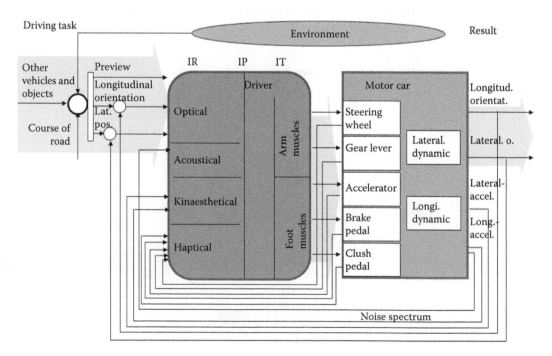

FIGURE 11.3
(**See color insert.**) Closed-loop driver—car.

traffic participants, as well as environmental and weather conditions. Here, the desired lateral position of the car on the road and its longitudinal position—equivalent to the desired speed—are determined in detail. The task of the driver is to detect the necessary information from the visual environment and to transform it in adequate operation of the control elements so that the actual lateral and longitudinal position of the car corresponds totally to the desired position; this is called the "result." The driving task can be reduced to the demand that every contact with standing or moving objects has to be avoided in the traffic field. The described task corresponds with the "stabilization task." To accomplish this, the driver has to determine the desired course and to decide in the immediate surrounding field of around 200 meters how the vehicle should move in location and time. This part of the task is called the "guiding task." The "navigation task" is the precondition for executing the guiding task. This task presents, in general, how the existing road network should be connected in order to reach the desired destination. The actual state of the car has to match with all these levels of tasks.

The description above does not encompass all tasks that have to be accomplished during driving. According to Geiser (1985), the total driving task can be divided into many subtasks. The *primary driving task* is described above, that is, the actual driving process, aimed at keeping the car on the road.

Besides this task, the driver has to accomplish additional tasks. These additional tasks typically present themselves along with the primary driving task and are dependent on the traffic and on environmental conditions. Furthermore, tasks that are necessary to inform other traffic participants about intended maneuvers are also part of a driver's task list. For example, operation of the direction signals, the windshield wiper, the light switch, the horn, and, in the case of a manual car, the gear lever and clutch pedal is also part of these tasks. Assistance systems like speed control or the autonomous cruise control (ACC) system also have to be operated on this level. All these control elements have to be used depending directly or indirectly on the driving task. Therefore, they are assigned as *secondary tasks*. Looking closer, they can be divided into reactive tasks and active tasks; reactions to a change of external conditions, like dipping the headlight for oncoming traffic or switching on the wipers in response to rainfall, are reactive tasks that can principally be automated. Active tasks are those by which the driver shows his intention (e.g., using the horn).

Tasks that have nothing to do with the driving tasks but aim to improve the needs of comfort, entertainment, and information are called *tertiary tasks*. The use of the heating/climate system, radio, telephone, and, in the future, Internet and communication with office and home technologies also belong to these tasks.

Although, owing to technical development, the load of information processing in secondary and tertiary tasks caused by the design of the equipment is currently being researched, investigation and design of the primary task are still of upmost importance, promising a reduction of accident frequency and improved operation of the car.

11.3 Information Processing: The Eye as a Window into the Brain

While driving a car, the driver must take in a lot of information, which he must evaluate to make decisions and to act suitably. To be able to understand these connections, it is necessary to point out the internal processes of the person in terms of the global frame discussed in the opening paragraph of this chapter. For this description, the standard categorization of human information processing in perception, processing, and realization of information is used.

11.3.1 How Does Information Enter the Brain?

If a person is in a room, he will always have the impression of being completely aware of everything around him. Without thinking too much about it, an accurate assessment about the surrounding environment can be made. This even includes a more or less exact idea of the areas that cannot be perceived with a current field of vision (i.e., the area of the room behind where a person stands). As the observer, a photographic-like picture of this room seems to represent the impression of a room in its detailed richness, even if the feeling of spatial distances and "being in this space" are limited or even missing.

On the contrary, objectively, it is known that at a very fundamental physical/physiological level, the human eye is only capable of seeing sharp in the central visual field (fovea centralis); this, however, only corresponds to a viewing angle of approximately 2 to 3 degrees. In this area of the eye, the number of receptors is also the densest; only in this area can color vision occur. The number of color receptors (cones) decreases steadily toward the periphery. At the periphery, there are fewer possibilities to connect the receptor cells, meaning that only some combinations of neuron cells (complex and hyper-complex) are capable of detecting edges or angles. On the other hand, motion receptors are more commonly found here. As a matter of fact, it is well known that the above-described impression of the subjective feeling of "being in the world" is a construct of our brain caused by successive scanning of the moving eye. However, this also entails that important things can be overlooked. If it is believed that one already knows the outcome of an event (for static objects this is quite natural) on the basis of previous experience, one would likely turn away.

While the environment has three dimensions, the picture on the retina has only two. Despite this, we are nevertheless able to perceive a three-dimensional environment. Therefore, most questions of visual perception deal with the question of depth perception. Depth perception occurs by interpretation of the interocular distance overlapping and slightly different visual fields of both eyes. Figure 11.4 represents the geometrical constellation of the picture of spatial circumstances on a two-dimensional picture surface. With the knowledge of the interocular distance and the focal length of the eye, while fixating on an object in each of the pictures, the suitable spatial position can be calculated. This is something that our brain has learned to do quite efficiently (typically during adolescence) and does so simply and mostly automatically. Admittedly, the spatial visual ability by stereoscopy finds its limit with a distance of approximately 40 meters.

Helmholtz (1866), with his treatise on physiological optics, laid the groundwork for a description of visual perception. Nowadays, these descriptions have come to be known as the laws of the optics in physics and as a description of the visual process in biology. To be able to understand the process of visual information perception while driving a vehicle, the knowledge of a simplified visual process is not sufficient. The aim of the following paragraph is not to describe in detail all processes of visual perception, but rather to describe in detail single parts of the process to lend an idea of how visual information is perceived while driving a vehicle.

What are the essential steps of the visual process? Visual perception begins with the reflexing of beams of a light source (e.g., the sun, floodlight) on physical objects or light beams that are emitted immediately by an object (e.g., floodlights of oncoming vehicles,

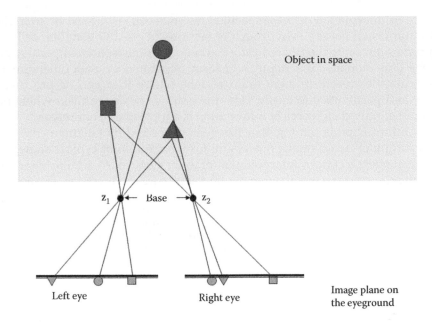

FIGURE 11.4
(See color insert.) Principle of the stereoscopic picture of a spatial constellation at two picture surfaces.

back lights, signal lamps to the traffic control). Light bundled up by the lens is caught in the retina by sensory cells. A two-dimensional picture of the outside world—like with a camera—is created, as shown in Figure 11.4. Although it is not yet known exactly how, generally speaking the light quants are converted into electric signals, which travel over the visual nerve into the brain. The retinal image can be seen as a two-dimensional needle picture (Gibson 1950). A good idea of how this happens was illustrated by Lindsay and Norman (1972): the connection types of the lateral inhibition and the negative feedback are already realized at the lowest level of perception immediately in connection with the receptor cells. If several neurons are interconnected at one neuron cell, there are cells that emit only an increased impulse rate if a certain pattern configuration on the sensory surface exists; these are the so-called complex cells. Also, these complex cells are again interconnected to hyper-complex cells, which show an increased impulse rate only with even more complexly arranged stimulus configurations. It can be imagined that in the manner shown here, a whole series of specific detectors can be formed. The following specific detectors have been discovered experimentally at the level of the hyper-complex cells: edge detectors and motion detectors, angle detectors, and detectors for specific lengths.

Werblin and Roska (2008) discovered that about a dozen quite different representations of the visual scene can be detected in this manner. Each of these representations contains another partial aspect of what happens in front of the eye. The abstractions are updated consecutively, adapted to the outside events, and contain the following information:

1. Object outlines (comparably of an outline drawing)
2. Speed and motion direction of the objects of the visual scene
3. Shady and bright areas

Each piece of information of these specified nervous cells is passed on to higher brain regions by the visual nerve's own groups of nervous fibers, the ganglion cells. A single ganglion type represents the filtered information of various spatiotemporal aspects of a visual scene like: motion, color, depth, and form. Separated by each other, partial information singularities reach different brain regions where they can be processed partly consciously and partly unconsciously. How the brain draws a seamless whole picture of reality from the individual pieces of information is a topic of current research.

How this information is put together has been described by Guzmán (1969). Guzmán invented a computer-based image processing for recognition of typical angle configurations, which suggest a certain interpretation of a flat picture. At similar viewpoints, the human brain seems to interpret the monocular flat picture on the retina. Figure 11.5 shows some examples of such configurations and their preferential interpretation. Figure 11.6

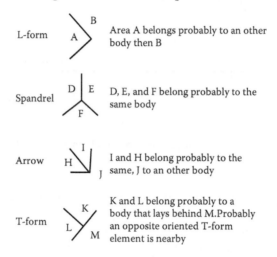

FIGURE 11.5
Typical angle configurations and their interpretation.

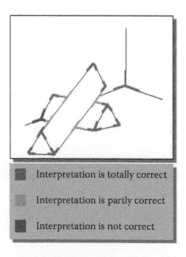

FIGURE 11.6
(**See color insert.**) Example of the application of typical angle configurations.

demonstrates how one applies this interpretation: two wooden logs, placed in a corner, that lie on top of each other are recognized. This interpretation cannot be denied if one firmly decides to see only a tangle of lines.

An analysis of neural processing by simple, complex, and hyper-complex cells shows that along with the increasing degree of complexity of the cells, caused by the type of incoming information, specificity too increases in terms of which information is extracted, leading, then, to the excitement of another cell specific for it. In the course of the analysis, less and less ganglions respond to a given signal. The high spontaneous activity rate at the low level of the neural processing becomes increasingly lower the higher the level of information processing. The cortex is in a state of relative rest, only interrupted sporadically by short spells of activation if relevant external signals appear. However, it seems to be a basic rule of the nervous system to find changes and differences and to consistently suppress remaining events. The latter can be seen as a higher-level adaptation mechanism.

The description of the perception process discussed until now is founded on the basis of physiological investigations. In contrast, the main idea described in the following is based more on psychological experiments. The "Pandemonium" model presented by Oliver Selfridge (1959) can be thought of as the further course of perception in the following manner: the cells that extract the simple qualities as discussed are switched to even higher cells in such a way that these react optimally only when a certain pattern corresponding to the specific interconnection is projected on the sensory surface. At the same time, several cells can be stimulated by the same stimulus configuration. Then, during further perception, that cell is selected which permits an integrated interpretation agreeing with contents according to memory. This becomes clear in Figure 11.6: "T-shaped" angle configurations suggest that the surface of the wooden log lying below is a part of a body that is identical with the room ground (see Figure 11.5). On account of other impressions and in favor of an integrated perception of the outside world, this interpretation is suppressed.

The described process refers not only to the perception of static surroundings but also to those of motion. Important in the technical environment is the seeing of a motion; it represents a sensory quality of the modality "seeing." Real motion perception takes place with the help of neuron systems "specific for motion" which are built up in all higher developed mammals mainly in the visual cortex. According to Rock (1968), the optical perception of movement can be understood well if the following working principles are assumed:

- The eyes never perceive the individual motion course of picture points on the retina, but always the mathematical components of it. The principle for motion perception is that equal components form a bounded unity and are distinguished in this manner from divergent components.
- If after selecting bounded unities from the picture field on the retina movement vectors are left, new bounded unities of a higher order are formed. These new unities are perceived in relative motion to the already formed unities.

Helmholtz (1866) introduced the concept of motion parallax. According to his definition, it describes the perspective shift of distant objects in different depths as a result of an observer's change in position. According to Helmholtz (1910), the motion parallax contains information about the distance between the observer and the object. This is valid for the case in which the observer moves toward the objects (see Figure 11.7) as well as for the case in which the observer moves along the objects (Figure 11.8).

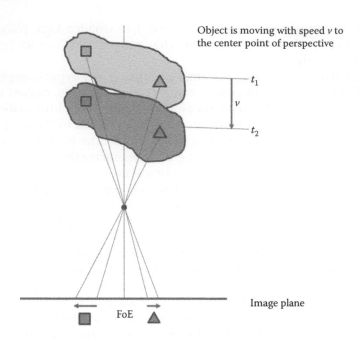

FIGURE 11.7
(See color insert.) Motion parallax: Objects with a different distance to the observer, which moves at the same speed, generate pictures of different speed on the image plane (retina) from which conclusions about the distance can be drawn. A unique point (focus of expansion, FoE) is given here on the straight connection between the focus of the central perspective and the point where the motion takes place.

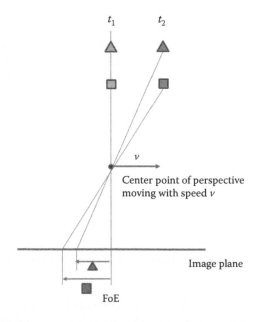

FIGURE 11.8
(See color insert.) Motion parallax: The observer moves past in objects of different distance with a speed v (e.g., as with the look from the window of a moving train). The farther away the observed objects are the less they move. The look on a point in the horizon shows no motion (focus of expansion, FoE).

11.3.2 The Optical Flow

In 1958, Gibson extended Helmholtz's definition of motion parallax and introduced his theory of visual control of locomotion by means of optical flow. Optical flow is the expanding or contracting visual field projected on the retina, which is caused by the motion of the observer (Gibson 1950). The representation of the speed vectors of all visible objects in a visual scene is understood here as the visual field. In other words, optical flow is the transformation of the surfaces of the surrounding optic array during locomotion (Gibson 1966), that is, the gradient of locomotion (Goldstein 2002). The optical flow is the relative motion between the observer and the visible space points projected on the picture surface (Chatziastros 2003). In the literature, several different definitions of optical flow can be found, which describe in different terms, the phenomenon observed by Gibson. In this text, the formulations of Gibson (1950, 1966) and Goldstein (2002) are referred to.

Optical flow characterizes the totality of optical changes in the visual scene (Chatziastros 2003) and represents the generalization of the motion parallax between a few objects on all objects of the visual field.

As already described, optical flow represents information produced by the motion of the observer. Between the locomotion of an observer and the optical flow, a reciprocal interrelation exists (Goldstein 2002). Optical flow is generated by the motion of the observer and serves information to the observer, which helps him to control and steer further motion. Figure 11.9 illustrates the relation that motion is the pre-condition of the perception of optical flow and perception is the basis of motion.

Figure 11.10 shows the optical flow of a simple movement situation, which can be derived from Helmholtz's considerations of the motion parallax in Figure 11.7. The points represent single elements of the environment; the lines describe their motion direction and, by the length, also the speed of the elements. In the center of the optical flow, neither a motion nor a motion parallax is visible (Warren et al. 2001). Hence, this point is called the focus of expansion (FoE) or "singular point" of the flow picture. FoE is the point from which the speed vectors seem to expand or contract radially depending on the direction of the movement. FoE indicates the movement direction of the observer in the case of a straight movement (Gibson 1950; Wann and Wilkie 2004; see also Figure 11.7).

Motions of an observer can be disassembled in translatory and rotatory components. A translatory motion generates a symmetrical flow field (see Figure 11.11). If the observer moves toward the FoE, the flow vectors point away and an expanding flow field is

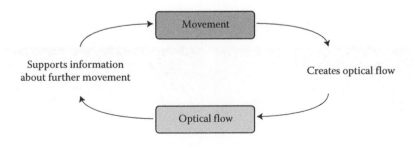

FIGURE 11.9
Reciprocal interrelation between locomotion and optical flow. Locomotion generates an optical flow, which presents information about the locomotion and thus steers the motion. This represents an important principle for our interaction with the environment. (After Goldstein, B. 2002. In *Wahrnehmungspsychologie*, 327–43. Heidelberg: Spektrum Akademischer Verlag.)

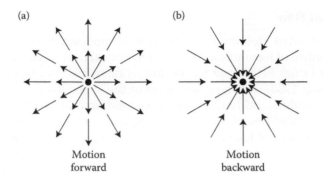

FIGURE 11.10
Optical flow (a) in the case of a motion forward and (b) in the case of a motion backward. (After Goldstein, B. 2002. In *Wahrnehmungspsychologie*, 327–43. Heidelberg: Spektrum Akademischer Verlag.)

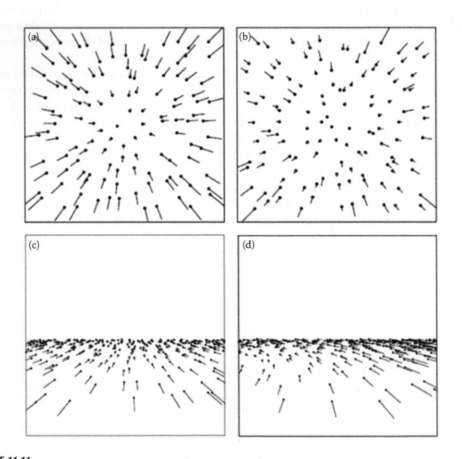

FIGURE 11.11
Optical flow on the picture surface when (a) driving vertically on a wall, (b) driving through a point volume, (c) driving straight ahead, and (d) driving in a curved journey. (After Chatziastros, A. 2003. Visuelle Kontrolle der Lokomotion. Dissertation. Germany: Justus-Liebig-Universität Gießen.)

generated, as shown in Figure 11.11a. If the observer moves away from the FoE, the flow vectors point at the center of the optical flow, generating a contracting flow field, as shown in Figure 11.11b.

The speed of the single elements and thereby the length of the vectors of the translatory flow picture depend on the distance of the environmental elements to the observer. With a linear translation, the angular speed of the elements is determined by the following relation:

$$\frac{d\theta}{dt} = (\sin\theta)^2 \cdot \frac{v}{x}$$

where v is the forward velocity of the observer, x is the distance of the elements vertically to the motion direction, and θ is the angle between the motion direction and the direction to the element of the visual scene (see Figure 11.12). The shorter the distance of elements to the observer, the greater the forward velocity and the higher the velocity in the optical flow.

The flow field, which is generated by a rotatory motion, contains parallel velocity vectors, each of which orient in the same direction. The rotatory or lamellar flow field contains no FoE. The length of the flow vectors in the rotatory flow field is independent of the distance of the elements to the observer; which is why the rotatory flow field, in contrast to the translatory flow field, gives no motion information to the observer. A cornering can be understood as the sum of translatory and rotatory motions. Analogously, the generated flow field can be seen as the overlap of translatory and rotatory flow fields (Figure 11.10d).

Self-generated movements of eyes, for example, caused by a glance sequence movement or a head movement, also generate a rotatory flow field (see Figure 11.13, middle). Nevertheless, this is separated from the movement of the whole body as described by the *reafference principle* of von Holst (1957), which explains some constant phenomena of perception. In the case of the *direction constant*, one needs to ask why when the eyeball rotates to the right, no subjective shift of the environment is recognized—even though the picture on the retina moves to the left by this movement. On the basis of the reafference principle, this effect is clarified by the fact that with every movement an internal model regarding the action exists (efference copy; see Figure 11.14). With a self-generated eye movement to the right, one expects that the picture will move to the left. If the picture really does move

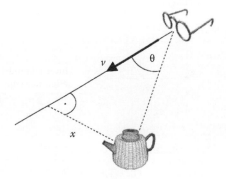

FIGURE 11.12
The angle velocity of an object (here teapot), is determined by the forward velocity v of an observer, the passing distance x, and the eccentricity θ of the object. (After Chatziastros, A. 2003. Visuelle Kontrolle der Lokomotion. Dissertation. Germany: Justus-Liebig-Universität Gießen.)

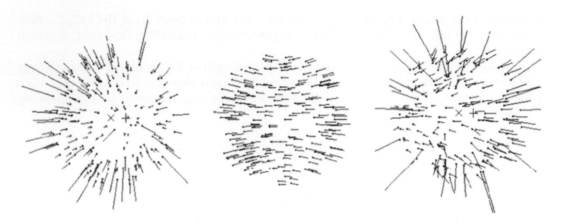

FIGURE 11.13
Generation of a retinal flow (on the right) as the sum of the flow field of a straight-ahead translatory motion (on the left) and the flow field of an independent eye movement (middle). (After Lappe, M. 2009. Visuelle Wahrnehmung von Bewegung. *Skriptum zum Seminar Visuelle Wahrnehmung von Bewegung,* Universität Münster. http://wwwpsy.uni-muenster.de/imperia/md/content/psychologie_institut_2/ae_lappe/freie_dokumente/einfuehrung1.pdf.)

to the left, actual and expected movements annihilate each other, and the environment is perceived as static. If the retinal picture moves without an autonomously initiated movement, movement is perceived as an objective fact. This can be illustrated by simply poking the corner of the eyeball from the outside with the fingertip. The comparison between the afference and the built-up picture in the brain is an unconscious process. Only after receiving inconsistent information will the process become conscious.

The resultant flow field from a translatory motion and an eye movement, from a translatory and a rotatory motion, or from a combination of all three motions does not differ in form. In all three cases, a complicated flow field is generated (see Figure 11.13, right). Because the optical flow, in this case, is only pictured on the retina and not on an image plane, this is referred to as *retinal flow.*

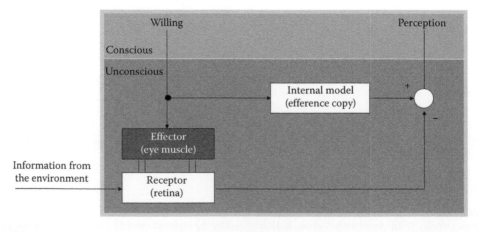

FIGURE 11.14
(See color insert.) Reafference principle. (After von Holst, E. 1957. *Studium Generale* 10 (4):232.)

From a translatory flow field, the processing of relatively simple information occurs without much effort. With the addition of a rotatory flow field, significant changes in the structure and the picture of the flow field occur, given the movement was self-initiated or rotatory. This necessarily also causes an increase in the amount of effort needed to process and perceive information from the flow field. Basic abilities in performing this operation are typically learned in the adolescent years of one's development. In terms of von Holst's (1957) reaference principle, a separation is made between motion initiated by the person and motion caused by "external influence." In other words, von Holst (1957) claimed that we are able to take the information provided by a given scene and filter out the effects that are caused by either the retinal flow field (movement of the eyes in the head), or the movement of the whole head, or even self-initiated rotary movement of the whole body.

Whereas the FoE with a translatory flow field can be equated with the actual movement direction, this is not possible with a complicated flow field. This raises the question: how does one handle a complicated flow field and in which way can this be processed? Are learnt abilities sufficient or are additional methods applied? To be able to answer these questions, numerous models have been developed.

In the preceding paragraph, which information the optical flow contains was explained. To be able to formulate a theory of the control of locomotion on the basis of optical flow, nevertheless, it must be ensured that the provided information can also be taken up and processed by the human brain. If this was not the case, the information about locomotion control would not be available at all. Therefore, how physiological processing of the optical flow works in the eye and in the brain, must be understood. Generally speaking, visual perception is the ability to detect, process, discriminate, and interpret visual stimuli. Visual perception can also be part of associating visual stimuli with former experiences, something beyond the pure absorption of information. Perception in general, and particularly here in visual perception, has already been investigated quite in depth. In the next section, perception will be briefly discussed on the basis of these already established investigations (see Fikus 1989; Mühlendyck 1990; Goldstein 2002).

The area in which the optical flow is on the retina is absolutely relevant for the perception of optical flow and the reception of information from the optical flow. As the receptor cells on the eye are connected in different eye regions, differently for complex and hypercomplex cells (e.g., in the fovea centralis preferred to edges and angle detectors and in the eye periphery preferred to movement detectors), which part is hit on the retina by the optical flow information can make a difference.

Peripheral or indirect sight describes a part of visual perception. In contrast to foveal vision, where an object must be positioned precisely at the center of fixation in order to have the maximum visual sharpness, peripheral vision provides rough, blurred, and optically distorted visual impressions, outside of the point of fixation (Goldstein 2002). The peripheral system covers more than 999 thousandth of the visual field. However, for the processing of information, only 50% of the visual nerve and 50% of the surface of the visual center are available to the peripheral system. The remaining 50% are left for the highly resolving but very slow fovea system. On account of this unequal relationship between the covered visual field and the amount of available resources, the properties of both foveal and peripheral perception differ. Moving outward from the fovea centralis, visual sharpness, color perception, sensibility to light, and the perception of contrasts decrease, whereas dynamic sensibility, temporal resolution, perception of brightness and darkness, as well as perception of movement and orientation increase (Goldstein 2002).

11.3.3 Information Processing

In terms of data processing from a cognitive perspective, one is able to perceive and interpret the environment around them via the provided visual information. Additionally, on the basis of this perception about the environment, one is able to optimally react to the environment. An essential precondition for information processing is the memory that includes, on the one hand, "internal models" that represent acquired knowledge and, on the other hand, a "decision mechanism" used in the decision-making stages of a concrete action. Therefore, the most important question is: how does the human brain link the external, ever-changing stimuli to its proper reaction? The following section will give an overview of this issue.

11.3.3.1 Human Memory

Because human memory is so fundamental to the current argument, we must have a more in-depth understanding of the working principle of memory. Memory can be roughly divided into sensory memory, short-term memory, and long-term memory. Sensory memory represents the lingering of the sensory cells and the complex and hyper-complex cells connected with them. Therefore, the capacity of the sensory memory corresponds to the capacity of the sensory organs. The retention time of sensory memory is not more than 200 milliseconds. The processes in short-term and long-term memory are very complex and only partly understood. For our purposes, only a simplified model of memory is needed, which is detailed enough to understand the principles of information processing during car driving. Figure 11.15 serves as a basis for explaining this model. Information that is received from the sensory organs and pre-selected by the complex and hyper-complex cells ("sensory memory") stimulates many neuron cells that may be distributed over different areas of the brain.

Some of the distributed cells may be closed to a circle. Such a circle represents active memory (Palm 1990). As long as one cell stimulates the other one, the information that is represented by this specific circle is actually present. This specific circle of connected cells represents the short-term, working, or primary memory, which typically keeps information active in our consciousness for between 3 and 15 seconds. Over time, when an

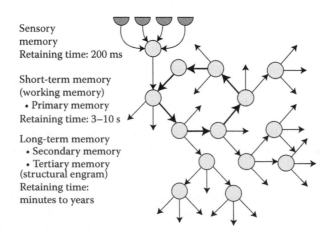

Sensory
memory
Retaining time: 200 ms

Short-term memory
(working memory)
• Primary memory
Retaining time: 3–10 s

Long-term memory
• Secondary memory
• Tertiary memory
(structural engram)
Retaining time:
minutes to years

FIGURE 11.15
A principle picture of human memory.

external or internal stimulation is received by the sensory organs, synapses can gradually be changed. So, certain circles that represent the repeated content are preferred over other neuronal connections. A structural engram is generated. When these circles are stimulated by an adequate external or internal (e.g., by active reflecting) stimulus configuration, the former experience is "remembered" again. We call this structural engram "long-term memory." Selfridge's Pandemonium model thought the ability of pattern recognition could be explained as an example of this process. In the course of time, these engrams can again disappear or be buried. We call this type of long-term memory "secondary memory." Its retention time can be between half a minute and years. Additionally, contents that are typically always remembered are stored in the "tertiary" type of long-term memory; for example, one's own name or the ability to walk, to ride a bicycle, or to swim belongs to this memory type. To realize a transition from primary memory to secondary memory, repetition and motivation play an important role. This process is controlled in the brain by the hippocampus and the limbic system.

Especially in connection with the dynamic properties of an automobile, the reaction time of human information processing is important. Through tracking experiments and the modeling of human properties by control theory methods (e.g., the research by McRuer and colleagues; see References), we know that the reaction time of unconscious, skill-based behavior (Rasmussen 1987) is around 200 milliseconds. However, when we want to understand the interaction between the driver and the car, not only this reaction time is important but also the subjective time horizon—the temporal context that the driver bases his actions on.

11.3.3.2 Internal Models

As shown in the previous paragraphs, categorization in information perception and processing is not in any specific order. Thus, essential elements of information processing are described by von Holst's principle in the same manner as aspects of information perception. The difference between information perception and information processing is only that more and more complicated efference copies are formed by a protracted learning process, beginning from infancy, which become "internal models." In Figure 11.16, Figure 11.15 has been extended by the model M_B (both figures are otherwise identical). An example of this is driving along a curve: when one comes to a rightward curve, it is not at all natural to know how much steering is needed to solve this driving task adequately. On account of a complicated learning process, the driver of an automobile forms an internal model M_A of how his vehicle reacts to steering and accelerator movements. Additionally, he already owns an internal model M_B, which indicates the actions he has to carry out in a given traffic situation. By his receptors, in particular the eye, but also by the acoustic, kinesthetic, and haptical canal, he takes up the given situation and derives from it an action sequence given by model M_B (model M_B can conclude only for simple-situation action sequences such as following a street course; in more complicated cases, decisions become necessary; see below). On account of this action sequence, with the help of model M_A, the driver has an expectation of the change of information from the outside world. If this change agrees with the actual ones, the whole process ordinarily remains unconscious. Only a divergence between the model idea and the feedback from the environment (if, for example, the steering behavior of the car on a smooth street is quite different from the usual) penetrates into the consciousness and makes the decision processes necessary, which then activate, perhaps, motor processes that were not included in the originally used model M_A (see Section 11.3.3.3).

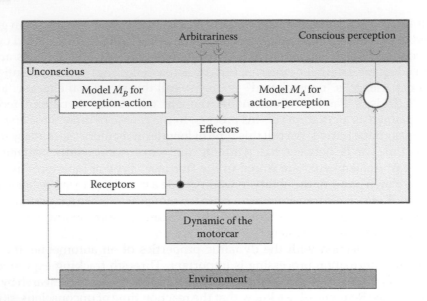

FIGURE 11.16
(See color insert.) Behavioral structure of more highly skilled activities in the example of automobile driving.

When working according to an internal model, the time necessary for this process can be estimated. It lies in the area of the already mentioned physiological response time of approximately 200 milliseconds. Additionally, external stimulus configurations (information perception) can excite certain absolutely "fuzzy" internal models. Among the rest, this effect depends on the different degrees of the affiliation of perceived stimulus configurations to sets and upper sets in the respective mental representation. This "similarity effect" can be the cause of errors, realistically causing inadequate situational actions to be derived.

11.3.3.3 Decision Mechanism

A discrepancy between the determined expectation represented in model M_A and the impressions of the real outside world received by the receptors penetrates into the consciousness and, in certain situations, requires a decision for an action, which seems possible also by the given stimulus configuration (similarity effect). Thus, an enlargement of the model, shown in Figure 11.16, of information processing is necessary as shown in Figure 11.17. An essential component of this enlarged model is the decision mechanism whose function consists of the ability to select between a large number of internal models. It corresponds to the above-mentioned working memory (i.e., short-term memory) and, therefore, is subjected also to its restrictions (see below).

How can this process be more exactly described? The action remains unconscious as long as the expected information is equal enough to the observed one. So, we can drive in certain situations without exertion and perform additional actions simultaneously, like speaking with the passenger, using the phone, listening to the radio, and so on. Only when a significant deviation is recognized between the observed and expected information does such information comes to consciousness (in our example, the information would come to consciousness if, for example, the car suddenly drives over black ice). Then, by using the active part of our brain, we look for an alternative and seek another action-reception

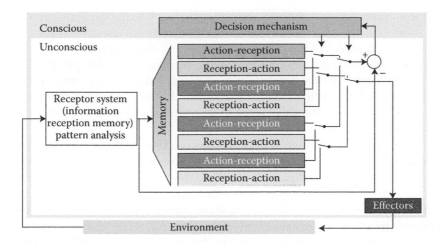

FIGURE 11.17
Model of human information processing.

model that proposes another solution, hopefully with a better outcome estimation. When we have found such a model, we proceed with the corresponding action on the effectors. It is obvious that this procedure needs time (taking our previous example, the car could already fell into a ditch after going over the patch of black ice by the time a better action is found). However, this "seeking" has another limitation commonly found in psychological experiments. Miller (1956) first discovered that human memory can handle only up to 7 ± 2 chunks (also referred to as "psychological units," "representation units," or "internal models"). These expressions are intentionally a bit unclear. This capacity for chunks can be increased by practice and experience, both of which allow for more efficient action planning in difficult situations. This, for example, could account for the difference between an experienced driver and a novice, which can be derived from the traffic accident curves. It has been shown that, on average, around 7 years after one obtains a driver's license, drivers reach a low, stabile level of accident probability. This 7-year period seems to be the amount of time needed to learn enough to be able to face nearly every situation in driving, responding to it in a correct way.

As already shown, the internal models can be subdivided into two main parts. One part contains the linking of perception configuration and the motor actions they derive from it (perception-action model). The other part contains an idea about the expected perception configuration on account of this action (action-perception model). By the decision mechanism, one of these models can be selected as indicated symbolically by switches in Figure 11.17. According to Figure 11.17 in the decision situation, if a preference for an action-reception reception-action pair is not yet fixed, the parallel switches for perception-action and action-perception models are separated. Now the decision mechanism sequentially selects ("in thoughts") every possible action-perception model and checks the size of the subjective benefit on account of the expected perception. Then, the model that promises the biggest subjective benefit given the circumstances (context) is selected for further action. Now, in the model represented in Figure 11.17, the switches are laid on the chosen action-perception model as well as on the accompanying perception-action model. At this point, the way is free for innervations of the effectors (musculature), which are supplied with a movement program according to the chosen model. By the action of the effectors, the configuration of the environmental stimuli changes, which is taken up by the receptors and is transferred to a comparative spot comparing this feedback to the expectation of the action-perception model. If the action leads to success, no difference appears in the comparative spot. However, with repeated repetition, the chosen model couple is stored as especially suitable for the stimulus configuration; that is, the respective "switch position" is taken as a new (i.e., learnt) higher action-perception model. Deviations at the comparative spot are consciously perceived and influence the decision mechanism in such a manner that when an individual border is exceeded, the decision structure is changed and can be shown in a new switch combination.

In many cases, a decision between several possible actions becomes necessary only by fact that different events are to be expected depending on a judgment of the external circumstances (i.e., context or "states of the world"). In terms of everyday life, humans are able to estimate objective probabilities of events through an observation of the frequency of events (Sheridan and Ferrell 1974). The expected subjective benefit consists of the subjective estimate of the states of the world and of the estimate of the benefit.

The discussed connections are illustrated in the example presented in Figure 11.18: the picture shows a traffic situation, different possible situations, and the possible reactions of road users. For a reaction to take place, a probability for each of the considered states of the world is estimated. In Table 11.1, the first line is a hypothetical estimate of a driver who is not especially in a hurry. In the left column, different possibilities are shown and, for each of these actions, a benefit is given. The benefit of every matrix element can be calculated by multiplying the probabilities of different possible situations and the benefit of the respective action. An unfavorable result of an action (e.g., collision with another road user) is to be considered as a "negative benefit" (i.e., damage). The sums in the last column show the respective mean benefit of a certain action, which incorporates the decision of the driver in favor of waiting ("straight ahead braking"). Table 11.2 shows the identical situation when the driver is in a great hurry and values any actions guaranteeing a quicker arrival. In this case, the decision falls in favor of overtaking ("accelerate to the left"). By comparing the results, it can be seen that depending on the mood of the driver (i.e., allocation of benefit), different actions are taken in an otherwise identical situation. If one analyses the person's

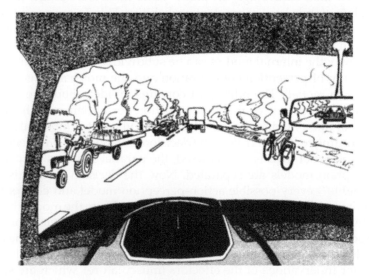

FIGURE 11.18
Example of a traffic situation in which a decision is necessary.

TABLE 11.1

Decision Matrix for a Patient Driver

Action without Haste	Cyclist Breaks Rank 0.3	Cyclist Remains on the Right 0.7	Oncoming Car Takes over 0.3	Oncoming Car Keeps His Lane 0.7	Truck Brakes 0.1	Truck Keeps Speed 0.9	Σ
Straight-ahead brake 0.4	0.12	0.28	0.12	0.28	0.04	0.36	1.2
Break to the left 0.3	0.09	0.21	0.09	0.21	0.03	0.27	0.72
Straight-ahead accelerate 0.1	−0.03	0.07	−0.03	0.07	−0.01	0.09	0.16
Accelerate to the left 0.2	0.06	0.14	0.06	0.14	−0.02	0.18	0.44

decision, one must note that the decision is heavily influenced by internal models (which can be wrong), and that the instantaneous benefit is in the foreground. Additionally, important factors could also remain disregarded because the decision mechanism is limited by short-term memory capacity (see Table 11.3). Human information processing is influenced by other factors like motivation, watchfulness, time pressure, and so on. Through motivation, the actual subjective benefit is determined.

According to the model ideas of human information processing, a rough distinction can be made between highly skilled actions, which need no decision, and decision-making processes. The former are not limited in their complexity by the capacity of short-term memory, whereas the latter are limited by this restriction and are more time consuming. If we derive actions from the internal representations stimulated by sense organs, the internal models, the categorization introduced by Rasmussen (1986) is helpful because it allows

TABLE 11.2

Decision Matrix for an Impatient Driver

Action with Haste	Cyclist Breaks Rank 0.3	Cyclist Remains on the Right 0.7	Oncoming Car Takes over 0.3	Oncoming Car Keeps His Lane 0.7	Truck Brakes 0.1	Truck Keeps Speed 0.9	Σ
Straight-ahead brake 0.1	0.03	0.07	0.03	0.07	0.01	0.09	0.30
Break to the left 0.2	0.06	0.14	−0.06	0.14	0.02	0.18	0.48
Straight-ahead accelerate 0.4	−0.12	0.28	−0.12	0.28	−0.04	0.36	0.64
Accelerate to the left 0.3	0.09	0.21	0.09	0.21	−0.03	0.27	0.66

TABLE 11.3

Decision Matrix When a Driver Is Patient, Taking into Account Limited Decision Depth Caused by Tiredness, Time Pressure, Excessive Demand, and So On

Action without Haste	Cyclist Breaks Rank 0.3	Cyclist Remains on the Right 0.7	Oncoming Car Takes over 0.3	Oncoming Car Keeps His Lane 0.7	Truck Brakes 0.1	Truck Keeps Speed 0.9	Σ
Straight-ahead brake 0.4							
Break to the left 0.3			0.09	0.21	0.03	0.27	0.42
Straight-ahead accelerate 0.1			−0.03	0.07	−0.01	0.09	0.12
Accelerate to the left 0.2							

finding a relation to treatment time. Rasmussen calls unconscious reactions to complicated stimulus patterns "skill-based behavior." This takes place on the basis of the background noise of the brain. The response times are typically around 100 milliseconds. The stimulus situations are treated according to "rule-based behavior," which needs a certain deliberate cognitive allowance but can be treated according to "proven patterns." The treatment time for such actions is around 1 to 2 seconds. However, for difficult, new situations, solutions can be found only by deliberate reflexing and weighing of possible results, that is, by "knowledge-based behavior." This can take several seconds to hours, days, and even more.

As shown, an essential aspect of the decision process is that an action is selected on the basis of which action will lead to the largest benefit in all circumstances. This must be often weighed out compared with possible damage (i.e., negative benefit). Thus, decision-making processes are also influenced by a person's willingness to risk and by his behavior in risk situations. The person subjectively estimates the risk of the result from the expected benefit to a desirable outcome. One decides on the action if the possible risk is lower than what can be personally accepted as the risk limit. Figure 11.19 shows different possible combinations of the subjective estimate of risk and objective risk. Basically, a subjectively higher estimated risk compared with the objective risk always represents a safe state.

Personally accepted risk is subjected to short-term and long-term changes. Moreover, individual differences account for much variance in behavior (e.g., a reckless motorcyclist undergoes not necessarily risk-prone difficult academic examinations).

In connection with risk, two basic problem fields arise with regard to the driving behavior:

- Many forms of failure can be traced to the fact that in the absence of experience opportunity (i.e., stimulus configuration in information perception), no adequate estimation of risk in relation to a situation (subjective risk) is possible (e.g., a close distance to the driver ahead might subjectively feel useful because it forces the driver ahead to clear the road; however, the risk would only be experienced when the driver has previous near-collision experiences).

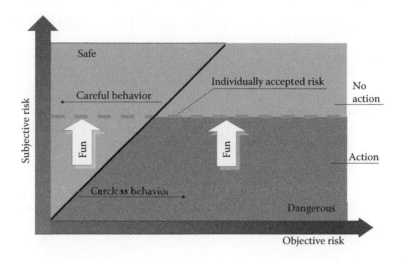

FIGURE 11.19
(**See color insert.**) Example of different combinations of subjective risk estimate, objective risk, and the safety of the action arising from it.

- According to the theory of "risk homeostasis" (Wilde 1982; O'Neill 1977), by reducing the objective risk (e.g., by technical measures) the person changes his behavior in the direction of "more dangerous" so far that the subjective estimation of the risk again becomes identical to the personally accepted risk (e.g., through better streets and chassis, cars are driven at higher speeds today than in earlier times).

In connection with this, the following question arises: What causes fun while driving? Many examples from the area of sports, arts, and pleasure show that for an individual fun arises from the experience of mastering a challenging task or completing a task successfully, implying that sometimes borderline risky behavior is touched upon. When we compare different areas of fun, then we see that an essential aspect of fun is reaching the individual border of performance, that is, being able to master the system. An example is a quotation from the German motor magazine *Auto-Motor-und-Sport*: "With switched off ESP (i.e., the electronic anti-skid system) the Porsche Turbo can be delightfully drifted diagonally." Thus, the intervention of active safety systems can lead to a decrease in fun while driving. Moreover, drivers wish to be supported in boring or cumbersome tasks (traffic jams, passing construction sites or bottlenecks) but engage in situations of free driving (Totzke et al. 2008). This has to be taken into account when specifying the human–machine interface for driver assistance. Therefore, there is an increased chance to take part in illegal behavior in order to experience fun while using a vehicle. If we want to enhance traffic safety, we must provide solutions so that fun can be found also in the safe area of the primary driving task.

11.3.4 Information Realization

Information realization aims to transform the action sequences generated in information processing to reality. Only mechanical movement caused by muscular strength is available for it. The principles of this transformation are demonstrated by the working principle of the so-called knee-jerk, which applies to all interactions controlled by the spinal cord.

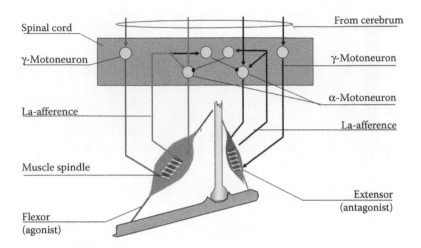

FIGURE 11.20
(See color insert.) Control circuit muscle spinal cord (here length servomechanism).

Motion programs, defined by the cerebrum, are given the essentials in two ways as a forcing function to the subordinated control circuit of the knee-jerk.

Quick movements and rough motor activity are innerved by α-motoneurons, the precise motor activity by γ-motoneurons. Figure 11.20 schematically shows a system-analytic-oriented representation of this information transformation.

The axons of the α-motoneurons, which are located in the spinal cord (as far as they innerve the musculature of the body periphery), form synapses with the cross-striped muscle fibers and are accessible by voluntary movements. According to the antagonistic principle, the basic structure of all higher developed animals, an antagonistic muscle (e.g., extensor), belongs to every agonistic muscle (e.g., flexor), which is capable of compensating the movement of the latter. This interconnection pursues both the goal of a controlled cooperation of agonist and antagonist and the controlled transformation of a posture motion activated by the cerebrum into reality. The axon of the motoneuron branches out in the muscle and innerves several muscle fibers. All muscle fibers innerved by an α-motoneuron form a "motor unity": because the muscle works according to an "all-or-nothing-principle," a measured-out muscle contraction is possible only in steps by innervations of a different number of motor unities. The muscle spindles stored in the muscle fibers serve as a length-measuring sensor and react to stretching with a raised impulse rate in the Ia-fibers. Because a stretch or compression of the whole muscle also causes a stretch or compression of the muscle spindles, the length change of the muscle is fed back by the Ia-afference.

The Ia-afferences are switched in the spinal cord exciting α-motoneurons of the identical motor unit of the agonistic muscle and over an inserted neuron hampering α-motoneurons of the antagonistic muscle. An activation or excitement of the α-motoneuron sent by the cerebrum causes a contraction, for example, of the flexor. The exciting impulse rate of the Ia-afference is reduced by the contraction, so that the muscle movement in a new neutral position (this corresponds to a certain posture) comes to a stop. This process is supported by the hampering interconnection of the Ia-afference on the α-motoneuron of a corresponding motor unit of the extensor, while there the spontaneously available tension is loosened. If by given innervations of the α-motoneurons, for example, the flexor is stretched by an external load, the exciting Ia-afferences provide for the increased strain of the extensor and their hampering interconnection for a declining effect of the flexor. The outlined control circuit is able to maintain the position required by the cerebrum and, to a great extent, it is able to do this despite consistent external changes and according to a temporal course mandated from the cerebrum. ("length servomechanism"; see Schmidt 1976).

The γ-innervations outlined in Figure 11.20 are capable of pre-stretching the muscle spindles in such a manner that even with smaller length changes of the muscle more changes of the Ia-afference arise (measuring range adjustment). Through the interconnection with α-motoneurons, a strain of the agonist and a suitable relaxation of the antagonist cause a movement that stops in a position determined by γ-innervations. Therefore, precise movement can be controlled by γ-innervations, whereas α-innervations stimulate more the quick and coarser movement.

Because γ-innervations go out from the cerebellum, which itself receives afference from the vestibular organ, the posture-keeping system is also procured by it. By this system, if extreme misalignments are detected, for example, of body weight, uneven floor, or effects of acceleration forces in a moved system, a stable and straight posture is aimed at. Beyond γ-innervations, the posture-keeping system is superimposed permanently on the arbitrariness of motor activity. Therefore, under extreme conditions in the automobile, it is possible that the posture-keeping system, innerved by the cerebellum, interferes with precise motor activity, which is innerved as γ-innervations.

Besides the just-described control circuit of the length servomechanism, a parallel control circuit is also realized, which one could call "strength servomechanism" (see Figure 11.21). In this control circuit, the tendon elements (Golgi elements) work as the measuring sensor that measures the stretch of the tendons by which the muscles are attached to the skeleton and thus measures the strength transferred by the muscle. The Ib-fiber and an inserted neuron have a hampering effect on the α-motoneuron.

If the muscle works statically against an immobile obstacle, by this control circuit a strength idea, as a forcing function of the cerebrum, is transferred into a defined real strength by α-innervations. This interconnection also shows a protective effect, by

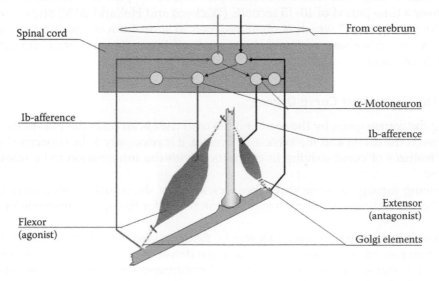

FIGURE 11.21
(See color insert.) Control circuit muscle spinal cord (here strength servomechanism).

receiving an influence from the outside; the Ib-afference becomes large in such a way that α-innervations decrease and the muscle gives way to external tension.

While driving through curves, the interconnection mechanism described here plays a decisive role for the feeling of steering (see Wolf 2009). The combination of motion perception by optical flow, the accompanying acceleration forces, and the restoration of the forces perceivable in the steering system together form the internal model for cornering. Consequently, every above-threshold deviation leads to decision-making processes, and thus in a given traffic situation possibly causes a dangerous delay in reaction.

11.3.5 Feeling of Time

Driving is motion and motion is a change of position in time. Therefore, it is of interest to understand action in motion in relation to the person in time. What do people feel with regard to the actual time or the time recently experienced? This question is important for all spoken connections because we live in the "now and today," and have memories of the past and expectations for the future, aspects that deal substantially with our memory. German psychologist Pöppel (2000) was intensely concerned about this question. In accordance with many neurological cerebral experiments, he found that our (conscious) thinking is clocked in 40-millisecond intervals. Furthermore, what is especially interesting is his scientific discovery about what we feel as "being present." Pöppel suggested that we experience presence as absolutely real, although, in contrast to a strictly logical consideration, it is merely the infinitely short dividing line between the past and the future. He found that the concept of being present can be divided into three areas: that which we feel immediately as presence corresponds to a duration of about 2 seconds. The immediate past, however, also belongs to the presence feeling, which Pöppel calls "presence of the past." It corresponds to a time period of a few seconds (we can repeat, for example, a just-spoken short sentence any time word by word; this is not possible for sentences that have been said more than half a minute ago). Furthermore, the "presence of the future" means that the expectation of what will follow now immediately belongs to the presence feeling. This whole area from presence of the past to presence of the future ranges over a time period of 10–15 seconds (Wickens and Holland 2000) and corresponds to the "forgetting time," which is often assigned to short-term or working memory. We can only act when we have an internal imagination about what we should do in the next immediate moment.

11.3.6 The Dynamic of Curve Driving

Tracking the course given by the road and the road user is an essential part of the interaction between the driver and the vehicle. Therefore, it is necessary to be concerned with the specific features of curve driving in connection with the information to be mastered by the driver.

For driving through a curve, three feedback levels of the vehicle motion were given by Fiala (1966), according to Crossman and Szostak (1969), for the optical information canal:

1. *Pre-information by prevision on the street ("floodlight orientation")*: Only by the information gained from the anticipation of the driver is one able to form an internal desired course for a given situation. All experiments (see below) show that the driver looks ahead at a distance within about 2 seconds in time (see "presence of the presence"!).

2. *Vehicle direction ("direction orientation")*: The skilled driver can estimate the motion direction of the vehicle on the basis of the optical flow and thus makes the vehicle's longitudinal direction according to the tangent of the seen curve.

3. *Lateral distance ("fog orientation")*: The skilled driver, like the unskilled one, immediately sees the distance to the edge of the road and tries to keep a safe distance to both sides.

In addition to these optical feedback channels, the kinesthetic perception of the transversal acceleration plays an important role. On the basis of his internal models, the driver knows which transversal acceleration he has to expect in connection with a seen curve and with a given speed. If this seems too high to him, he reduces speed immediately.

The dynamism of optical feedback can be calculated from the geometry of curve driving (see Figure 11.22 for an explanation).

By the steering wheel angle λ and a steering system translation relation u, a wheel angle $u \cdot \lambda$ in the front wheels results. A curve radius r_K is determined with the wheel base l. If the vehicle drives on this radius, a curve of the length $r_K \cdot \varphi_F$, the vehicle direction changes compared to the original direction by the angle φ_F. At the same time, it has the deviation a from the original straight-ahead course. In terms of feedback for a driver in an uncritical situation, one can carry this out without the description of effects of higher order, like slip angle, transversal slip, and so on. When there is a small angle φ_F, the lateral distance of the vehicle, relative to the desired course, can be derived from Figure 11.22:

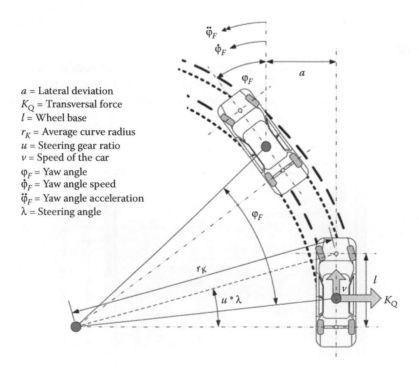

a = Lateral deviation
K_Q = Transversal force
l = Wheel base
r_K = Average curve radius
u = Steering gear ratio
v = Speed of the car
φ_F = Yaw angle
$\dot{\varphi}_F$ = Yaw angle speed
$\ddot{\varphi}_F$ = Yaw angle acceleration
λ = Steering angle

FIGURE 11.22
(See color insert.) Geometry of curve driving.

$$\frac{\mathrm{d}^2 a}{\mathrm{d}t^2} = \frac{v^2 \cdot u}{l} \cdot \lambda$$

Therefore, by the steering wheel angle λ, the driver determines the acceleration of the distance a to the roadway edge. From an ergonomic perspective, this is the difficultly in having a hand-controlled acceleration (Bubb 1993). In addition to that, the influence of the steering wheel position depends squarely on the just-driven speed.

The temporal change of direction orientation φ can be derived from Figure 11.22:

$$\frac{\mathrm{d}\varphi_F}{\mathrm{d}t} = \frac{v \cdot u}{l} \cdot \lambda$$

The change of the direction orientation is determined with the steering wheel angle λ, and this change depends only on the speed. As the driving of a vehicle is a so-called compensatory task, this is very easy to master (Bubb 1993). A skilled driver will try to grasp the direction of the longitudinal motion of the vehicle from the optical flow and to steer only this.

Figure 11.23 shows the driver's view. One can imagine his behavior in such a way that he virtually "points" with the steering wheel in the direction in which he wants to drive. This is visualized by the white points on the steering wheel in Figure 11.23. Consequently, the sighted point is closer with a "direct" steering system than with an "indirect" steering system. With a speed-dependent steering system, one can understand that the steering system is direct with low speed and is indirect with high speed. By means of the forcing factor k_0, one can lay out this dependence in such a way that the deviation b_{2s} must be sighted, which corresponds to a prevision of 2 seconds. The following formula states this connection: $b_{2s} = k_0 \dfrac{1}{v} \cdot u \cdot \lambda$

With this interpretation, one simplifies the driving curve and reduces the square speed dependence, while steering according to the lateral distance. Today, such speed-dependent steering transformations are offered by some car manufacturers (e.g., BMW and Audi).

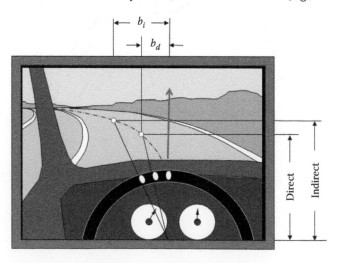

FIGURE 11.23
(See color insert.) Point of view of the driver.

11.4 Data Capturing at the Input/Output

As already mentioned, the eye can perceive sharply only a small angle area of 2 to 3 degrees and only by visual movement an internal picture of the outside world is composed in the brain; it is quite a natural everyday experience to understand the direction of attention of a person by observing their gaze direction. By capturing the line of sight, we have a so-called peer tube into one's behavior. Of course, this peer tube supplies no foolproof knowledge about what is actually seen and which internal models of the observed person are really stimulated. However, there is a distinction between the external "physiological fovea" and the internal "psychological fovea," which can be observed indirectly by asking (see Zinchenko and Virgiles 1972). Both attention directions must not necessarily be identical; the difference can amount up to 2 degree (Kaufman and Richards 1969), even if a high correlation with a certain temporal delay between both can be assumed generally.

Besides this differentiation between internal (psychological) attention and external, overt (physiological) attention direction, glance behavior control is also to be considered (see the experiments by Remington 1980). We speak of *distraction* if a changing stimulus in the peripheral field of vision causes us to look there, and of *averting* (at a physiologically relatively low level) if we voluntarily look at a new object of instantaneous attention (AOI). Only the latter is of interest to the current question; actually, both appear similar and are mutually exclusive to each other.

In spite of all general restrictions, glance analysis can tell us something about instantaneous attention. At least the following statement can be a basis for a practicable experimental approach: "What is not in the field of vision cannot be grasped subjectively and plays, therefore, no role inaction generation."

As already shown in the first paragraph, a conclusion on the internal processes in the brain can take place only if a synchronous recording of all input and output information takes place in one given situation. In this section, the technical preconditions are explained.

11.4.1 Input Side: Acquiring Eye-Tracking Data

Different gaze-capturing systems are available that work according to different principles, such as head-based and touch-free methods. Additionally, electrooculogram is also available, which by means of surface electrodes mounted near the eye registers the potential difference between the cornea and the skin. In the angle area of 40 degrees, this method supplies good results. However, it is very susceptible to artifacts by electrical tension variations dependent on the time of day, eye blinking, and facial musculature.

11.4.1.1 Head-Based Methods

A visual field camera is mounted to a slide-proof helmet, which is placed on the head of the subject. The camera's picture is superimposed to the line of sight of the eye, in a connected computer. With regard to the capture of the eye movement, the following procedures can be used:

- *Limbus, pupil, or eyelid registration*: The eye is lit up wide extensively with infrared light. The second eye camera, mounted on the helmet, receives the picture of the eye over a mirror that reflects only infrared light and is completely permeable by visible light. The eye picture is magnified by a corresponding calibration procedure (zoomed) that can be overlaid immediately to the visual field picture. In another form of this technology, the position of the dark pupil in the eye picture is received by picture processing technology.

- *Cornea reflex method*: An infrared light source linked with the helmet directs a focused ray on the eye. The facet-like surface of the eye reflects this ray which is caught by a camera, also mounted on the helmet (Purkinje picture technology). After a calibration procedure, the detected position of its picture can be overlaid onto the visual field picture and indicates the actual line of sight.

- *View axis measurement (point of regard measurement)*: An infrared light beam is directed on the eye and generates a reflex. The second camera mounted on the helmet captures this reflex and the momentary position of the dark pupil. By means of picture processing, the positions of both objects are grasped. From their relative location, the position of the eye and the line of sight can be calculated in the computer and overlaid onto the visual field picture.

In contrast to procedures based on picture processing technologies, the simple superimposed method is very robust against disturbances. However, it requires a human interpreter to evaluate the frames. In contrast to this method with picture processing technologies, it is also possible to capture both eyes as well as the convergences of the gaze axes. Indeed, picture processing is very sensitive to variations of light and, thus, rather less just for the application in the free field.

11.4.1.2 Touch-Free Methods

With the touch-free methods, one or two cameras firmly mounted in the space observe the test person. An infrared beam is directed at the head of the test person and this generates a reflex in both eyes. The pictures of both observation cameras are analyzed in a computer by means of picture processing. To find the eye position, the head position and the posture of the head are registered by another procedure (also on optical base or, if necessary, by means of an electromagnetic head tracking system). Similar to the helmet-based procedures described above, the respective position of the reflex and the pupil is determined in every camera picture. Depending on the system, this happens only in one eye (ETS system) or in both eyes (Facelab system). From their relative position and the position of the eye, also calculated by picture processing, the line of sight of the eye or both eyes in space can be determined. With the ETS system, these lines of sight are marked consecutively in the picture of a camera firmly fixed in the scenery (e.g., vehicle). However, the Facelab system working with two cameras and taking up both eyes supplies only the coordinates of the line of sight. Therefore, if the surroundings are firm (e.g., working on a console) and the positions of the possible observation points (AOIs) are known, a fully automatic evaluation is possible. However, because of the many interlocking picture processing processes, both methods are very sensitive to light variations. Although both described procedures would be helpful just for in-vehicle application, their application is rather difficult.

The results reported here were gained with the system DIKABLIS. It belongs to the limbus, pupil, or eyelid registration; however, it can be combined with some opportunities that allow touch-free methods. In the following, this system will be described a little more exactly. The device consists of three components: the head unit, the radio system, and the recording computer.

The head unit examines the data of the field of vision and the left eye. The components of the head-based eye movement-capturing unit are based on a comfortable lightweight titan frame, which allows a non-slip surface. The field camera, which sits concentric between the eyes, receives the surrounding sphere of the experimental subject. The camera grasps what is in the visual space of the experimental subject (visual field). The ocular camera, which is mounted in front of the left eye, takes a black-and-white photo. To receive a high-contrast picture, the eye is filmed in the infrared area.

These data reach the reception station by radio transmission and go from there to the recording computer, where recording software is run. Here, calibration procedures are carried out and the data are examined. In a preshow window, the position of the eye (eye video) and the visual area of the test person (field video) can be seen any time. Therefore, an online view of the line of sight is always possible. The glance data are evaluated on the basis of the ISO standard (ISO/TS 15007-2:2001). In this standard, exactly how eye-tracking experiments should be realized is described, in addition to determining and defining the necessary identity values. Because of this, results can be compared across several experiments. According to the ISO standard, the following data are to be recorded or calculated:

- Total glance time
- Glance frequency
- Time off road-scene-ahead
- Total glance time as a percentage
- Fixation probabilities
- Link value probabilities
- Maximum glance duration
- Mean glance duration

In Tables 11.4 and 11.5, the identity values are represented with the help of which one can estimate the attention of the driver by single glance of objects or scene signs. Table 11.4 summarizes the measures related to the glance frequency, whereas Table 11.6 shows

TABLE 11.4

Measures for the Attachment of Attention from Glance Frequencies

Attachment of Attention		
Identity Value	**Description**	**Unit**
Glances related to Area of Interest (AOI)		
Absolute glance frequency	The absolute number of glances at an AOI within a scene is defined.	[]
Relative glance frequency	The number of glances at an AOI divided by the sum of all glances within a scene.	[%]
Average glance frequency	The average of the absolute glance frequency within a scene.	[]
Standard deviation of glance frequency	Indicates information about whether the number of glances within a scene is steadily distributed across all attached AOIs.	[]
Glance frequency	How often, per second, a glance to an AOI takes place. The number of glances at an AOI within a scene is divided by the glance duration.	[1/s]
Percentage of glance portion	The whole resting time on the AOI is divided by the duration of the observation period.	[%]

TABLE 11.5

Retention Time-Based Identity Values and a Description of Their Relationship with Attention

Attachment of Attention		
Identity Value	Description	Unit
Retention time		
Retention time	The retention time is defined the "time span from the moment when the driver fixes a target for the first time until the eyes walk to another target" (EN ISO 15007-1:2002 (D)). It excludes, therefore, transient saccades.	[s]
Cumulated retention time	All single retention times on an AOI during the observation period, summed up.	[s]
Relative cumulated retention time	The accumulated retention time of an AOI is divided by the sum of all accumulated retention times during an observation period.	[%]
Average retention time	Average of all retention times on an AOI during the observation period.	[s]
Standard deviation of the retention time	The standard deviation of the retention time during an observation period.	[s]
Maximal retention time	The longest (maximum value) single retention time on an AOI during an observation period.	[s]

the identity values derived from the retention time. As base identity values, the reported viewing identity values from the documents of ISO 15007-1, ISO 15007-2, and SOW J-2396 can be enumerated here.

11.4.1.3 Indicators for the Driver's Load

Table 11.6 summarizes all indicators for the driver's load. These values were determined on the basis of the X/Y coordinates of the pupil center, recorded by DIKABLIS. These coordinates are looked at for a defined period and they give a good sense of the driver's load. According to Saito (1992), visual search decreases with rising load. In addition, the amplitude of the average saccade angle decreases with higher load (Menn, Studer, and Cohen 2005). The portion of the environmental glances can be concluded on the basis of the load: the less the load, the more one permits himself to look around. This was shown by the realization of tertiary tasks (Schweigert 2003).

11.4.2 Output Side

Data only from the input side are not sufficient to interpret human behavior and to discuss the test results. Recording the steering movement of the test person doesn't provide a sufficient statement about the behavior in certain situations. Only temporal synchronization of the steering movement can supply expressive information. The situation is to be understood in such a way that it should describe the whole event space of the test person, that is, the existing traffic situation, the relation of the streets, the mood of the driver, and so on. A detailed statement is possible only by the simultaneous consideration of these parameters. It requires the synchronous representation of all data, which is guaranteed by the presented eye movement-capturing device DIKABLIS. The classification of the traffic situation must be distinguished, in principle, by the street situation (i.e., objective traffic situation of the involved vehicles), the driving situation (i.e., the situation that is shown objectively to the

TABLE 11.6

Identity Values Based on the Movements of the Pupil for a Defined Period

Driver's Load		
Identity Value	**Description**	**Unit**
Saccade values		
Visual seeking activity	This describes the amplitude of the average saccade angle per time unit. The searching activity is calculated, while the corresponding distance segments of the angles of all singular saccades are summed and are then divided by the duration of the observed segment. Identity value according to Saito (1992).	[°/s]
Average saccade angle	The average is computed from the angles of all singular saccades.	[°]
Standard deviation of the saccade angle	The standard deviation of the saccade angle during an observation period	[°]
Saccade frequency	The saccade frequency describes the relation of the number of saccades in the observation period to the temporal expansion of the observation period.	[1/s]
Amplitude of the average saccade angle	This identity value describes the amplitude of the average saccade angle.	[°]
Surrounding looks		
Percentage of surrounding looks	Here all glances that do not belong to the real driving task are defined. Example: glances to the right and left of a roadway (i.e., to trees, shrubs, etc.).	[%]
Percentage of surrounding looks within a curve	Definition as above; for a left turn all looks on the left side within the curve (bend area) are considered therefore (on the left of the roadway). For right curves, therefore, right sided.	[%]
Percentage of surrounding looks outside a curve	Definition as above; for a left turn all right-sided looks (on the right by the roadway) are observed therefore outside the curve (bend area). For right curves, therefore, on the left side.	[%]

driver), and, finally, the driver's situation (i.e., the subset of the driving situation that the driver perceives individually caused by his properties and abilities). A difference between the driving situation and driver's situation can possibly lead to an accident.

Therefore, in this research area, simulator experiments are especially informative because the whole traffic scenery can be recorded synchronically, including all reactions of the driver, because it is generated artificially. With suitable simulators (e.g., with the driving simulator of the Institute of Ergonomics, University of Technology, Munich) it is even possible to control the traffic events by a participant's behavior, such that he or she will always encounter the desired traffic situation to be investigated (Wohlfarter and Lange 2008). All this is much more difficult in the real experiment because many practical elements are involved. This is especially the case for elements that require an exact position of the vehicle on the street. Information on movement direction and speed of the other road users can be received only rudimentarily (often only by video observation), much less than that which can be influenced by the experimenter. Therefore, in addition to being a safety precaution for the test persons, simulator experiments dominate this research area.

11.5 Human Glance Behavior While Driving a Motor Car

The time capacity required for an ideal fulfillment of the primary driving task is dependent on numerous factors; some examples would be its dependency on the individual characteristics of the driver, the traffic density, the roadway state, and the weather. The more complicated an actual driving situation, the greater the time needed for the primary driving task; the remaining time is available for secondary and tertiary tasks. In general, a minimization of the time required for these additional tasks increases the safety benefit.

11.5.1 Results of Driving in Longitudinal Traffic

While driving, when we observe glance behavior by an eye tracking system, we can distinguish between "scanning" and "processing" (see Figure 11.24; Cohen 1985). Scanning glances have a rather short duration—on average 400 milliseconds. By scanning the edges of the road, other traffic participants and traffic signs are perceived. Processing glances means that not only special AOIs are fixated, such as the instruments, the mirror, and the display of the car, but also objects in the environment that are not relevant for traffic. The processing glances need, on average, twice the time of scanning glances (see Figure 11.25).

In our own experiments, we have worked closer with scanning and processing glances while curve driving. The experiments were carried out in the simulator of the Institute of Ergonomics, which permits a very realistic feeling to the test driver by means of the Silab software and 180° projections. The Silab software brings the experimental subject straight into a certain situation, regardless of the behavior shown before. Markov's analysis with the significance test of Liu (1998) allows one to see the regularity of glances, which nevertheless appear in all experimental subject—despite the fact that the glance sequence is dependent on the individual and the actual situation. As the most important part, anchor points are identified out of the area of the tangent point: the close, middle, and distant

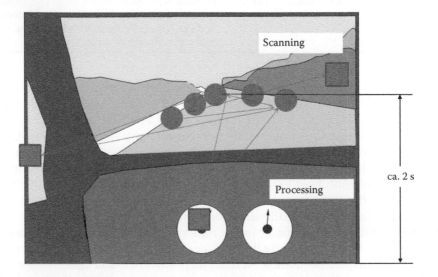

FIGURE 11.24
(**See color insert.**) Glance behavior: By "scanning", the course of the road is received. By "processing", specific areas of interest are glanced.

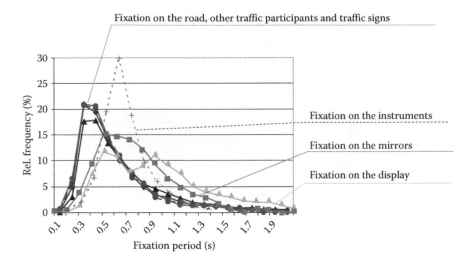

FIGURE 11.25
(**See color insert.**) Experimental results of eye tracking experiments. (From Schweigert, M. 2003. Fahrerblickverhalten und Nebenaufgaben Dissertation an der Technischen Universität München.)

street area, the speed indication, road signs, and, if available, a vehicle moving ahead, oncoming traffic, and a broken down vehicle are all available in the simulation.

With curve driving, rough segments can be distinguished: "glance behavior during curve approaching and orienting," "glance behavior in the curve," and "glance behavior with leaving the curve." The typical behavior is illustrated in Figure 11.26. In the approaching phase, the driver looks first at the speedometer to ensure the speed is adequate for the estimated curve radius. The next glance is directed to the tangential point of the curve (when turning left, this is ordinarily the middle stripes; when turning right, the right street edge). Among other things, it serves to anticipate the curve and is done on average 2 seconds before curve entry. The anticipation time is extended (the tangent point is fixed earlier) with increasing restriction of the view. The next glance checks the distance to the right street edge (when following a right curve, this can also be the first distance to the left middle stripe). Then, the next glance ensures the distance to the respective opposite side. Now, a controlling glance at the speedometer follows once more.

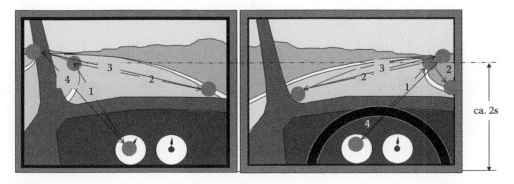

FIGURE 11.26
(**See color insert.**) Typical gaze sequence in a left curve and a right curve.

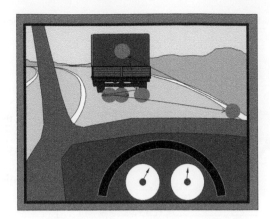

FIGURE 11.27
(See color insert.) Typical gaze sequence driving behind a car ahead.

The following driving situations distinguish themselves by a distinctive glance connection by the vehicle moving ahead. This appears increasingly with a truck moving ahead (see Figure 11.27).

The fact that the presence of present has a duration of 2 seconds has much importance for glance behavior. All experiments with glance behavior in car driving show that, normally, information is scanned only at a distance of 1 to 1.5 seconds and a maximum of 2 seconds ahead (distance = speed × preview time; Donges 1978; Yuhara et al. 1999; Guan et al. 2000; Schweigert 2003); several experimental results show we accept taking the view from the road for up to 2 seconds (e.g., Zwahlen, Adams, and DeBald 1988; Gengenbach 1997; Schweigert 2003). Gengenbach (1997) showed that the scanning rate decreases immediately before and after averting; the loss on information is compensated by an increased scanning rate (see Figure 11.28).

In a further investigation, the influence of tertiary tasks and different layouts of such tasks on glance behavior was observed in more detail by Rassl (2004). His subjects had

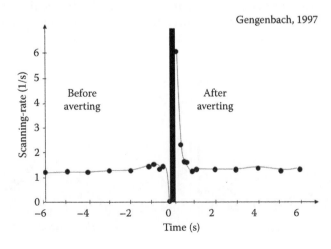

FIGURE 11.28
(See color insert.) Scanning rate before and after averting glance from the road.

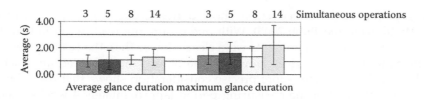

FIGURE 11.29
(See color insert.) Glance attention in connection with tertiary tasks.

to choose one of 3, 5, 8, and 14 options by a central control element (similar to the BMW i-drive controller), while driving. It is of interest that the selection needs on average about 1.2 seconds and there is no significant difference between these deviation times depending on the number of presented options. However, when we look at the maximum duration of distracted glances, the instance of the 14 options is significantly different from the others. The maximum distraction time in this case is an average of 2.2 seconds. As Figure 11.29 shows, one distraction time of 12 seconds was even observed.

That is not a singular event! In the research by Rassl (2004), another part of the experiment showed a 16-second distraction. Furthermore, with the operation of the ACC system, we also found distraction times of 12 seconds. The psychological explanation for these long dark periods is given by the experience of presence. Normally, after 2 seconds of distraction we become worried and turn our glance back to the road. However, when in the beginning of the distraction we have the impression that the surrounding scene will not majorly change and when the distracting task becomes attractive, in such rare cases we use the total time span between the presence of the past and the presence of the future. In none of these cases do we subjectively recognize the long distraction time from the road because our internal model shows us the supposed road scene.

In another investigation of the Institute of Ergonomics, five measuring drives were carried out in order to investigate the acceptance of head-up display (HUD) and ACC, the effectiveness of it, and the originating habituation effects. During the drives, the test persons had to carry out tasks with the ACC operation. The first measured drive (without HUD) carried out served as a baseline drive in order to record glance behavior and the retention time of the experimental subjects by customary indication tools. After the baseline drive, the subjects carried out measured drives with activated HUD after a week. In the period between the measured drives, subjects became accustomed to the car equipped with HUD and ACC. For an objective evaluation, the glance data of the subjects were recorded over the course of the habituation phase and were compared with the baseline drive. The evaluation of the ACC system took place by the registration of the operating time and errors. In addition to the objective data, a subject's subjective acceptance was reported by questionnaires.

A comparison of the glance frequencies on the HUD and the instrument panel or central information display (CID) showed that the HUD was immediately and completely accepted by all subjects. Already by a subject's first contact with the display technology, which was still at that point unknown for them, the HUD dominates relative to the customary indicators with an average 85% of the glance proportion. For the period in which an operation of the ACC system has taken place, the dominance of the HUD becomes even clearer. Also, the navigation information is read by all subjects preferentially from the HUD. The use of the CID limits itself mainly to the representation of the navigation map (adjustment in the CID: navigation map and arrow view).

An investigation of the effectiveness showed two groups of subjects with different behavior (Wohlfarter and Bubb 2005). With one group, the reading periods of the HUD at the end of the series of experiments were clearly lower than the reading periods of the instrument panel (baseline drive). However, the other group showed an exact contrary glance behavior. Nevertheless, more precise consideration shows that the subjects of the second group at the end of the measuring period (approximately 4 weeks) have not yet completely concluded their individual habituation phase. Therefore, from the observed behavior it is to be assumed that after a further habituation period, the glance times on the instrument panel would be shorter. In summary, the HUD is accepted subjectively and objectively by all subjects immediately and completely, while the effectiveness and efficiency compared to the customary indicators depend on the individual development. In general, the experiments clarify the advantage of the visualization of speed, navigation, and ACC information with the help of the HUD compared with customary indicators. However, by contrast, it also becomes recognizable that a high density of information generates a considerable visual and mental workload in the subjects with the HUD. This has to be considered for further developments, in particular for the question: "What should be indicated in the HUD?"

From this investigation, a more precise idea regarding the habituation effects of the HUD were revealed such that with new applications, the corresponding internal models of the respective test person must first be founded and then trained. In this investigation, as well as in others (e.g., Weinberger 2001), it appears that drivers need at least 4 weeks to become acclimatized.

In a further investigation in the driving simulator of the Institute of Ergonomics, 35 test persons were escorted through a cross-country and city journey (Wohlfarter 2012). Glance investigations were carried out with regard to peripheral vision. After special scenes, the test persons were questioned about the task. In one scene, the test persons had to read text on an advertising board with the additional task of maintaining the current speed limit. The scene, shown in Figure 11.30, was in a slight right curve. A road sign was on the right side ("60 km/h in the case of wetness").

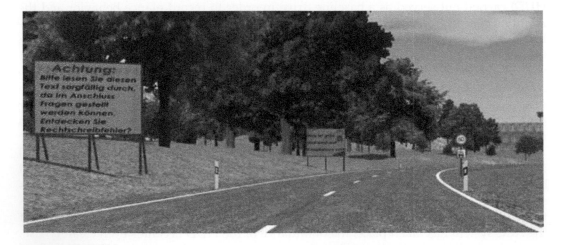

FIGURE 11.30
(**See color insert.**) The advertising board is on the left side; on the right, the tempo limit sign is seen. It is completely cleared and visible at every moment.

The limit "60 km/h in the case of wetness" was correctly recognized only by 14.3% (5 test persons) of the drivers. Even though the traffic sign is only ordinary, it is empty and never covered (see Figure 11.30). In this scene, the workload is obviously very high for many test persons. Within the glance analysis, when fixation was maintained on the advertising boards nearly no controlling glances on the roadway take place as they are to be expected according to "normal" glance behavior (see Figure 11.25). This confirms that lane keeping by peripheral perception in spite of cornering is possible; however, this also increases the angular distance to the traffic sign and reduces perception.

Thirteen subjects fixated on the speed limit sign of "60 km/h" by one or more glances. However, only 40% of them correctly recognized the additional sign "in the case of wetness." It can, therefore, be derived that the additional sign "in the case of wetness" is not identified as an important element. The drivers, who have perceived only the speed limit, were not even aware of the existence of an additional sign (questionnaire after the scene). This information was sorted out as non-relevant by the perceptual system. This example shows that visual attention is necessary for the perception of details. The results of this experiment point out how effective it would be to have the support of technology in traffic sign recognition and its representation in the instrument panel or in the head-up display. In a further investigation, 23 subjects were observed in a field test with the eye-tracking system DIKABLIS. The subjects drove through selected road segments and had to follow a given driving route. The road segments were very varied from simple right-before-left situations to the crossing of big intersections in town areas. The evaluation of constrictions (single-line street by parking vehicles) shows how single information units on the edge of the street must be refreshed in shorter distances to make sure important elements are not overlooked. Figure 11.31 shows the saccade frequencies for the different heading types.

On the heading segments "highway" and "multi-lane with marks," identical numbers of saccades are required (significance 0.356). On all other roadway types, they differ significantly from each other. Therefore, the saccade frequency depends on the visual claim

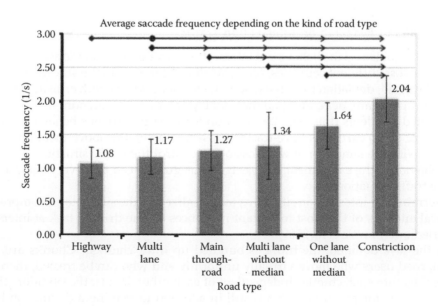

FIGURE 11.31
(**See color insert.**) Mean saccade frequency of all subjects dependent on the heading type.

of the heading type; the higher the visual claim, and thus the more linked to information perception, the greater the saccade frequency (this is a result that has already become visible in connection with glance averting and the renewed glance attention on the street; see Figure 11.28). With highways, as well as with multi-lane town traffic with road markings, no additional information except the roadway and the surrounding traffic is required to fix the driving strategy. This means that the situation is regulated by road markings and the surrounding traffic flow. With main through-roads, the available driving space is narrower; that is, the danger potential by other road users rises. Therefore, information from the environment with higher frequency must be refreshed. It is also necessary to grasp much secondary information, such as pedestrian, oncoming traffic, traffic lights, and so on. Consequently, the driver has to follow several sources of information for an estimation of the situation. Another aspect that has an influence on mental load is the familiarity of a situation. If the driver comes, for example, to unusual situations, which appear to him as if important information is missing (e.g., missing middle stripe), he looks to his surroundings for a visual aid that supports him in assessing the situation. On account of the searching glances, an increased saccade frequency results, as found with certain heading types such as "multi-lane oM: multi-lane without mark" and "single-lane oM: single-lane without mark." The relatively high saccade frequency of two saccades per second is due to the need for the driver to be able to orient himself according to the left and right edge of the road to avoid collisions. By this behavior, the driver can change his control behavior. Now, the lateral distance and longitudinal orientation of the vehicle is controlled. As discussed in Section 11.3.6, the driving task changes from easy to-be-mastered speed control to more difficult to-be-used acceleration control. It was shown that this effect appears when a leading car drives ahead on a narrow road because it causes one to concentrate on the longitudinal orientation. At the moment, experiments by Israel (2012) show that this effect is made available, permanently, by the indication of the safety distance in the form of a crossbeam virtually lying on the roadway in the corresponding distance ($x_s = v \cdot t_S$, where $t_S = 1.5$ s), realized by the so-called contact-analogous HUD (Bubb 1981).

11.5.2 Results of Research on Intersection Traffic

A particular problem is the behavior at intersections. Depending on the accident statistics, especially across different countries, accidents due to longitudinal traffic (driving against the vehicle ahead, deviation from the roadway, etc.) or accidents with cruising traffic come first. In Europe, again, depending on the country, intersections account for 30–60% of all injury-related accidents (InterSafe 2009). To understand the driver's behavior at intersections, Plavšic (2010) carried out eye-tracking research using the above-mentioned driving simulator. With the simulator, it was possible to control the traffic situation as a function of the behavior of the experimental subjects; it was guaranteed that every subject came to the same traffic situation.

To determine the intersection situations to be realized in the simulator, a comprehensive theoretical analysis of the most important influences on the driving task at intersections was carried out (Plavšic et al. 2009).

To fix the task demand, the traffic is bundled up into "chunks." Chunks are, on this occasion, road users who move virtually uniformly and who can be treated, therefore, as a whole; the more such chunks, independent of each other, in a traffic situation, the more complicated it is for the driver. This is still in addition to making a distinction between chunks, which the driver has to react to immediately and that which he only has to observe. On the basis of these facts, Plavšic (2010) developed a procedure with which the complexity of a traffic situation can be quantified. Thus, it is possible to have an order of rank of the difficulty of the scenarios used in the experiments.

This resulted in a test course consisting of 10 intersection situations; maneuvers (on the left, right, and left), priority regulation (having priority of way, letting the right of way, stop sign, and right-pre-left regulation), and the presence of a car ahead were varied. The difficulty of a task in every situation was evaluated by the identification of the most important influences. The investigated intersection situations and their assessment are outlined in Figure 11.32.

A task analysis was carried out for every intersection scenario. The production of a cognitive driver model and the definition of an ideal driving behavior were the bases for this analysis. In general, ideal driving behavior can be described as behavior corresponding to legal regulations. Nevertheless, there is a range of correct behavior for every traffic situation. To define the driving task at intersections, the intersection area was divided into five phases: approaching, slowing down, driving through, bending, and leaving the intersection. In every area, a rule-based decision was necessary.

With regard to glance behavior, it was necessary to analyze how well the observed glance behavior fit to the normative task. For normative behavior, Plavšic (2010) refers to categories outlined by Schweigert (2003):

- Continuous monitoring of the motion of one's own vehicle (mostly by the peripheral view).
- Continuous anticipation of the behavior of other road users (explorative scanning).
- Situations that require an eye movement (behavior at intersections and with obstacles).

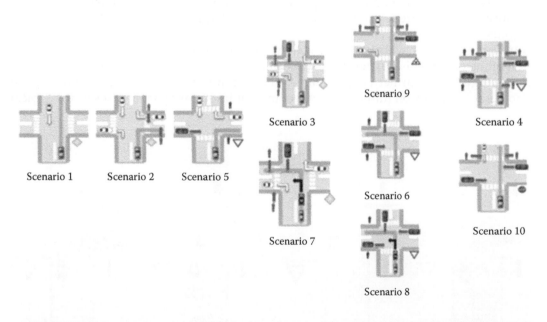

Scenario 1   Scenario 2   Scenario 5   Scenario 3   Scenario 9   Scenario 4

Scenario 7   Scenario 6   Scenario 10

Scenario 8

Increasing difficulty of task

FIGURE 11.32
(See color insert.) Investigated intersection situations ordered according to the degree of task difficulty.

On this basis and further categorizing the necessary glances as "essential," "important," "previewing," and "irrelevant," trigger points are put for the separate scenarios that lay down normative glance behavior. Then, the behavior observed with DIKABLIS is reflected in it.

The experiments were carried out with 24 subjects (average age: 27 years; 3 women and 21 men). After the subjects had finished the first test drives, the separate scenes were demonstrated to them for a judgment. The experiment was then repeated under time pressure, and the subjects made a separate subjective judgment.

The results of the experiments are divided into subjective data (received by the evaluation of the questionnaires) and objective data (driving simulator, DIKABLIS). With the *subjective data*, according to the NASA TLX questionnaire, it appears that crossing an intersection is a very challenging task. In addition, a significant difference appears in the load between the baseline and the drive under time pressure. No other differences could be ascertained according to the subjective estimation of task difficulty, orientation, misjudgment, and the risk of a collision in the different scenarios.

The *objective data* refer to the recording and the analysis of the eye movements, specifically, the difference between the observed behavior and the theoretical ideal behavior. In addition, the following values were analyzed by means of eye tracking: glance duration, glance frequency, percentage of time, and maximum glance duration on 16 predefined AOIs.

As a result, it can be said that the presence of other road users was the strongest "performance-shaping factor" of visual behavior. If more than four objects were present in the scene, visual behavior was determined almost completely by the objects in the scene (bottom-up processes). This glance behavior was independent of the maneuver carried out or the priority regulation. The consequence was that in complicated scenarios the views in priority-entitled directions were often omitted. In Figure 11.33, the difference between the glance sequences with and without other traffic is shown. In contrast, the top-down controlled glance behavior, characterized by an active searching, is dependent on given intersection characteristics. In this case, the maneuver itself had a stronger influence than priority regulation. Furthermore, the same subjects committed the same error, missing the opportunity to focus on traffic signs or leaving out important partial tasks or the typical

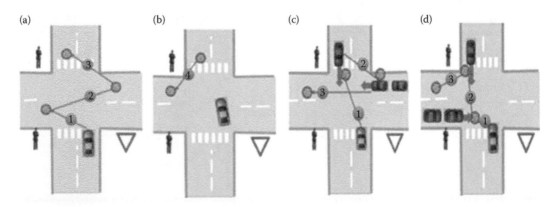

FIGURE 11.33
(See color insert.) Typical glance sequence in scenario 6: (a) Drive through if no other road users exist. (b) Bend if no other road users exist. (c) Drive through with oncoming and traffic crossing from the right. (d) Drive through with oncoming and traffic crossing from the left.

number of glances in certain phases. This supports the hypothesis that a high portion of errors is of a systematic nature and could also be prevented.

A description of the most important results per segment is shown in the following. Detailed results can be seen from Plavšic (2010).

- *Approaching phase*: In the approaching phase, the drivers mostly focus on the middle (1 to 2 seconds) of the "driving tube" or the wider (>2 seconds) "driving tube." In approximately 60% of the cases, the focus was directed only upon the right side of the roadway. The most important tasks in the approaching phase are anticipatory tasks. In connection with this, perception of the traffic signs and the suitable adaptation of the driving behavior have top priority. Indeed, only approximately 60% of the subjects have directly focused on the controlling traffic sign, with the exception of the stop sign. Nevertheless, the most serious error was non-adapted speed.

- *Slowing-down phase*: The accidents, which occurred in the third and fourth phase, were mostly already predetermined by errors committed in the slowing-down phase; the discrepancy between ideal and actual behavior was very high in this phase. The most serious errors were omitting glances in the direction of weaker road users (e.g., pedestrians). Only 15% of the subjects made sure that other traffic participants maintain priority regulation. The influence of time pressure was the strongest in this phase, which was often responsible for failing to complete important tasks.

- *Bending phase*: The glance behavior in this phase is characterized by focusing the point, which is in the middle of the roadway (anchor point). Focusing this point serves to better stabilize the car during the bending maneuver (see also the results shown in Figure 11.26). The typical glance sequence during bending to the right was a short glance to the left and then a glance to the right. In 40% of the cases, a glance to the oncoming direction was also observed. The typical glance sequence on a leftward bend was a glance to the left, to the right, then in the oncoming direction, and then to the left again. If the test persons had priority, they only glanced to the left approximately 25% of the time. The influence of the other road users was very strong in this segment. In many cases, the drivers carried out the wrong glance sequences and this often resulted in the priority-entitled traffic participants being overlooked.

- *Leaving the intersection*: The errors committed in this segment were not as critical as those in the other phases.

The presence of the present, with a duration of 2 to 3 seconds, encourages us to not always keep our gaze on the road. Schweigert (2003) carried out glance research in enlarged experiments. He found out that glance was also directed to non-traffic relevant objects in 89% of all observed traffic situations, under normal non-stressing conditions. When the traffic situation becomes more difficult, first we reduce the glance to these non-traffic relevant objects, then to specific AOIs, and then we reduce the attention to traffic signs, tachometer, and mirrors. When the situation becomes very complex, it can be observed that the driver, in 41% of all cases, counts on the behavior of other traffic participants according to the rules. When the situation becomes still more complex, in 7% of the situations, the driver omits even the glance to primary necessary information (see Figure 11.34). Thus, voluntary glances, not found by traffic situations, can be seen as an indicator of mental load under

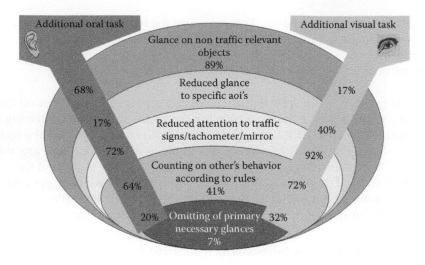

FIGURE 11.34
(**See color insert.**) Percentage of faulty glance behavior. (From Schweigert, M. 2003. Fahrerblickverhalten und Nebenaufgaben Dissertation an der Technischen Universität München.)

these conditions. Schweigert (2003) made experiments with additional oral and visual tasks that were comparable under the aspect of attraction of attention. By these additional tasks a further reduction of free glances is observed. In Figure 11.34, a change in relation to the non-interfered situation is indicated. It can be observed that an additional oral task, on average, has a little less influence than an additional visual task.

11.6 Modeling of Internal Representation

11.6.1 Outside World and Internal Representation

How can we complete our image of our surroundings from the information captured by these results? Figure 11.35 helps to understand this process. By scanning at the level of the sensory memory, information is taken in and stimulates internal models that are stored as a general concept in the form of a structural engram in our long-term memory.

By this stimulation the corresponding internal model is "awoken" and becomes, in this way, a part of the working memory. This can be made clearer if we take the example discussed earlier of driving on a leftward road bend. The information received by scanning stimulates a general internal model of the concept of a road with a bend to the left. By adapting this concept to real stimuli in the working memory, we can see the real width and the real curve of this road. Further scanning stimuli give us information about traffic participants on this road. The scanned information of these objects also stimulates internal models of their behavior. As we can see, only a short glance is enough to recognize the speed and the course of an oncoming car or the expected behavior of a pedestrian. As our gaze can only scan a scene sequentially, it is possible that relevant objects are not observed. The combination of all this information gives us a feeling of the presence of the situation; we believe only this internal image to be reality.

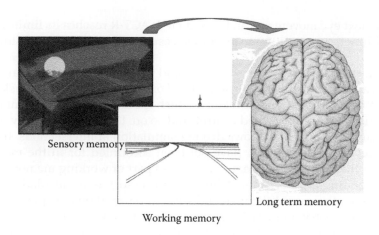

Sensory memory

Long term memory

Working memory

FIGURE 11.35
(See color insert.) Stimulation of internal models by external stimuli.

As a function of the subjective perceived complexity of the scene, the need arises for other controlling glances. Thus, the result of the study by Schweigert (2003) is that in uncritical situations, gazes are also increasingly directed to objects that have no relevance to the driving task. With increasing complexity, the glance upon driving-relevant objects is continually reduced. With increasing complexity of the traffic situation, the gaze is reduced to objects relevant to the traffic situation. When the situation is highly complex, even this view is omitted and it is assumed that other traffic participants, who are not observed, behave according to a prediction the driver makes, which corresponds to his or her experience (equal to the internal model). Because driving subjectively occurs in the present, the time span of the "presence of the present" of approximately 2 seconds plays a dominant role for the "permissible averting time." Indeed, for example, a tertiary task (or events in the outside world, beyond the real driving task; e.g., while driving past a scene of an accident) can capture so much attention that this interferes with the major task and will cause a certain "forgetfulness" of the primary driving task.

In terms of improving the system so that accidents do not occur, the question of how gaze behavior is represented within the internal picture of the outside world must be answered. This is, of course, to be considered on the basis of the fact that this gaze behavior is responsible for a corresponding, corrected, and refreshed internal picture of the outside world.

11.6.2 Models of Driver Behavior

To get an idea of the cognitive process while steering a vehicle, which concretizes the outlined beginning of Section 11.5.1, and to understand a more complicated traffic situation (and, if necessary, to predict possible mistakes), different calculative driver models have been developed. In the following, a scanty overview will be given on the relevant driver models that could serve this purpose.

First, the ACR-R (adaptive control of thought-rational) is considered. Its original intention was to develop a user's model that allows a simulation of human interaction with different interfaces. With this model, a special ACT-R driver model is prepared, which allows a model of the driving task on three-lane highways, including lane changes and simultaneous phoning. Other road users can be involved, provided they drive in the same direction. By means of the attention module EMMA (eye movements and movement of attention), the next eye movement can be predicted. ACT-R reaches its limits because of its expansive arithmetic expenditure to its borders, especially if complicated situations are to be simulated.

Additionally, the model Soar (state, operator and result) contains a mechanism for problem solving, learning, motor behavior, and visual orientation, and a multitask mechanism. For Soar, the model DRIVER was developed which is built up from different modules like visual orientation, navigation, speed control, and so on. DRIVER is the only model within the cognitive architectures that allows driving simulation at intersections. Indeed, at this point newer developments of Soar have not been accounted for in the model DRIVER, which, among other things, considers forgetting as part of working memory.

QN-MHP (queuing network-model human processor) is a calculative architecture, which connects mathematical theories and simulation methods of queues (QN), with a processor of human behavior (MHP); the latter is based on the model GOMS (goals, operator, methods, selection rules). Additionally, a driver model derived from QN-MHP was created, which takes into account real time and orientates itself to a great extent to the driver's behavior—specifically, in the perception, processing, and realizing of information. This model permits the simulation of second tasks. Future developments will refer to speed controlling, taking into account the influence of traffic as well as the vestibular organ and auditory inputs. Presently, nevertheless, the model works with a constant speed of 72 kilometers per hour and can only be used by the University of Michigan.

COSMODRIVE was developed in France at INRETS with the aim of explaining the information processing of the driver. At the moment, it is not available to the general public, apart from the fact that a large portion of the literature is only available in the French language.

PARDIC is based on the structure of COSMODRIVE. It can simulate critical situations that arise from visual distraction. Otherwise, identical restrictions are valid for this system as per COSMODRIVE.

ACME was developed by Deutsche Luft-und Raumfahrt with the aim of making available a model of the driver in a real-time simulation, which allows one to model critical driver states in different traffic situations and which can ultimately be used for the development of assistance systems. The biggest disadvantage of the system is that it is not open for external users. Moreover, it is still in a state of development.

The program PELOPS was developed by BMW in connection with RWTH (University of Technology of Aachen). Its purpose is to simulate the interaction between the driver, the vehicle, and their surroundings. In particular, it can simulate traffic flow with high exactness, even in complicated stop-and-go situations. Indeed, it is completely specified on the longitudinal traffic.

Finally, the program SSDRIVE models on a real-time basis the driver's vehicle interaction with a special focus on driver error. It is also not accessible publicly.

11.6.3 Recommendation for the Simulative Model of Driver Cognition

Plavšic (2010) developed recommendations for the concept of a new driver model from experiences with available driver models. The object of this model is the support, during the development of driver's assistance systems, at the guidance level; it should simulate driving errors and predict and explain why such errors occur. Recommendations are made for the level of details and the complexity of the program expenditure. In terms of further development, the ergonomic demand arises for a program to be simply learnable. According to Plavšic, the raised demands are fulfilled by the so-called

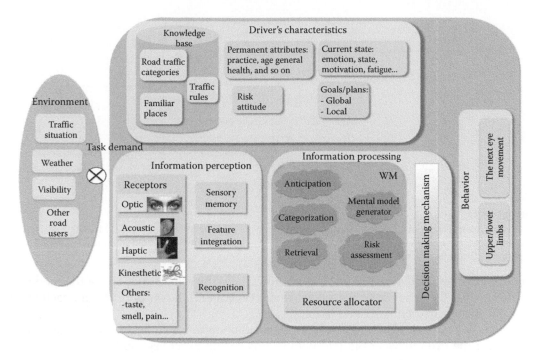

FIGURE 11.36
(**See color insert.**) Multi-agent system. (From Plavšic, M. 2010. Analysis and Modeling of Driver Behavior for Assistance Systems at Road Intersections, Dissertation. Munich: Lehrstuhl für Ergonomie, Technische Universität München.)

multi-agent's system. Thus, a structure is to be realized as it has been already demonstrated in Section 11.2 in its principles (Figure 11.36).

The agents themselves can be divided into four groups:

- Information perception agent: optical, acoustic, and vestibule information
- Information processing agent: categorizing, generating of mental models, anticipation, risk evaluation, and decision making
- Information realizing agent: eye movement, movement of the upper and lower extremities

Each of the separate agents in Figure 11.36 is to be realized individually. As an example, the modeling of the perception agent is shown in Figure 11.37. There is in each case an agent for the driver's characteristics, containing aspects like knowledge, durable attributes, present state, and so on.

Then a driving process can be shown in the form of a cycle with different transitional opportunities (Figure 11.38). Now, for each of the states, a separate agent can be assumed. Exemplarily, this is shown for the case of free driving (state 1) in Figure 11.39.

In Figure 11.38, the behavior at intersections is shown. In every segment shown, the normative and the observed usual behavior are modeled (more details can be found in the study by Plavšic 2010).

The driver behavior will be modeled in each case at the level of the driving situation, including deterministic and probabilistic descriptions. In the first step, the knowledge of

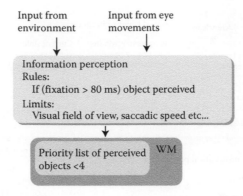

FIGURE 11.37
(See color insert.) Modeling example for the information perception agent. (From Plavšic, M. 2010. Analysis and Modeling of Driver Behavior for Assistance Systems at Road Intersections, Dissertation. Munich: Lehrstuhl für Ergonomie, Technische Universität München.)

the driver is modeled as a fuzzy value that influences the other functions of the model. In the following, the behavior of the eye movement agent and the output rules for each of the possible inputs are demonstrated in detail.

In Plavšic's model, driving error is of particular importance and special attention to modeling the eye movement is laid before considering exact segments. In particular, in

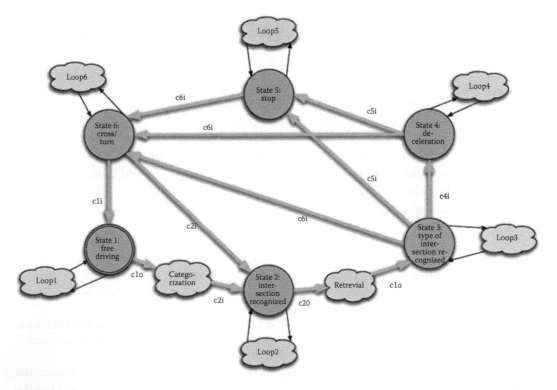

FIGURE 11.38
(See color insert.) Temporal and causal distribution of states in an example of crossing the intersection. (From Plavšic, M. 2010. Analysis and Modeling of Driver Behavior for Assistance Systems at Road Intersections, Dissertation. Munich: Lehrstuhl für Ergonomie, Technische Universität München.)

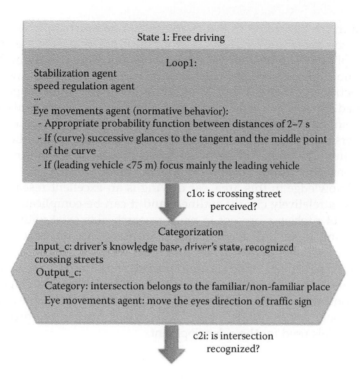

FIGURE 11.39
(See color insert.) Cognitive state 1: Free driving. The loop occupies all the agents within one state and is named so because of its repetitiveness. Categorization agent belongs to state 1. (From Plavšic, M. 2010. Analysis and Modeling of Driver Behavior for Assistance Systems at Road Intersections, Dissertation. Munich: Lehrstuhl für Ergonomie, Technische Universität München.)

this connection a so-called error watcher is realized, which can calculate the difference between normative behavior and observed behavior, in the experiments.

On the basis of the described analyses and properties, currently at the Institute of Ergonomics, a driver model is provided which is modularly built up and whose realization will last for a longer period. The construction orientates itself on ergonomic-software principles, especially with regard to its demand for expandability, modularity, and a simple configuration.

11.7 Conclusion

It is a triviality to ascertain that our actions are initiated and controlled by the brain. However, the cognitive foundations that form the basis for action—including action modification and the motives for right and wrong actions—are all but trivial. With the help of the methodologies already active in neurophysiology and neuropsychology, one attempts to shed light on an otherwise unclear situation. Just as in connection with controlling machines, which move vast amounts of energy, basic knowledge about these action backgrounds is of extraordinary meaning because one hopes to thereby make a contribution to safety by designing ergonomically.

It was shown in the beginning of this chapter that one must apply neurophysiological knowledge to come to realistic conclusions about the functionality of the brain. Under the aspect of the application for real design, one must go out from a shell model. This model contains, in its most internal core, the physiology of synaptic transients and the knowledge of neural connections. In the next shell, the knowledge of allocation of specific processing areas is contained. However, in order to develop concrete design proposals, ideas of the so-called internal models for specific situations must be developed. To come here by realistic attempts, the persistent synchronous capture of the input and output behavior is necessary in experiments. Therefore, it is necessary to record eye movements in connection with overt behaviors and to virtually "peer tube" into the brain.

To speed up knowledge in this area, car driving is an excellent research topic. This is because the task is relatively clearly outlined, and it can be complicated also arbitrarily. Both basic kinds of problems present in neuroresearch also exist with human–machine interaction: tracking tasks and decision tasks. Forming internal models for mastering these tasks is demonstrated in detail. All things summed, a general model is derived for behavior in driving situations, which is an important condition for developing ergonomic solution proposals. In the close future, this model will be further developed and solution proposals will continue to be derived. In the next step, it is indispensable to value the effectiveness of these solution proposals, again, in the experiment and to further refine at the same time the models used for their development.

References

Bubb, H. 1977. *Ergonomie des Mensch-Maschine-Systems Habilitation*. Münich: Institut thr Ergonomie, Technischen Universität München.

Bubb, H. 1981. The influence of braking distance indication on driver's behaviour. In *Human Factors in Transport Research*, edited by D. J. Oborne and J. A. Levis, Vol. II, 338–46. London/New York: Academic Press.

Bubb, H. 1993. Systemergonomie. Teil 5. In *Ergonomie*, edited by H. Schmidtke, 305–458. Münich, Wien: Hanser Verlag.

Chatziastros, A. 2003. Visuelle Kontrolle der Lokomotion. Dissertation. Germany: Justus-Liebig-Universität Gießen.

Cohen, A. 1985. Visuelle Informationsaufnahme während der Fahrzeugsteuerung in Abhängigkeit der Umweltmerkmale und der Fahrpraxis. *Schweizerische Zeitschrift für Psychologie* 44 (4):249–88.

Crossman, E. R. F. W., and H. Szostak. 1969. Man-machine-models for car-steering. In Fourth Annual NASA—University Conference on Manual Control. Washington, DC: National Aeronautics and Space Administration.

Donges, E. 1978. Ein regelungstechnisches Zwei-Ebenen-Modell des menschlichen Lenkverhaltens im Kraftfahrzeug. *Zeitschrift für Verkehrssicherheit* 24:98–112.

Epping, B. 2009. "Sie sind doch Ihr Gehirn—wer sonst?" Portrait. Wolf Singer. *Spektrum der Wissenschaft* 09/2009:74ff.

Fiala, E. 1966. Lenken von Fahrzeugen als kybernetische Aufgabe. *Automobiltechnische Zeitschrift* 68(5):156.

Fikus, M. 1989. *Visuelle Wahrnehmung und Bewegungskoordination*. Frankfurt am Main: Deutsch.

Geiser, G. 1985. Mensch-Maschine-Kommunikation im Kraftfahrzeug. *ATZ* 87:77–84.

Gengenbach, R. 1997. Fahrerverhalten im Pkw mit Head-Up-Display. Gewöhnung und visuelle Aufmerksamkeit. VDI Fortschrittsbereiche Reihe 12: Verkehrstechnik/Fahrzeugtechnik, No. 330.

Gibson, J. J. 1958. Visually controlled locomotion and visual orientation in animals. *British Journal of Psychology* 49:182–94.

Gibson, J. J. 1950. *The Perception of the Visual World*. Boston: Houghton-Mifflin.

Gibson, J. J. 1966. *The Senses Considered as Perceptual Systems*. Boston: Houghton-Mifflin.

Goldstein, B. 2002. Kapitel 9: Wahrnehmung und aktive Motorik. In *Wahrnehmungspsychologie*, 327–43. Heidelberg: Spektrum Akademischer Verlag.

Grau, A. 2003. Momentaufnahmen des Geistes? *Gehirn & Geist* April 2003, 76–80.

Guan, H., Z. Gao, K. Guo, and Q. Li. 2000. An optimal preview acceleration model for velocity control in driver vehicle-environment system. In *Proceedings of the 5th International Symposium on Advanced Vehicle Control (AVEC 2000)*, Ann Arbor, Michigan, August 22–24, 2000, pp. 525–30.

Guzmán, A. 1969. Decomposition of a visual scene into three-dimensional bodies. In *Automatic Interpretation and Classification of Images*, edited by A. Gresselli, 243–76. New York: Academic Press.

Helander, M. 1988. *Handbook of Human-Computer Interaction*. Amsterdam: North-Holland.

Helmholtz, H. v. 1866. *Handbuch der phsiologischen Optik, Bd. 1: Anatomische Beschreibung des Auges*. Hamburg: Voss.

Helmholtz, H. v. 1910. *Handbuch der pysiologischen Optik, Bd. 3: Die Lehre von den Gesichtswahrnehmungen*. Hamburg: Voss.

InterSafe. 2009. InterSafe, Subproject of PReVENT (Preventive and Active Safety Applications Integrated Project). http://prevent.ertico.webhouse.net/en/prevent_subprojects/intersection_safety/intersafe/

ISO/TS 15007-2:2001. Road vehicles—Measurement of driver visual behaviour with respect to transport information and control systems. Part 2: Equipment and procedures. http://www.iso.org/iso/iso_catalogue/catalogue_tc/catalogue_detail.htm?csnumber = 32149

Israel, B. 2012. Potenziale eines kontaktanalogen Head-up Displays für den Serieneinsatz. Dissertation. Münich: Technischen Universität München.

Jürgensohn, G. 1997. *Hybride Fahrermodelle*. Dissertation an der Technischen Universität Berlin, ZMMS Spektrum, Band 4. Würzburg: Pro Universitäts Verlag.

Kaufman, L. and W. Richards. 1969. Spontaneous fixation tendencies for visual forms. *Perception and Psychophysics* 5:85–8.

Lappe, M. 2009. Visuelle Wahrnehmung von Bewegung. *Skriptum zum Seminar Visuelle Wahrnehmung von Bewegung*, Universität Münster. http://wwwpsy.uni-muenster.de/imperia/md/content/psychologie_institut_2/ae_lappe/freie_dokumente/einfuehrung1.pdf

Lindsay, P. H. and D. A. Norman. 1972. *Human Information Processing. An Introduction to Psychology*. New York and London: Academic Press.

Liu, A. 1998. Chapter 20: What the driver's eye tells the car's brain. In *Eye Guidance in Reading and Scene Perception*, edited by G. Underwood, 431–52. Oxford: Elsevier Science Ltd.

McRuer, D. T. 1980. Human dynamics in man-machine-systems. *Automatica* 16 (S):237–53.

McRuer, D. T. and H. R. Jex. 1967. A review of quasi-linear pilot models. *IEEE Transactions on Human Factors in Electronics* HFE-8 (3):S.231–49.

McRuer, D. T., H. R. Jex, W. F. Clement, and D. Graham. 1967. Development of a Systems Analysis Theory of Manual Control Displays. Report Nr. TR-163-1, System Technology Inc.

McRuer, D. T., R. E. Magdaleno, and G. P. Moore. 1967. A neuromuscular actuation system model. *Third Annual NASA-University Conference on Manual Control*, NASA SP-144, 281.

McRuer, D. T., R. W. Allen, D. H. Weir et al. 1977. New results in driver steering control models. *Human Factors* 19 (4):S.381–97.

Menn, M., N. Studer, and A. Cohen. 2005. Eye movement behaviour when driving through the Gotthard tunnel: A pilot study. In *Proceedings of the 13th European Conference on Eye Movements (ECEM13)*, Bern, August 14–18, 2005.

Miller, G. A. 1956. The magical number seven plus or minus two: Some limits on our capacity for processing information. *Psychological Review* 63:81–97.

Mühlendyck, H. 1990. *Augenbewegung und Visuelle Wahrnehmung*. Stuttgart: Enke.

O'Neill, B. 1977. A decision-theory model of danger compensation. *Accident Analysis & Prevention* 9:157–65.

Palm, G. 1990. Assoziatives Gedächtnis und Gehirntheorie. In *Gehirn und Kognition*, 164–74. Heidelberg: Spektrum der Wissenschaft Verlagsgesellschaft.

Parasuraman, R., ed. 2003. Neuroergonomics: Research and practice [Special Issue]. Guest editorial: Neuroergonomics. In: *Theoretical Issues in Ergonomics Science* 4 (1–2):1–3.

Plavšic, M. 2010. Analysis and Modeling of Driver Behavior for Assistance Systems at Road Intersections. Dissertation. Munich: Lehrstuhl für Ergonomie, Technische Universität München.

Plavšic, M., M. Duschl, M. Tönnis, H. Bubb, and G. Klinker. 2009. Ergonomic design and evaluation of augmented reality based cautionary warnings for driving assistance in urban environments. In *Proceedings of the 17th World Congress on Ergonomics (International Ergonomics Association, IEA)*, Beijing, China, August 9–14, 2009.

Pöppel, E. 2000. *Grenzen des Bewußtseins—Wie kommen wir zur Zeit und wie entsteht Wirklichkeit?* Frankfurt a.M. und Leibzig: Insel Taschenbuch.

Raichle, M. E. 2010. Im Kopf herrscht niemals Ruhe. *Spektrum der Wissenschaft* 06/2010:S60ff.

Rasmussen, J. 1986. *Information Processing and Human-Machine Interaction. An Approach to Cognitive Engineering*. New York: North-Holland.

Rasmussen, J. 1987. The definition of human error and a taxonomy for technical system design. In *New Technology and Human Error*, edited by J. Rasmussen, K. Duncan, and J. Leplat, 23–30. New York: Wiley & Sons Ltd.

Rassl, R. 2004. Ablenkungswirkung tertiärer Aufgaben im Pkw—Systemergonomische Analyse und Prognose. Dissertation. Münich: Technischen Universität München.

Remington, R. W. 1980. Attention and saccadic eye movements. *Journal of Experimental Psychology: Human Perception and Performance* 6:726–44.

Rock, I. 1968. The basis of position-constancy during passive movement. *American Journal of Psychology* 81:262–5.

Rockwell, T. H. 1971. *Eye Movement Analysis of Visual Information Acquisition in Driving: An Overview*. Raleigh: North Carolina State University.

Saito, S. 1992. Does fatigue exist in a quantitative measurement of eye movements? *Ergonomics* 35:607–15.

Schmidt, R. F. 1976. Motorische systeme. In *Physiologie des Menschen*, edited by R. F. Schmidt and G. Thews. Berlin/Heidelberg/New York: Springer-Verlag.

Schmidtke, H. 1993. *Ergonomie, 3. Auflage*. Wien: Carl Hanser Verlag München.

Schweigert, M. 2003. Fahrerblickverhalten und Nebenaufgaben Dissertation an der Technischen Universität München.

Selfridge, O. 1959. Pandemonium: A paradigm for learning. *Symposium on the Mechanization of Thought Processes*. HM Stationary Office, London.

Shannon, C. E. and W. Weaver. 1949. *The Mathematical Theory of Communication*. Urbana, IL: University of Illinois Press.

Sheridan, T. B. and W. R. Ferrell. 1974. *Man-Machine-Systems, Information, Control and Decision. Models of Human Performance*. Cambridge, MA: MIT Press.

Timpe, K.-P. 2001. Fahrzeugführung: Anmerkungen zum Thema. In *Kraftfahrzeugführung*, edited by T. Jürgensohn and K.-P. Timpe, 9–27. Berlin: Springer.

Totzke, I., V. Huth, H.-P. Krüger, and K. Bengler. 2008. Overriding the ACC by keys at the steering wheel: Positive effects on driving and drivers' acceptance in spite of a more complex ergonomic solution. In *Human Factors for Assistance and Automation*, edited by D. de Waard, F. O. Flemisch, B. Lorenz, H. Oberheid, and K. A. Brookhuis, 153–64. Maastricht: Shaker.

von Holst, E. 1957. Aktive Leistungen der menschlichen Gesichtswahrnehmung. *Studium Generale* 10 (4):232.

Wann, J. P., and M. Wilkie. 2004. How do we control high speed steering. In *Optic Flow and Beyond*, edited by L. M. Vaina, S. A. Beardsley, and S. K. Rushton, 401–17. Dordrecht, The Netherlands: Kluwer.

Warren, W., B. Kay, W. Zosh, A. Duchon, and S. Sahuc. 2001. Optic flow is used to control human walking. *Nature Reviews Neuroscience* 4:213–6.

Weinberger, M. 2001. Einfluss von ACC-Systemen auf das Fahrverhalten. Dissertation. Münich: Technische Universität München.

Werblin, F. and B. Roska. 2008. Wie das Auge die Welt verfilmt. *Spektrum der Wissenschaft* 5:41–7.

Wickens, C. D. and J. G. Hollands. 2000. *Engineering Psychology and Human Performance*, 3rd ed. Upper Saddle River, NJ: Prentice Hall.

Wiener, N. 1948. *Cybernetics or Control and Communication in the Animal and the Machine*. New York: MIT Press.

Wilde, G. J. S. 1982. The theory of risk homeostasis: Implications for safety and health. *Risk Analysis* 2(2):209.

Wohlfarter, M. 2012. Modellierung der Informationsaufnahme und -verarbeitung beim Führen eines Pkws. Dissertation in progress. München: Lehrstuhl für Ergonomie, Technische Universität München.

Wohlfarter, M. and H. Bubb. 2005. Akzeptanz und Effektivität von Fahrerassistenzanzeigen im Head-Up-Display am Beispiel ACC und NAVI. In *Abschlussbericht: Teil 1 Ergebnisse der Untersuchung*. München: Lehrstuhl für Ergonomie, Technische Universität München.

Wohlfarter, M. and C. Lange. 2008. Fahrsimulator-Forschungsumgebung am Lehrstuhl für Ergonomie. *Ergonomie Aktuell* 9 (Summer):8–16.

Wolf, H. 2009. Ergonomische Untersuchung des Lenkgefühls von Personenkraftwagen. Dissertation. München: Technischen Universität München.

Yuhara, N., L. Tajima, S. Sano, and S. Takimoto. 1999. Steer-by-wire-oriented steering system design: Concept and examination. *Vehicle System Dynamics Supplement* 33:692–703.

Zinchenko, V. P. and N. Y. Virgiles. 1972. *Formation of Visual Images: Studies of Stabilized Retinal Images*, translated by Consultants Bureau. New York: Plenum Press.

Zwahlen, H. T., C. C. Adams, Jr., and D. P. DeBald. 1988. Safety aspects of CRT touch panel controls in automobiles. In *Vision in Vehicles II*, edited by A. G. Gale, 335–44. Amsterdam: Elsevier North-Holland Press.

12

Potential Applications of Systems Modeling Language and Systems Dynamics to Simulate and Model Complex Human Brain Functions

Waldemar Karwowski, Tareq Z. Ahram, Chris Andrzejczak, Magdalena Fafrowicz, and Tadeusz Marek

CONTENTS

12.1 Introduction

Modeling is a universal technique to understand the real world through abstraction. A model is a representation of a selected part of the world. The success of the model is measured in different ways and according to the model user's expectations. To model the human brain, it is important to understand how the brain's components (systems) function and the mechanisms of handling information in order to try to improve our understanding of its processes and the mechanisms of communication (Ramos, Ferreira, and Barcelo 2012). The human brain is an organ that contains many contrasts. It is compartmentalized, but certain functions seem to span large areas.

The human brain is composed of seemingly simple neurons, yet the connections between these neurons are intricate and immensely complex. It consumes about one-fifth of the body's energy supply, and has priority access to blood, requiring high levels of sugar and oxygen to operate. It is also protected by a complex defense system, ranging from being bathed and supported in its own unique filtered blood, cerebrospinal fluid, to having a physical and chemical barrier that is selectively permeable to only the most necessary and safe chemicals required for its function. Originally thought to dissipate heat from the body much as a radiator does for a car's engine, the brain is now known to be responsible for controlling vital life functions as well as efficiently processing information.

From the systems design viewpoint, the main issue in human factors and ergonomics (HF/E) discipline is to determine the requisite and absolutely essential compatibility of the artifact–human system, and use it as a reference point for system improvements. Cognitive engineering aims to assure such requisite compatibility in the functioning of the artifact–human system with respect to complex and uncertain (cognitive and perceptual) inter-relationships between system users, machines, and the environment. Such analysis must account for the natural nonlinear dynamics of cognitive and perceptual processes of the human brain. This chapter examines some of the critical issues and methodological needs for future development of systems engineering brain cognitive and perceptual models. The modeling paradigm with respect to cognitive systems dynamics performance is also discussed.

12.2 Human Factors

The science of HF/E aims to discover and model how people interact with their environments and perceive their surroundings, given the specific human characteristics, limitations, and performance capabilities. In doing so, ergonomics faces the problem of increased complexity of the system and the related human and system-based dynamics. Dynamics and fuzziness is not only a state of the human mind but also the essence of human development and existence, and a necessary condition for human learning, growth, and survival. Systems dynamics methodologies allow accounting for complex and natural human and human–machine fuzziness, and provide the necessary framework for successful modeling efforts in the human perception and HF/E discipline. To develop the proper relationship between people and the outside surroundings (natural and artificial, i.e., technology-based), the intrinsic dynamics and fuzziness of human perception must be treated by system designers and engineers as natural requirements of their everyday activities.

The human world is complex and exhibits inherent uncertainty and vagueness. Therefore, to study the behavior of human systems it is necessary to develop dynamic and approximate modeling approaches. Karwowski (1991) (see also Karwowski and Salvendy 1992) suggested that perceptual fuzziness should be looked upon as the natural model of people at work and those human-made systems that interact with people, embedded into traditional descriptions of human sensory, information processing and communication, or physiological functioning processes. In this context, complexity and fuzziness are not just products of the human mind that can be described and comprehended only through formal mathematical theories. Fuzziness, as a basic quality of human understanding, is also the essence of human development and existence, and a necessary condition for human learning and growth.

While the contemporary HF/E discipline attempts to model and describe how people interact with their outside environment, the common understanding is that human beings are too complex to be fully understood or described in all their characteristics, limits, tolerances, and performance and perceptual capabilities, and that no unified or comprehensive mathematical models are available to describe and integrate all the above-mentioned measures and findings about human behavior. The mathematical models currently used in modeling human perceptual capabilities suffer from the measuring problem, which includes difficulties in encoding and describing the varying task load and human workload, the state of social and physical environments, and design and measurement of the information flow in people and machines (Karwowski et al. 1999). The unified methodology of human perceptual systems engineering, dynamics, and fuzzy sets is viewed as a powerful modeling tool that can overcome some of the above problems to model human cognitive and perceptual components.

Neuroergonomics can be defined as the study of the brain and behavior at work (Parasuraman 2003). Parasuraman (2003) stated that the field of neuroergonomics combines two disciplines: neuroscience, the study of brain structure and function; and HF/E, the study of how to match technology with the capabilities and limitations of people so they can work effectively and safely. "The goal of merging these two fields is to use the startling discoveries of human brain and physiological functioning both to inform the design of technologies in the workplace and home, and to provide new training methods that enhance performance, expand capabilities, and optimize the fit between people and technology" (Parasuraman and Rizzo 2007). Research in the area of neuroergonomics has been nourished in recent years with the emergence of noninvasive techniques for monitoring human brain function that can be used to study various aspects of human behavior in relation to technology and work, including mental workload, visual attention, working memory, motor control, human–automation interaction, and adaptive automation.

Cognitive ergonomics is defined as the science that aims to assure compatibility in the artifact–human functioning with respect to complex and uncertain interrelationships between system users, machines, and the environment (Guastello 1995; Karwowski et al. 1999; Wells et al. 2011; Ahram and Karwowski 2011a). Such analysis must account for natural nonlinear dynamics (chaos) and the fuzziness of human cognitive processes. Uncertainty because of vagueness of human decision making and thoughts is inherent to any complex system, and to the human perceptual processes. To study complex artifact–human systems it is necessary to use modeling approaches that are approximate in nature. Systems engineering and fuzziness is a useful model for human language and categorizing processes. Fuzziness describes an event ambiguity and measures the degree to which an event occurs, not whether it occurs or not (Zadeh 1973; Kosko 1992). Systems engineering and systems dynamics modeling provide useful frameworks for modeling a variety of complex tasks, situations, artifacts, and environments, and their interactions with people. As this type of complexity occurs at all levels of human interactions with the outside environment, ranging from physical to cognitive tasks, it can be used as the natural model of human sensory, information processing, communication, or physiological functioning. The potential advantages for systems engineering and systems dynamics modeling applications in human sciences are as follows:

- To model human language and categorizing inter-related perceptual processes.
- To augment conventional statistical techniques in analysis of fuzzy and complex decision making.
- To supplement for statistical techniques such as reliability analysis and regressions, and structurally oriented methods such as hierarchical clustering and multidimensional scaling.

In view of the above, systems engineering, fuzzy logic, and systems dynamics methodologies can provide a useful modeling framework for the applied neuroergonomics, human cognition and perception, and especially for modeling a variety of complex human brain functions, systems, and artifacts, and their interactions with the environment.

12.3 Overview of Human Brain Functions

The human brain is divided into two hemispheres connected with fibers, which interpret the world differently (Di Carlo, Khoshnevis, and Udwadia 2009; Ramos, Ferreira, and Barcelo 2012). The left-brain thinking or the L-mode is the analytical, quantitative, verbal, rational, linear, step-by-step thinking. The right-brain thinking or the R-mode is the integrative, qualitative, holistic, creative, and visual thinking. The brain consists of four main structures: the cerebral cortex, famous for its many folds and valleys; the cerebellum; the brainstem, responsible for many automatic processes; and the limbic system. These brain elements have direct analogs in other animals, with simpler elements such as the brain stem actually serving as the entire brain in animals lower on the evolutionary ladder. The brain's evolutionary history can be broken down into the reptilian brain (the oldest), the limbic brain, present in most mammals, and the neocortex, first found in primates but most developed in humans (Jacobs et al. 2007). There are also four major elements of the cerebral cortex; these are the frontal lobe, the temporal lobe, the parietal lobe, and the occipital lobe. The brain has two hemispheres connected by the corpus callosum, which is responsible for transferring information between the two hemispheres.

Brain functions have largely been mapped, and it is mostly known what functions each of the major regions perform. Many such findings came about by studying human subjects who have experienced damage to various areas of the brain; areas that have known damage can then be linked to resulting behavior (Kolb 2003). More modern investigative measures use advanced noninvasive imaging techniques that can visualize activity during given behaviors. For example, the frontal lobe is responsible for movement of body parts and for higher cognitive tasks such as speaking and planning. The parietal lobe concerns itself with sensory information coming from the skin. It also serves a role in spatial recognition and reasoning associated with mathematics. The occipital lobe is known to process visual information. The temporal lobe contains elements that operate on memory and navigate through space. Emotions are known to activate areas of the amygdala.

Human perception is a dynamic nonlinear process under control of the observer who is consciously aware of the observed phenomena. The process of conscious perception is a fuzzy one, with ambiguity due to both physiological thresholds for physical stimuli and pattern recognition and judgment requirements. For example, at what frequency an intermittent light will be perceived as just flickering is an ambiguous question and, hence, the eye flicker frequency is fuzzy and dynamic with environmental conditions, not a random phenomenon, as it refers to the degree of noticeable flickering rather than the question of whether it occurs (Karwowski and Salvendy 1992). It should be noted here that the psychophysical laws, which relate the magnitude of change in physical stimuli (ΔI) that will just be noticed by an observer, are also fuzzy laws. According to the Weber–Fetchner law, the magnitude of change in a physical stimulus that will be just noticed by an observer is a constant proportion of the stimulus. Although defined in terms of the magnitude of ΔI that will result in a judgment of a difference in the levels of physical stimuli 50% of the time (so-called just-noticeable difference), this law refers not to the probabilistic statement of whether the perception of change will occur, but to what level of the difference in physical stimuli such a change will be observed (Karwowski and Salvendy 1992).

The degree to which many sources of object stimuli and different dimensions of the same objects can be processed by the human brain exemplifies the fuzzy dynamic nature of human perceptual processes (see Figure 12.1). The human ability to process information from different stimulus objects at one time is limited. However, several dimensions

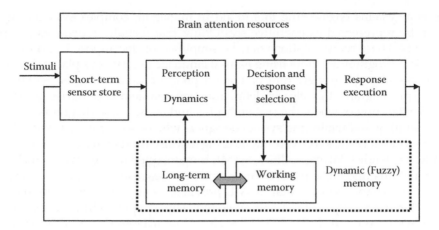

FIGURE 12.1
An example system dynamics model of human information processing.

of a single object can be processed in parallel (Wickens 1987). Therefore, we ask the most important question: To what degree can the human brain process several sources of object stimuli and different dimensions of the same objects? The answer to this question indicates the need to consider the fuzzy and dynamic nature of human perceptual processes. A similar question can be posed with respect to stimulus-central processing capability. For example, in the human–machine system, the displayed information can be arranged along a continuum that defines the degree to which that information is spatial–analog (i.e., information about relative locations, transformations, or continuous motion), linguistic–symbolic, or verbal (i.e., a set of instructions, alphanumeric codes, directions, or logical operations) in nature.

The border between these two systems (i.e., the verbal–spatial), however, is ambiguous and subject to human perception dynamics and fuzzy interpretation. Although the distinction between the short-term (working) memory and the long-term memory has been universally accepted, the degree to which the memory is short or long is also a fuzzy and dynamic category (see Figure 12.1). The same applies, and even more so, to the classification of spatial and verbal perceptual memory systems.

12.4 Systems Modeling Language

The field of systems engineering is concerned with the whole, the complexity, the multi-disciplinarity, the holistic thinking, the synthesis and, consequently, it seems natural to identify these concerns with the R-mode, which is normally neglected in engineering curriculum (Di Carlo, Khoshnevis, and Udwadia 2009). The Object Management Group (OMG) and the International Council of Systems Engineering (INCOSE) have joined efforts and developed an extension of the unified modeling language (UML) for systems engineering: the systems modeling language (SysML) (OMG SysML 2011), which was released in 2007. This visual SysML, which supports the specification, analysis, design, and verification of complex systems, is considered as the next de facto modeling language for systems engineering.

SysML is a systems engineering tool to aid in managing complex systems. At its core, SysML can be represented as cognitive scaffolding that visually represents complex systems elements. These representations may be simplified or decomposed, and often contain pseudo-code, a programmer's tool using natural language to serve as a placeholder for actual code. Pseudo-code will strongly hint or suggest programming elements. SysML also provides powerful diagrams that clearly define functional system boundaries, providing at-a-glance understanding of where the system begins and ends. These diagrams are especially useful for defining and reminding system designers who or what interacts with the system. SysML is a subset of UML, a software engineering tool also used to manage complex systems. Specifically, it extends UML capabilities. SysML is maintained by the OMG, which publishes updates, maintains, and implements changes, and provides resources and training materials.

The capabilities and benefits that SysML provides to any application managing complexity are far from fully utilized and exploited. This chapter will describe the benefits SysML can bring to the fields of neuroscience and neuroergonomics, especially from an applied view. The overarching theme of this chapter is that SysML manages complexity, and good management of said complexity offers measurable, discrete, and easily applicable avenues of understanding complex brain functions. The human brain, being one of the most complex entities currently in existence, could be better understood with some of its complexity managed. Benefits of modeling the human brain in SysML are not only academic, but applied as well. Authors such as Sarter and Sarter (2003) describe the benefits of predictors of performance through psychophysiological measures. These measures can be represented by diagrams and linked to their underlying brain structures, using simulation data to create useful, predictive models.

SysML is very powerful because it integrates, visualizes, and aids in enacting methods and processes from fields related to nonlinear dynamics, namely those from systems engineering, cognitive engineering, human systems integration (HSI) and HF/E. SysML is created and defined by the OMG. As mentioned, SysML is an extension to the UML, as defined in Figure 12.2. It builds upon and extends the capabilities of UML, a powerful graphical tool for modeling systems.

The capabilities and benefits that SysML provides to any application managing complexity are far from fully utilized and exploited. This chapter will describe the benefits SysML can bring to neuroscience and HF/E, especially from an applied view. The overarching theme of this chapter is that SysML manages complexity, and good management of said complexity offers measurable, discrete, and easily applicable avenues of mitigating risk. SysML is widely used as a visualization tool to promote complex system understanding to a variety of stakeholders.

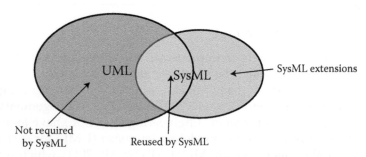

FIGURE 12.2
(See color insert.) Relationship between SysML and UML. (Adapted from OMG SysML. 2011. Retrieved october 26, 2011, from http://www.omgsysml.org/.)

According to Ramos, Ferreira, and Barcelo (2012), the object process methodology (OPM), which was founded by Dori in 2002, and the corresponding graphical and textual representations, object process diagrams (OPDs), and object process language (OPL) enlarge the domain of object-oriented-modeling tools for systems engineering (Dori 2002; Grobshtein and Dori 2009).

The provided bimodality (i.e., graphical and textual) facilitates the understanding of brain functions complexity as it is very similar to the power of both sides of the brain, that is, the right side that acts like the visual interpreter and the left side that acts like the language interpreter. According to Grobshtein and Dori (2009), this intuitive dual notation provides a single model that is comprehensible to the different stakeholders (both technical and nontechnical) involved in the development process. They are available at the software environment object process CASE tool (OPCAT). The OPM is based on three fundamental aspects of a system: the structure (how it is made), the function (what it does), and the behavior (how it changes over time). The function is enabled by the architecture of the system that combines the structure and the behavior. The graphics (i.e., OPDs) and the natural language (i.e., OPL) express these characteristics in a unified frame of reference that corresponds to an integrated single model.

SysML diagram types and their activities are outlined in Figure 12.3. The basic unit of SysML is a block. Blocks are denoted with bold type and encased in guillemets (≪ ≫). These blocks represent hardware. By connecting blocks, hierarchies are quickly formed. These hierarchies are enclosed in rectangles and called package diagrams. The HSI diagram components can be identified under both the behavior and structure diagrams. This can be done to compensate for a human capabilities diagram and task requirements with respect to human performance, which does not exist.

Johnson et al. (2007) described a more behavioral modeling approach using SysML diagrams. These authors claim that SysML succinctly defines system structure and behavior using the following diagram types:

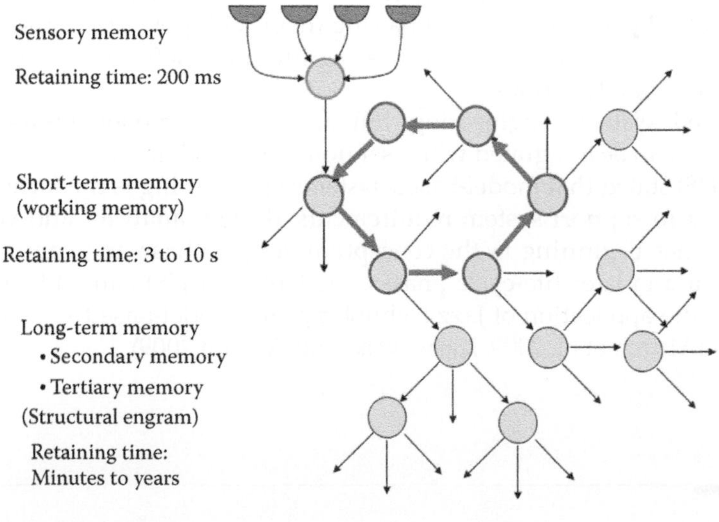

Sensory memory

Retaining time: 200 ms

Short-term memory
(working memory)

Retaining time: 3 to 10 s

Long-term memory
• Secondary memory
• Tertiary memory
(Structural engram)

Retaining time:
Minutes to years

FIGURE 12.3
(See color insert.) Extended SysML diagram taxonomy incorporated with considerations of human systems integration. (Extended model based on original framework by Reprinted from *A Practical Guide to SysML: The Systems Modeling Language*. Burlington, MA: Morgan Kaufmann, Friedenthal, S., A. Moore, and R. Steiner, Copyright 2008, with permission from Elsevier.)

- *Activity diagrams* describe inputs, outputs, sequences, and conditions that govern various system behaviors.
- *Sequence diagrams* describe the flow of control, commands, and responsibilities between actors and a system or its components.
- *State machine diagrams* model discrete behavior and guide developers and designers through finite state transitions in system states.
- *Parametric diagrams* model mathematical constraints against system properties.

Guillerm, Demmou, and Sadou (2010) demonstrated that SysML drives requirements integration by assigning various diagrams to visualize the requirements process:

- *The requirements*: Requirements diagram, Use Case diagram
- *The structure*: Block diagram (internal/external)
- *The behavior*: Statechart, Activity diagram, Sequence diagram
- *The constraints*: Parametric diagram

Relationships are easily defined and displayed. Requirements can be linked to other components of the model, affording simplified traceability and knowledge of responsibility. Modifications or changes to system properties are easily managed through these diagrams, making impact analysis straightforward.

One often-touted benefit of SysML through this work is that it offers traceability to requirements. Tracing requirements back to system functions is integral to the understanding of inner workings of the brain. Slicing is a technique developed to help manage complex software systems, which have been growing exponentially in recent times. It is traditionally used to aid in debugging software as only sections are looked one at a time, rather than the entire program. Slicing is applicable to neuroscience investigations as it narrows the investigative scope to only relevant elements regarding brain behavior. By using appropriate slicing activities and pairing them with powerful SysML visualization techniques, SysML can demonstrate practical significant benefits to the correctness of and understanding of brain functions.

In model-based systems engineering, human behavior model libraries and human behavior analysis can be integrated with user domain model libraries. Friedenthal, Moore, and Steiner (2008) stated that model-based systems engineering is the formalized application of modeling to support system requirements, design, analysis, and verification and validation activities beginning in the conceptual design phase and continuing throughout development and later life-cycle phases. Model-based HSI can add value to systems engineering by the application of Jazz technology and model-based systems engineering methodologies (Ahram et al. 2009; Karwowski and Ahram 2009).

12.5 Modeling Human Brain Functions Using Systems Engineering

SysML is a modeling language that aids in visualizing complex software or systems of systems, ideally suited to modeling and visualizing neuroergonomic and cognitive constructs. The brain and its capabilities may be simulated on one part of the model, while a computer system may be simulated on another (Ahram and Karwowski 2009; Ahram et al. 2009). The respective dynamics, strengths, and capabilities combined with the shortcomings of each system can be shown graphically, and task performance or decision making can be simulated, analyzed, and optimized.

Using real data on human perceptual and cognitive performance combined with the current understanding of brain structure and function, SysML along with systems dynamics can create cognitive models predicting perceptual task performance by implementing models of known structures, their interactions, and perhaps implement the results of fuzzy logic to create meaningful, visual, and quantitative models. Figures 12.4 and 12.5 show an example model of the dorsal/ventral streams in visual perception and brain left- and right-side structures. The SysML model breaks down brain perceptual and decision-making structures and their functions. It can be used for training or educational purposes in addition to the simulation of dynamic decision making. Simulations can be quickly made from this and related models (Ahram et al. 2009). Systems dynamics along with SysML will prove to be an exciting addition to the growing neuroergonomics set of toolbox capabilities.

This compartmentalized, yet interconnected, nature of the brain lends itself to modeling through SysML. The various diagrams and connecting elements of SysML can aid in understanding brain function, while the simulation aspects of SysML can actually begin to model, predict, and describe brain function across multiple layers of abstraction. A practical example is that SysML diagram elements can describe how individual brain elements working together can exhibit complex, visible behavior. The evolutionary history of the brain, with various structures and layers building on each other, forms a relationship that can be exploited by the various SysML diagrams and connection types.

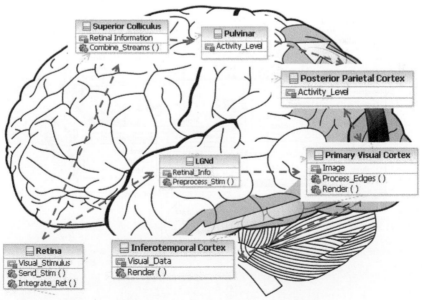

SysML Model of Dorsal/Ventral Stream in Visual Perception

FIGURE 12.4
(See color insert.) Generic overview of brain structures related to visual perception represented in SysML.

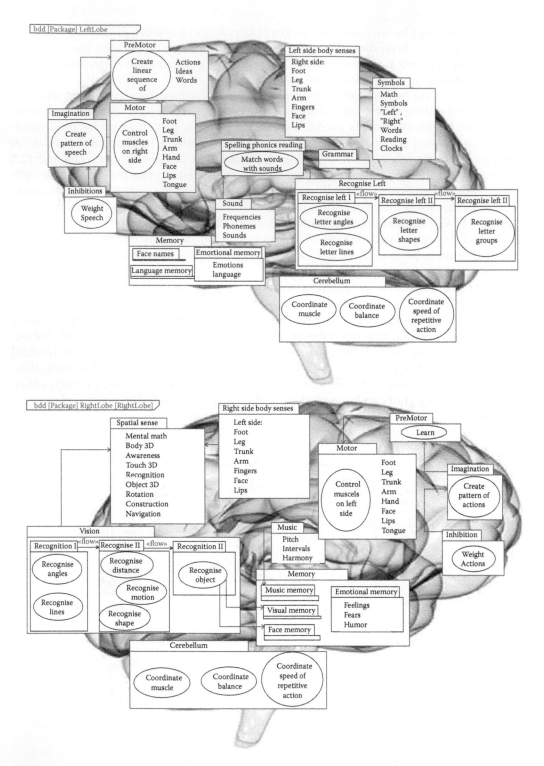

FIGURE 12.5
(See color insert.) SysML block definition diagram for the detailed brain left- and right-side structures.

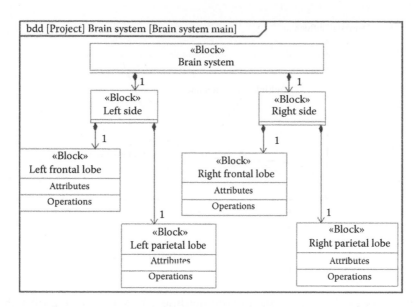

FIGURE 12.6
(See color insert.) An example SysML brain subsystem.

Class diagrams can represent different areas of the brain. They can contain the variables or information that is processed or manipulated at the respective area of the brain. Furthermore, relationships can be demonstrated through connections drawn between the diagrams themselves. In the example shown in Figures 12.5 and 12.6, the SysML block definition diagram depicts the individual brain left- and right-side structures, and the text below the structure labels describe processes (functions) or information (variables) that can be passed between them. The overall diagram displays and demonstrates the relationships of information flow in the dorsal and ventral streams within the brain responsible for visual representation.

Considering the uncertainty and complexity in the process of information interpretation, dynamic fuzzy systems can be a useful modeling approach for analysis and design of human–machine interactions. Shimizu and Jindo (1995) proposed a framework for dealing with ambiguities and nonlinearity of the human information processing relevant to modeling of human sensitivity. The conventional methods to quantify the relationships between human sensations and physical characteristics that influence them are typically the multivariate analysis techniques such as multiple regression analysis and quantification theory. However, when higher-order data are involved, it is much more difficult to find a model formula that suitably represents the nonlinearity factor. Moreover, many conventional methods have traditionally excluded the ambiguities that can arise in the process of recognizing and making subjective evaluations of the physical characteristics. The main advantage of dynamic fuzzy systems is that the ambiguities and nonlinearity (e.g., of human sensation) can be taken into account and quantified to derive correlations with the considered physical characteristics of the product. A dynamic fuzzy regression method can be applied for the evaluation of human perceptual sensitivity, for example, the perceived thermal sensation in a car interior. The nonlinearity of human sensation modeled through the traditional method of the multiple regression analysis is illustrated in Figure 12.7.

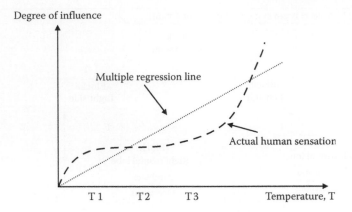

FIGURE 12.7
An example of nonlinearity of human sensation and perception. (After Shimizu, Y. and T. Jindo. 1995. *International Journal of Industrial Ergonomics* 15: 39–47.)

Although it is possible to treat the marked nonlinearity shown in Figure 12.8 by transforming the variables, it is difficult to determine how the variables should be transformed into the non-fuzzy regression. It was shown that 85% of the data items obtained through the subjective evaluations of the car temperature fell within the range of the predicted values obtained from the fuzzy regression analysis method. The results also showed that

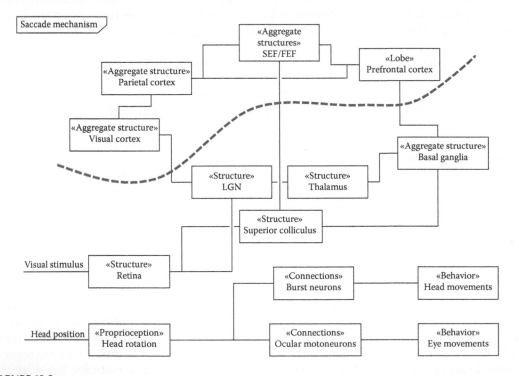

FIGURE 12.8
(See color insert.) A SysML package diagram describing the saccade mechanism for eye movements. (Modified from Ng, G. 2009. *Brain-Mind Machinery: Brain-Inspired Computing and Mind Opening.* New Jersey: World Scientific Publishing Company.)

dynamic fuzzy logic supported making predictions that take into account natural ambiguity of human perceptual sensations. Furthermore, the application of fuzzy regression analysis made it relatively easy to obtain results that were closer to the true subjective evaluations made by the people.

Decisions are typically followed by responses. The human response processes are intrinsically dynamic, even though the prevalent definition of the relationship between the choice reaction time and the degree of choice (the Hick–Hyman law) is based on the information content of a stimulus (S) in bits as follows: $RT = a + b(S)$. The very visible presence of human fuzziness cannot be overlooked in the paradigm of stimulus–response compatibility. This paradigm relates to the physical relationship (compatibility) between a set of stimuli and a set of responses, as it affects the speed of human response. As pointed out by Karwowski and Salvendy (1992), the spatial relationship between arrangements of signals and response devices in human–machine systems with respect to direction of movement and adjustments are often ambiguous, with a high degree of uncertainty regarding the effects of intended control actions.

Figure 12.8 describes the structures involved in saccade movements, those rapid movements of the eye that occur when shifting the eyes' focus. Consciously desired saccades are dictated by a flow of activity from the cerebral cortical areas and the basal ganglia to the superior colliculus. The eyes are constantly darting around seeking information, and unwanted saccades result when novel, dynamic, or high-magnitude information is presented to the eyes. These unwanted saccades can be suppressed to focus attention on one desired spot (Hikosaka, Takikawa, and Kawagoe 2000).

The dashed line in Figure 12.8 is a representation of the cerebral cortex, and shows the relative positions of the brain structures to each other within the cortex. The other diagrams found outside of this boundary reside outside of the cortex, with the lateral geniculate nucleus residing inside of the thalamus, which is found between the cerebral cortex and midbrain. The basal ganglia are connected to the cerebral cortex but are actually found at the base of the forebrain.

The hierarchical nature of the brain, and specifically its function, is described in Figure 12.9. The overall diagram is presented as a package diagram (a container) with context diagrams embedded within it connected to each other. The context diagrams are responsible for showing what belongs in the system. They are linked together showing the structure of the brain's internal mechanisms directly responsible for rapid-eye movements, or saccades.

The brain is shown as a system, and the context diagrams help define the boundaries of this system. This specific example demonstrates how context diagrams within the brain can define which systems are responsible for a given function or cognitive mechanism. This example defines only which brain structures are required to run the saccade mechanism; it does not explicitly exclude structures that are not required. Diagrams that are more complex could then describe how this particular brain mechanism relates to outside actors, actions, or other bodily systems; however, these are not represented here.

Figure 12.10 provides a broad overview of information exchanges in the brain, both internal and external, showing visible behavior. Information from the sensory organs is processed within the limbic system, specifically the thalamus. Memories are created, and depending on the circumstances, properties, and nature of the information it is stored, ignored, or processed further.

For example, the skin is constantly sending information about clothes touching it; however, this information is quickly disregarded and not even remembered until specifically called or acted upon. A particularly pleasant scent or visage is processed and likely stored

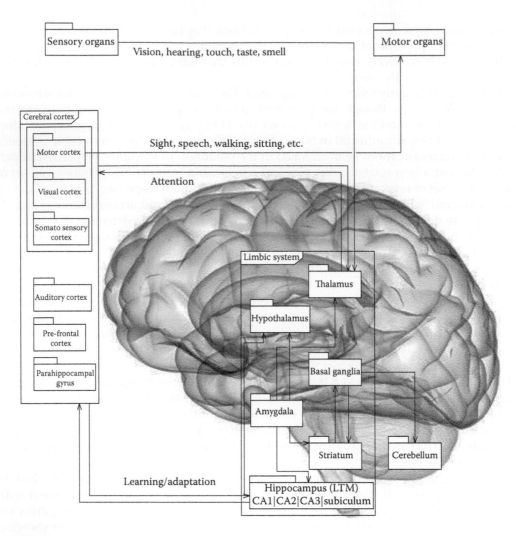

FIGURE 12.9
Brain architecture in SysML. (Modified from Ng, G. 2009. *Brain-Mind Machinery: Brain-Inspired Computing and Mind Opening.* New Jersey: World Scientific Publishing Company.)

long term. Imagine a scent such as that of the house you grew up in and see the associated memories that are quickly elicited. Visual information that is incomplete or not ready to be used immediately will be processed further. A blurry face or a math problem is an example of such a stimulus.

Activity from the amygdala regarding emotions may enhance or detract the memorability of an item. There are various theories of memory, some mutually exclusive or only applicable in certain domains or situations, further illustrating the problem of complexity investigation the brain presents.

Knowledge and data are best used to make predictions about future outcomes. Using SysML to logically link brain structures and processes to behavior is a possible course of action. Figure 12.11 describes the hierarchical arrangement of brain processes and their associated roles in certain behaviors using SysML block definition diagram as an example of behaviors decomposed by brain structures. Both musical aptitude and reading

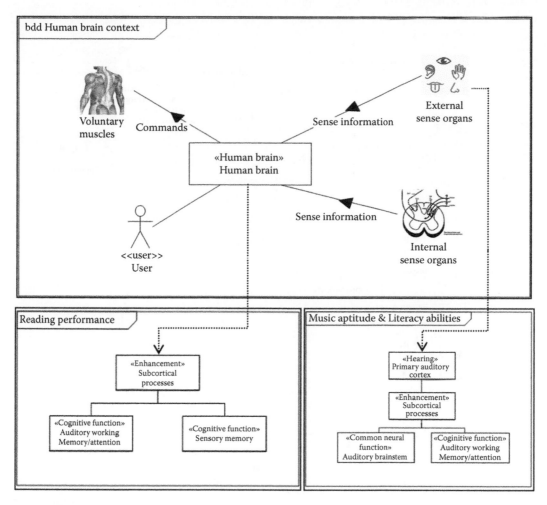

FIGURE 12.10
(**See color insert.**) SysML block definition diagram for example behaviors decomposed by brain structures.

performance rely on subcortical processes. Music aptitude differs from reading performance slightly by using more of the auditory brainstem, which handles low-level automatic processes. Reading performance involves more of sensory memory, as patterns for words must be recognized, recalled, and put to use toward building and understanding of the text.

12.6 Systems Dynamics Modeling of Complex Human Perceptual Functions

Systems dynamics modeling of human perception is a novel graphical approach to make the modeling of dynamical perceptual systems accessible by combining the relations

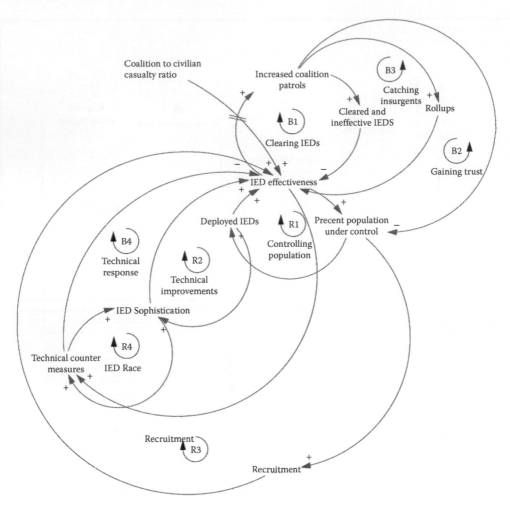

FIGURE 12.11
(See color insert.) An example systems dynamics model in the context of warfare technology concept decision making. (After Choucri, N. et al. 2006. Understanding and modeling state stability: Exploiting system dynamics. In *Proceedings of the 2006 Institute of Electronics Engineers Aerospace Conference*, Big Sky, MT, March 4–11, 2006. USA: Institute of Electrical and Electronics Engineers.)

we perceive in such systems. According to Fuchs (2006, 2010), the simple ideas behind systems dynamics models correspond to a basic form of human thought. It makes use of a very few structures that are projected onto virtually any type of dynamical system and its processes; that is, it makes strong use of analogical reasoning (Fuchs 2002a,b). For example, Figure 12.11 shows an example systems dynamics model in the context of warfare technology concept. Systems dynamics applies to dynamic problems arising in complex social, managerial, economic, or ecological systems (i.e., any dynamic system characterized by interdependence, mutual interaction, information feedback, and circular causality). The field developed initially from the work of Forrester (1961, 1969) in his seminal book *Industrial Dynamics*, which is still a significant statement of philosophy and methodology in the field. Within 10 years of its publication, the span of applications grew from corporate and industrial problems to include the engineering, science, research and development, and the dynamics of growth in a finite world. Systems dynamics modeling is now applied in defense and theory-building in social science (Ahram and Karwowski 2011b; Ahram, Karwowski, and Amaba 2011), and other areas, as well as decision making (Systems Dynamics Society 2011; Ahram and Karwowski 2011a,b) and service engineering (Karwowski et al. 2010).

The name industrial dynamics no longer does justice to the breadth of the field, so it has become generalized to systems dynamics. According to Morecroft (2007), the modern name suggests links to other systems engineering methodologies. Systems dynamics emerges out of servo-mechanisms engineering, not general systems theory or cybernetics (Richardson 1991). Forrester (1969) provided the following framework for systems dynamics structure: closed boundary, which includes feedback loops, levels, rates, goal, observed condition, discrepancy, and desired action. According to the Systems Dynamics Society (2011):

> The importance of levels and rates appear most clearly when one takes a continuous view of structure and dynamics. Although a discrete view, focusing on separate events and decisions, is entirely compatible with an endogenous feedback perspective; the system dynamics approach emphasizes a continuous view. The continuous view strives to look beyond events to see the dynamic patterns underlying them. Moreover, the continuous view focuses not on discrete decisions but on the policy structure underlying decisions. Events and decisions are seen as surface phenomena that ride on an underlying tide of system structure and behavior. It is that underlying tide of policy structure and continuous behavior that is the system dynamicist's focus.

Complex systems develop because of the natural tendency of components and subsystems to resonate and synchronize (Robertson-Dunn 2009). This form of complex assembly develops because of existing nonlinearities such as those aspects related to growth needs and increased interaction between various human perceptual and cognitive components. As energy levels rise, structures that require high energy to form can be created and become very stable because the energy levels needed to destroy them are no longer present (Robertson-Dunn 2009).

Research into complex systems has examined the understanding of specific systems rather than looking at the phenomenon as a whole (Norling, Powell, and Edmonds 2008). The modeling paradigm described in this chapter is based on a wide range of evidence and an approach that focuses on the behavior of complex systems in general. Emergent, self-organizing, complex systems are non-stationary, non-equilibrium, non-homogeneous, and non-linear. They are formed via processes that are episodic, during which structures are created and energy stored in those structures. Structures can be formed by removing or applying energy. All complex systems including human cognitive and perceptual processes are dynamic and are capable of displaying some form of oscillation (Sterman 2000; Robertson-Dunn 2009). The oscillation may be either the result of an external, driving force or a characteristic of the system itself.

In the case of falling energy levels for human perception dynamics, neural structures can arise and develop more connections that reflect particular relationships between components and subsystems or a new acquired knowledge based on human perceptual capacities. When the energy levels cycle above and below particular values, structures already formed can be transformed and/or participate in other more complex structures increasing the nonlinearity and dynamics of such human perceptual system.

It is a characteristic of complex systems that the perceptual components of a system can be influenced and changed by the system itself. This happens when system-designed behavior leads to accumulation of high levels of energy that result in the components being impacted.

The self-organizing nature of complex systems can be the result of one or more phenomena such as energy wells and resonance due to the human perceptual and learning process itself and can be assisted by the presence of existing structures that can facilitate the development of specific, more likely, or more efficient structures including those responsible for decision making (Robertson-Dunn 2009). Although this might look like the phenomena of design in general human-designed systems, in reality it is simply a catalytic effect or a preference for that which already exists. A summary of the analysis of complex systems is given in Table 12.1.

Many of the nonlinear features and behaviors of the complex systems are typically disregarded in exchange for a simple system understanding (Gleick 1987; Karwowski 1991). In the traditional view, simple systems were thought to behave in simple ways, whereas only complex behavior implied complex causes. It should be noted here that complex human perceptual and cognitive systems are the rule rather than the exception in ergonomic and neuroscience studies (Karwowski 1991); owing to the interaction and continuous exchange of information with the surrounding environment, such systems could experience turbulence and coherence at the same time, with abrupt changes in behavior. It is plausible that many such systems exhibit the "Feigenbaum phenomenon" (Feigenbaum 1980); that is, under certain circumstances these perceptual and cognitive decision-making systems develop chaotic behavior, which cannot be explained in the framework of traditional research approaches used in cognitive ergonomics or neuroscience of today.

Human cognitive and perceptual complex systems are the new scientific frontier that was emerging in the past decades with advances in modern computing technology and the study of new parametric domains in natural systems (Robertson-Dunn 2009). An important challenge involves unprecedented difficulty in predicting human behavior by their structure and the interaction strength between perceptual and cognitive system components. Complex perceptual and cognitive systems are shielded completely by their specific individual features. So these fuzzy and dynamic systems are a counter example to

TABLE 12.1

Principles of Complex Systems

Nonlinearities	Stable complex system structures are dependent on the nonlinear nature of the components and their interactions.
Emergence	Properties that emerge from a complex perceptual and cognitive system are consequences of its structure and development over a long period of time.
Hierarchies	Complex systems can act as components of systems that are more complex.
Creation	Complex systems are created via episodic energy interchanges with their environment or through the learning process where individuals acquire new knowledge.
Stability	Complex systems have structures that are stable within certain limits. They are created as energy levels vary—sometimes by the application of large amounts of perceptual and environmental needs, energy, and sometimes by setting or annealing.
Structures and complexity	A variety of structures, energy storage, and/or resonant frequencies are required for systems of greater complexity.
Interactions	Complex systems interact and synchronize with other systems via resonant and nonlinear mechanisms.
Human energies	Complex human systems can form on the basis of conceptual energy storage mechanisms and resonance mechanisms.

Source: Adapted from Robertson-Dunn, B. 2009. Meta modelling self organising, emergent and complex systems. Retrieved from: http://www.drbrd.com/docs/MetaModellingComplexSystems.doc.

reductionism, which have been influential in science with a Cartesian method that is only valid for complicated systems.

It is possible today to study complex cognitive and perceptual systems using systems dynamics and fuzzy nonlinear modeling that allow handling of some of their dynamical properties associated with natural system invariants in a way similar to the investigation of complex information systems. Because of their qualitative nature, independent of system state space dimension and generic imprecision, such dynamical models are capable of compensating a variety of system parameters and functional variations (Robertson-Dunn 2009).

12.7 Conclusions

Although tremendous advances have been made in neuroscience, reverse-engineering the brain is still a grand challenge (Nageswaran et al. 2010), with researchers proposing competing hypotheses and modeling approaches to explain the nature of coding and speed of processing by brain circuits and functions; better understanding can be exploited using SysML and systems engineering concepts to enable the simulation of large-scale, biologically realistic brain circuits. The capabilities and benefits that SysML provides to any application managing complexity are far from fully utilized and exploited. This chapter describes the benefits SysML can bring to neuroscience and HF/E especially from an applied point of view. The overarching theme of this chapter is that SysML manages complexity, and good management of said complexity offers measurable, discrete, and easily applicable avenues of mitigating complexity and nonlinearity of human brain functions. SysML is widely used as a visualization tool to promote complex system understanding to a variety of engineering problems.

The study of human cognitive capabilities faces the problems of system complexity, nonlinear dynamics, and related human and system-based fuzziness that increase the ever-present incompatibility between people and their living and working environments. As pointed out in this chapter, fuzziness and dynamics are not just a product of the human mind but the essence of human development and existence in the ever-more complex world where we live, and a necessary condition for human learning, growth, and survival in a challenging environment rich in computing technologies and fast processing mobile services. To develop a cohesive and durable relationship between people and the outside surroundings (both natural and artificial), the intrinsic dynamics of human perceptual and cognitive processing must be treated by system designers and engineers as natural system design requirements with complex interactions with the environment. Systems engineering methodologies, such as SySML and systems dynamics, allow incorporation of human cognitive complexity into the design process, and provide the necessary framework for successful modeling efforts in the human factors engineering discipline.

References

Ahram, T. Z. and W. Karwowski. 2009 Human–systems integration modeling using systems modelling language. In *Proceedings of the 53rd Annual Meeting of the Human Factors and Ergonomics*

Society (HFES), October 19–23, 2009, San Antonio, TX, Vol. 53, no. 24, pp. 1849–53. Los Angeles: Sage/HFES..

Ahram, T. and W. Karwowski. 2011a. Social networking applications: Smarter product design for complex human behaviour modeling. In *Proceedings of the 14th International Conference on Human-Computer Interaction (HCII 2011)*, Orlando, FL, July 9–14, 2011, *Lecture Notes in Computer Science: Human Centered Design*, Vol. 6776, pp. 471–80. Berlin and Heidelberg: Springer.

Ahram, T. Z. and W. Karwowski. 2011b. Developing human social, cultural, behaviour (HSCB) ontologies: Visualizing & modeling complex human interactions. Presented at the Office of Secretary of Defense, Human Social, Culture Behavior Modeling (HSCB Focus 2011), February 8–10, 2011, Chantilly, VA.

Ahram, T., W. Karwowski, and B. Amaba. 2011. Collaborative systems engineering and social networking approach to design and modeling of smarter products. *Behaviour and Information Technology* 30 (1): 13–26.

Ahram, T. Z., W. Karwowski, B. Amaba, and P. Obeid. 2009. Human systems integration: Development based on SysML and the rational systems platform. In *Proceedings of the 2009 Industrial Engineering Research Conference*, Miami, FL, May 30–June 3, 2009, pp. 2333–8.

Choucri, N., D. Goldsmith, S. E. Madnick, D. Mishtree, J. B. Morrison, M. Siegel, and M. Sweitzer-Hamilton. 2006. Understanding and modeling state stability: Exploiting system dynamics. In *Proceedings of the 2006 Institute of Electronics Engineers Aerospace Conference*, Big Sky, MT, March 4–11, 2006. USA: Institute of Electrical and Electronics Engineers.

Di Carlo, T., B. Khoshnevis, and F. Udwadia. 2009. Whole brain thinking in systems architecting. *Systems Engineering* 12: 265–273.

Dori, D. 2002. *Object-Process Methodology: A Holistic Systems Paradigm*. New York: Springer.

Feigenbaum, M. J. 1980. Universal behavior in nonlinear systems. *Los Alamos Science* 1:4.

Forrester, J. W. 1961. *Industrial Dynamics*. Cambridge, MA: The MIT Press. Reprinted by Pegasus Communications, Waltham, MA.

Forrester, J. W. 1969. *Urban Dynamics*. Cambridge, MA: The MIT Press. Reprinted by Pegasus Communications, Waltham, MA.

Friedenthal, S., A. Moore, and R. Steiner. 2008. *A Practical Guide to SysML: The Systems Modeling Language*. Burlington, MA: Morgan Kaufmann (Elsevier Science).

Fuchs, H. U. 2002a. *Modeling of Uniform Dynamical Systems.*, Zürich: Orell Füssli Verlag.

Fuchs, H. U. 2002b. A simple continuum model leading to the reciprocity relation for thermoelectric effects. Report, Zurich University of Applied Sciences at Winterthur, Switzerland. Retrieved from: https://home.zhaw.ch/~fuh/MATERIALS/Thermoelectricity.pdf

Fuchs, H. U. 2006. System dynamics modeling in science and engineering. Invited Talk at the *System Dynamics Conference*, University of Puerto Rico Resource Center for Science and Engineering, Mayaguez, December 8–10, 2006. Retrieved from https://home.zhaw.ch/~fuh/MATERIALS/PR_SDMSE.pdf

Fuchs, H. U. 2010. *The Dynamics of Heat*, 2nd ed. New York: Springer-Verlag.

Gleick, J. 1987. *Chaos: Making a New Science*. New York: Penguin Books.

Grobshtein, Y. and D. Dori. 2009. Creating SysML views from an OPM model. In *Proceedings of the 2nd International Conference on Model Based Systems Engineering*, Herzelya and Haifa, Israel, March 2–5, 2009, pp. 36–45.

Guastello, S. J. 1995. *Chaos, Catastrophe, and Human Affairs*. Mahwah, NJ: Lawrence Erlbaum Associates.

Guillerm, R., H. Demmou, and N. Sadou. 2010. Information model for model driven safety requirements management of complex systems. In *Proceedings of the First International Conference on Complex Systems Design & Management (CSDM '10)*, Paris, France, October 27–29, 2010, pp. 99–111.

Hikosaka, O., Y. Takikawa, and R. Kawagoe. 2000. Role of the basal ganglia in the control of purposive saccadic eye movements. *Physiological Reviews* 80 (3): 953–78.

Jacobs, D. K., N. Nakanishi, D. Yuan, A. Camara, S. A. Nichols, and V. Hartenstein. 2007. Evolution of sensory structures in basal metazoa. *Integrative and Comparative Biology* 47 (5): 712–23.

Johnson, T. A., C. Paredis, R. Burkhart, and J. Jobe. 2007. Modeling continuous system dynamics in SysML. In *ASME International Mechanical Engineering Congress and Exposition*, November 11–15, 2007, Seattle, Washington, USA.

Karwowski, W. 1991. Complexity, fuzziness and ergonomic incompatibility issues in the control of dynamic work environments. *Ergonomics* 34: 671–86.

Karwowski, W. and T. Z. Ahram. 2009. Interactive management of human factors knowledge for human systems integration using systems modeling language. *Journal of Information Systems Management* 26 (3): 262–74.

Karwowski, W., J. Grobelny, Yang Yang, and Wook Gee Lee. 1999. Applications of fuzzy systems in human factors. In *Handbook of Fuzzy Sets and Possibility Theory*, edited by H. Zimmermman, 589–620. Boston, MA: Kluwer Academic Publishers.

Karwowski, W. and G. Salvendy. 1992. Fuzzy-set-theoretic applications in modeling of man-machine interactions. In *An Introduction to Fuzzy Logic Applications in Intelligent Systems*, edited by R. R. Yager and L. A. Zadeh, 201–20. Boston, MA: Kluwer Academic Publishers.

Karwowski, W., G. Salvendy, and T. Ahram. 2010. A human-centered approach to design and modeling of service systems. In *Introduction to Service Engineering*, edited by G. Salvendy and W. Karwowski, 179 206. New York: John Wiley & Sons.

Kolb, B. 2003. Overview of cortical plasticity and recovery from brain injury. *Physical Medicine and Rehabilitation Clinics of North America* 14 (1): S7–25.

Kosko, B. 1992. *Neural Networks and Fuzzy Systems: A Dynamical Systems Approach to Machine Intelligence*. Englewood Cliffs, NJ: Prentice Hall.

Morecroft, J. 2007. *Strategic Modeling and Business Dynamics: A Feedback Systems Approach*. New York: John Wiley & Sons.

Ng, G. 2009. *Brain-Mind Machinery: Brain-Inspired Computing and Mind Opening*. New Jersey: World Scientific Publishing Company.

Nageswaran, J. M., M. Richert, N. Dutt, and J. L. Krichmar. 2010. Towards reverse engineering the brain: Modeling abstractions and simulation frameworks. In *Proceedings of the 2010 18th IEEE/ IFIP International Conference on VLSI System on Chip Conference (VLSI-SoC 2010)*, September 27–29, 2010, pp. 1–6.

Norling, E., C. R. Powell, and B. Edmonds. 2008. Cross-disciplinary views on modelling complex systems. In *9th International Workshop on Multi-Agent-Based Simulation*, Estoril, Portugal, May 12–13, 2008, pp. 183–94. Berlin and Heidelberg: Springer-Verlag.

OMG SysML. 2011. Retrieved October 26, 2011, from http://www.omgsysml.org/

Parasuraman, R. 2003. Neuroergonomics: Research and practice. *Theoretical Issues in Ergonomics Science* 4: 5–20.

Parasuraman, R. and M. Rizzo. 2007. Introduction to neuroergonomics. In *Neuroergonomics: The Brain at Work*, edited by R. Parasuraman and M. Rizzo, 3–12. New York: Oxford University Press.

Ramos, A. L., J. V. Ferreira, and J. Barcelo, J. 2012. Model-based systems engineering: An emerging approach for modern systems. *IEEE Transactions on Systems, Man, and Cybernetics, Part C: Applications and reviews* 42 (1): 101–11.

Richardson, G. P. 1991. *Feedback Thought in Social Science and Systems Theory*. Philadelphia: University of Pennsylvania Press. Reprinted by Pegasus Communications, Waltham, MA.

Robertson-Dunn, B. 2009. Meta modelling self organising, emergent and complex systems. Retrieved from: http://www.drbrd.com/docs/MetaModellingComplexSystems.doc.

Sarter, N., and M. Sarter. 2003. Neuroergonomics: Opportunities and challenges of merging cognitive neuroscience with cognitive ergonomics. *Theoretical Issues in Ergonomics Science* 4 (1–2): 142–50.

Shimizu, Y. and T. Jindo. 1995. A fuzzy logic analysis method for evaluating human sensitivities. *International Journal of Industrial Ergonomics* 15: 39–47.

Sterman, J. 2000. *Business Dynamics: Systems Thinking and Modeling for a Complex World*. New York, NY: McGraw-Hill.

Systems Dynamics Society. 2011. http://www.systemdynamics.org

Wells, W., W. Karwowski, S. Sala-Diakanda, K. Williams, T. Ahram, and J. Pharmer. 2011. Application of systems modeling language (SySML) for cognitive work analysis in systems engineering design process. *Journal of Universal Computer Science* 17 (9): 1261–80.

Wickens, C. D. 1987. Information processing, decision-making, and cognition. In *Handbook of Human Factors*, edited by G. Salvendy, 72–107. New York: John Wiley & Sons.

Zadeh, L. A. 1973. Outline of a new approach to the analysis of complex systems and decision processes. *IEEE Transactions on Systems, Man and Cybernetics* 3: 28–44.

13

Neuroethics: Considerations for a Future Embedded with Neurotechnology

Joseph R. Keebler, Grant Taylor, Elizabeth Phillips, Scott Ososky, and Lee W. Sciarini

CONTENTS

13.1 Introduction

Neuroethics is a burgeoning interdisciplinary field that integrates the sciences of biology, genetics, psychology, neuroscience, and philosophy (Churchland 2006). As technology continues to advance we must be vigilant about the way new devices and human–technology systems are integrated into society, workplaces, and the human condition. It is our intention to use this chapter to raise questions and concerns in some budding neuroscientific areas by exploring possible technological advancements, as well as current-day technology that can give insight into the way humans may interact with neurotech systems in the future. We begin by first examining the philosophical roots of "neuroethics"—specifically, the late American philosopher Robert Nozick's (1938–2002) "Experience Machine" thesis, a debate on whether humans would willingly immerse themselves in a false reality. These assumptions have been contradicted by a multitude of reports and studies on the rampant growth of video game and Internet addiction, which will be reviewed. We will then move into the areas of selection, neuro-entertainment, neuro-clinical diagnoses, and neuro-marketing, exploring a possible future where the value of brain information may surpass that of either words or actions.

13.1.1 Entering the Experience Machine

Imagine if you could have your mind inserted into a false reality. Not only could you go anywhere you want without physically traveling there, but you could be anyone you want, living any lifestyle or fantasy that you could possibly imagine. This type of false reality was coined the "Experience Machine" by Nozick (1974). Theoretically, upon entering the machine, one could be given the opportunity to access any and all accomplishments, positions, or powers imaginable. Although enticing, Nozick (1974) argued that human beings would not want to be immersed into the false reality of such an Experience Machine. He based this assumption on a simple principle related to achieving one's full potential. That is, individuals need to accomplish goals in life to self-actualize, and that being handed a false reality in no way leads to this sense of accomplishment (Nozick 1974). Although his reasoning is sound, there is a current technological trend that seems to demonstrate the opposite, with human beings quite willing to immerse themselves into false realities. One pronounced demonstration of this can be found in the modern trend of Internet and gaming addiction. Worldwide, people are socializing, interacting, and living through technology such as Second Life, World of Warcraft, and Facebook. Consequently, it could be argued that not only will people be willing to immerse themselves into the Experience Machine, but that it is already occurring in some form.

13.1.2 Technology Addictions as Insight for the Future

Many instances of Internet/computer/video game addiction and use demonstrate that Nozick may have been wrong. Although in no way do we intend to take a stance on the nature of video game addiction, or the ethics of video game use, this trend does demonstrate a unique human quality. Human beings, especially younger generations, have shown that they are entirely willing to immerse their lives into a virtual world for the pleasure and opportunity to become someone or something that reality does not or cannot allow them to be. The Experience Machine is here, at least in a primordial form, and we, as a race, are devoutly immersing ourselves into it. As Hancock states in his book *Mind, Machine and Morality: Toward a Philosophy of Human–Technology Symbiosis*: "At the other end of the spectrum, we encounter virtual addiction, where the alternative reality proves so seductive that an individual is tempted not to return to the real world" (2009, 110).

This is in stark contrast to Nozick's thesis. Throughout this chapter there will be a recurring theme of asking a relevant question: What are current methods of neurotechnology use, and, more importantly, should we continue to develop said technology given its current uses?

A useful way to approach these questions is to frame them in terms of Maslow's "hierarchy of needs" (1943), which states that a person must meet certain needs (physiological,

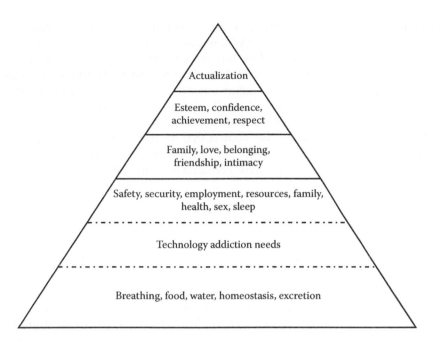

FIGURE 13.1
A modified version of Maslow's hierarchy of needs, including a level for technology addiction needs.

safety, love/belonging, esteem) to "self-actualize" or achieve true personhood and reach one's full potential in life. The lower the needs in the hierarchy, the more fundamental they are to human survival. As such, in times of hardship or distress, a person will abandon the higher needs to ensure that the lower needs are fulfilled.

By adding technology needs to Maslow's hierarchy, we get an entirely different route to self-actualization. Figure 13.1 shows a reconstruction of Maslow's hierarchy to fit with current technology addiction behavior. According to this reorganization, a new level has been added indicating modern technological needs. As such, some of the needs from the original levels have been reorganized. This reflects behavior that accompanies technology addiction. For example, sleep can be ignored or regarded as less important when an individual is experiencing a technology addiction. Thus, it is given a much higher place on the pyramid compared to the original hierarchy. Further, as technology becomes more pervasive in our everyday lives we may see trends where physiological needs are separated into immediate resources (air, water) whereas the needs that require more real-world interaction and time (sex, preparing food, sleep, *true* social interaction) are instead ignored or placed on a more distant tier of the hierarchy. Self-actualization is moved even more distal from the base and, owing to an inability for real-world growth, may be even less achievable than in a nontechnology-oriented lifestyle. Real-world needs such as esteem and love/belonging are instead replaced with online social interactions. They are fulfilled, but in a way that decomposes the rest of the need-based model. Although there isn't anything inherently "wrong" with interacting with computers and the Internet in this way, it demonstrates a human propensity for immersion into the Experience Machine. This is important for understanding how individuals will interact with technology in the future, especially as virtual technologies become more and more life-like.

Similarly, as neurotechnology becomes more immersive and realistic, what will humans regard as ethical use of this technology? Will we, as a race, allow ourselves to be upgraded, as if we were machines? Will we allow our lives to be fully shoved into false realities where our existence can be prefabricated? According to Nozick, the answer is simply "no." Nozick would argue that without real achievements in life, an individual has no purpose. According to modern-day research and media claims, though, the answer is not so clear. Can achievements in games or other virtual realities replace the need for achievements in life? Modern use of technology has shown that an Experience Machine may be more tempting then Nozick originally hypothesized. If we ask the question again, but instead phrase it for the present, "Will individuals consider entering an Experience Machine?," the answer is simply "yes."

13.2 Neuroethics in Entertainment

13.2.1 Brain–Computer Interface

The realm of entertainment presents a uniquely interesting challenge to the establishment of ethical guidelines for neuroadaptive systems. The addition of brain–computer interfaces (BCIs) to enhance experiences such as movies, websites, and video games underscores the need to consider privacy and addiction issues within the neuroethics discussion.

Current BCI technology provides very little by way of gleaning any significant personal data from its user; however, this should not discount the need to take a forward-thinking position toward ethical guidelines in these systems as they mature. Nijholt and Tan (2007) described a three-stage evolutionary process for technology applied to the development of BCIs. In the first stage, a proof of concept is built to demonstrate basic functionality and potential feasibility of the technology. In the second stage, termed emulation, the technology is used to replicate functions of existing devices. With respect to video games, for example, this would be the stage at which BCIs take the place of joysticks for movement or button presses. In the final phase, the technology becomes mature, no longer a novelty of the system. Computer mice or cellular phones are examples of technologies in mature phases. As researchers, designers, and eventual users of BCIs, we must consider the ways in which technology interaction might change as neuroadaptive systems mature.

Much of the research with neuroadaptive interfaces takes place within the medical domain. BCIs are approaching the second stage, emulation, in that domain. They are used to help the disabled by creating novel mobility platforms (Graimann, Allison, and Gräser 2007), to interact with computer systems (Lecuyer et al. 2008), or to treat neurological disorders like epilepsy (Illes and Bird 2006). With respect to entertainment, however, BCIs are still in the initial or proof-of-concept stage. Computer-based entertainment prototypes use BCIs to move avatars (Friedman et al. 2007) and manipulate objects within a virtual environment (Nijholt, Erp, and van Heylen 2008). However, at this time, these applications do not exhibit the complex interactions and advanced gameplay of a big-budget title on a major game console. Currently available is a toy-based on the Star Wars franchise that encourages users to "use the force" via worn sensors that measure various brain states in order to "levitate" a small ball inside an air chamber. Although both examples use brain interfaces for control, they do not necessarily exhibit neuroadaptive capabilities. It is needless to say that the data captured by such devices, at this time, provide little cause for concern with respect to a discussion of ethical guidelines for neuroadaptive systems.

13.2.2 Mind Games

Eventually neuroadaptive entertainment systems *will* mature beyond what can already be done with a mouse, keyboard, and joystick to create truly novel experiences, notably in gaming. Imagine, for instance, a game that is capable of monitoring your level of engagement, or flow state. The game might adjust the level of stimuli (adversaries, explosions, etc.) when it detects that your recorded level of enjoyment is not meeting a predetermined level. A game's difficultly can be adjusted in real time when game-based neuroadaptive systems detect your frustration, or even increase your tension as an added challenge. These examples of the potential uses of neuroadaptive systems in gaming are passive in nature, but not to the exclusion of active interaction game primitives (e.g., self-regulation of brain states) that will likely evolve alongside passive counterparts. For instance, a proof-of-concept game, Brainball (Ilstedt 2003), challenges users to control a ball on a surface through the act of relaxation. The games of the future, whether "video"-based or presented through some other medium (e.g., virtual reality), may prove to be more engaging and immersive than the already impressive current generation of video games.

Furthermore, an ethical discussion within gaming's new neuroadaptive frontier emerges in a place not unfamiliar to this domain: addiction. There are many types of games, and just as many reasons why people play games: challenge, socialization, role playing, and so on. Some of the reasons to engage in this activity, such as compulsion or distraction from reality, might be attributed to underlying factors such as depression (Chou, Condron, and Belland 2005). When game designers eventually possess the ability to individualize each player's experience on the basis of their brain data, then the argument is made that these games will become even more engaging (than they already are), thus presenting an even greater risk of addiction.

There are countless examples of players escaping reality (Ng and Wiemer-Hastings 2005) as a result of the time spent playing massive multiplayer games such as World of Warcraft, Everquest, and Ultima Online. These cases can often lead to the deterioration of real-life social interactions as well as an increase in suicidal thoughts (Kim et al. 2006). These cases are also no longer solely attributed to "hardcore games"; examples of addiction are prevalent in casual games such as Farmville, where microtransactions quickly add up to large expenditures (Driskell 2010). These games allow players to accumulate (virtual) wealth, power, and socialize with others, while also remaining under the cover of relative anonymity (Chou, Condron, and Belland 2005). It is difficult to imagine how the addition of neuroadaptive feedback loops within games will increase their influence over individuals looking to escape into these worlds. It is not unrealistic to envision video games (in the traditional sense) evolving into full-blown Experience Machines given sufficient BCI maturity.

One potential solution, then, is to propose that neuroadaptive interfaces should be developed to prevent, rather than widen, the pathway to this type of addiction. Instead of altering game difficulty when sensing frustration, the software may recommend the user take a break from the game. If a player is engaged in a flow state within the virtual environment of an MMORPG (massively multiplayer online role-playing game) for an extended period of time, the game may temporarily suspend a player's account as a safety precaution. The problem with such solutions is striking a balance between a user's choice to engage in an activity and the designer's intention to provide precautions for their safety.

In addition, many people make similar choices to indulge in other areas of life, despite the obvious hazards to their well-being. People may choose to smoke, drink, or eat to excess in an effort to satiate needs but destroy their bodies in the wake. Many legal outlets are available where people are able to gamble away money on sports or games of chance. Why, then, should those same experiences be restricted in entertainment if we choose to engage in them freely? It may be more appropriate to determine whether or not our free will is compromised by entertainment systems that actively monitor our states in order to keep us engaged, which might be the most pressing issue for the future of video games.

There are also confidentiality concerns with respect to brain data and gaming. Are entertainment software companies responsible to take action under specific, potentially critical circumstances? For example, if in the normal course of playing a video game it is detected that a player is feeling extremely violent and depressed, should the game console notify the police, or perhaps a psychiatrist? Currently, it is impossible to determine whether the violent feelings are simply the result of the immersive game experience, or indicative of a physical manifestation of violence toward others or oneself; it may never be possible to separate feeling from intent, or intent from action. Video games and the "causal versus correlated" argument surrounding violence are outside of the context of this discussion. What *is* important to note here is how ethical obligations apply to human safety with respect to brain data collected primarily for entertainment purposes.

13.2.3 Privacy in Social Entertainment: Oxymoronic?

Privacy issues within entertainment applications are particularly interesting because people are willing to provide personal data to create personalized entertainment experiences. Consider, for example, the type of personal data that is posted to online social networking websites, such as Facebook or Twitter. Photos, real-time location tracking, and demographic and contact information are some of the common items that might be found within a user's profile. Simultaneously, privacy controls allow users to restrict the type of information available to spammers and strangers. Because of ongoing privacy concerns over the protection of data on sites like Facebook (Acquisti and Gross 2006), the system seems counterintuitive at times and subversive at others. Users post personal information to their profile with the goal of connecting with other users, and this information is then put under lock and key (by constantly changing privacy settings) to keep their information confidential from other parties.

Looking toward the future, updates posted to our Twitter feed or Facebook page may someday result not from our fingertips on the keyboard, but rather from signals generated directly from our brains and translated to the virtual page. Given a sufficient resolution of brain scanning technology, we might log on to these sites to discover that a friend is feeling anxious today, or is experiencing feelings of love or enjoyment. Do our concerns over privacy change on the basis of how this information is generated and posted to our profiles? What if these posts were generated subconsciously, then posted automatically? (For example, "Status changed: Sara's brain scan indicates she is feeling cranky.") It might sound a bit far-fetched, but stranger things have been imagined for purposes of entertainment.

Going beyond the casual linkages found within many online social networks, neuroadaptive feedback might also be used as a new "dimension of compatibility" on more intimate applications like dating websites. Would we be appalled or relieved to learn the true nature of a person's interest in another's profile, or does it take all of the excitement out of getting to know someone and building relationships? Alternatively, neuroadaptive feedback might be used to help a user narrow down a list of potential profiles and even teach the user something about their own tendencies about which they may not have been completely aware.

Such an analysis by a dating website might reveal that a user prefers blondes to brunettes, or verbose profiles to sparse ones, or even subconscious sexual preferences.

13.2.4 There's Personal Data, Then There's Brain Data

We will assume that people are averse to the idea of divulging personal information to marketers and advertisers, but then we turn right around and post the minutiae of our lives into blogs, social pages, and multiplayer online video games. In the end, what becomes of all of the neruroadaptive data that is collected to improve our gaming experiences, strengthen our social networks, and invigorate our love lives? It would be naïve to think that it will all evaporate into the ether after being collected for the primary purposes described above. Data from our online interactions is being mined for purposes other than entertainment. The use of neuroadaptive systems may require some fine-tuning to omnipresent "privacy policies." We may not be opposed to having our brain data used for focus groups or video game usage statistics, but what about criminal investigations, background checks for employment, or targeted advertising ("Feeling depressed? Drugs can help!")?

Unlike verbal or written data, brain data happens spontaneously. We may not be able to conceal our thoughts, despite our intentions to keep them private. And, just as in the current environment of digital commerce, social networking, and multimedia interactivity/entertainment, a future with neuroadaptive systems will require users to stay informed about the capabilities of such interfaces. This will be especially important in entertainment contexts, where it may not be immediately apparent what type of brain data is being collected and how it might be utilized in the future. It is the responsibility of both those who provide the system/software/hardware as well as the individual who uses it to maintain an understanding of specifically what data will be collected, if it will be archived, and how it might be used.

13.3 Neuroethics in Selection

13.3.1 Genetic Information Nondiscrimination Act

Although no legal doctrine has been created to directly oversee the future of neurotechnology, litigation associated with genetic information may set a legal precedent. On May 21, 2008, then-president George W. Bush signed into the law, the Genetic Information Nondiscrimination Act (Hudson, Holohan, and Collins 2008). This bill was developed to prevent the discrimination of Americans on the basis of genetic information, specifically from insurance providers or employers. The bill was a direct response to the Human Genome Project, which set out to map the function of the roughly 25,000 genes in human DNA, and fully sequence the billions of base pair components that combine to form these genes. Consequently, the Human Genome Project provided the foundation for tremendous progress to be made toward our collective understanding of how genes interact to develop unique characteristics, with a great deal of research conducted to investigate the genetic foundation for diseases and disorders. Thanks to this research, for the first time patients can now have their genes sequenced to determine their precise susceptibility to specific diseases. Although the sequencing of genes can provide a great deal of insight into human predispositions, this process is still in its infancy and is currently incapable of providing a definitive diagnosis before a disease has actually developed. However, it can help by alerting patients that they are at an elevated risk for a particular disease and, subsequently, by educating them on what steps they can take to help avoid it.

Although this new ability has provided a valuable service to patients, fear has developed concerning its use by insurance companies to charge higher rates for coverage, or by employers to avoid hiring those with a genetic predisposition to diseases that may require costly medical procedures or time off work. The Genetic Information Nondiscrimination Act seeks to avoid this discrimination by making it illegal for insurance providers or employers to discriminate against those with a greater likelihood of developing a disease in the form of raising rates, denying coverage, or precluding employment.

The Genetic Information Nondiscrimination Act is, in accordance with previous non-discrimination legislation, intended to keep employers focused on hiring those best qualified for the position in question, rather than any ulterior motives based on gender, race, and so on. However, though the bill seems to specifically prevent discriminatory practices based on genetic markers of disease, it may be counterintuitive to its original goal of keeping employers focused on hiring the best and brightest for the job. More specifically, the language of the bill completely disallows the use of any genetic information in the hiring process. This ignores the equivalent potential of genetic markers to predict cognitive and emotional characteristics, as evidenced by the growing field of neurogenomics (Boguski and Jones 2004), which may be useful as employment selection tools.

13.3.2 Neuropersonality

Subjective measures of personality and general cognitive abilities have proven to be effective predictors of job performance, and are, therefore, valuable tools in the selection of employees (Hunter and Schmidt 1998). However, questions have been raised regarding the validity and reliability of these self-report measures, where inaccurate or intentionally misleading responses can be difficult to prevent. Morgenson et al. (2007) discuss these problems inherent in the use of self-report personality measures, concluding that more objective measures of personality must be developed if it is to be considered during the selection process. The field of neurogenomics has helped advance this cause by finding evidence for genetic markers of personality factors such as extraversion (Rettew et al. 2008), neuroticism (Wray et al. 2007), and agreeableness (Luo et al. 2007), which could provide valuable information linking personality and employability. Beyond personality, evidence has also been found for the genetic basis of cognitive abilities, such as attentional control (Rueda et al. 2005) and both spatial and verbal working memory (Ando, Ono, and Wright 2001). All of these relationships are the result of genetic variation responsible for the physical development of specific brain structures, as well as the production of neurotransmitters. Therefore, the genetic tests can provide a relatively simple method of detecting minute physical differences in specific brain structures or levels of neurotransmitters within specific brain regions, which may not be detectable through alternative measurement tools such as functional magnetic resonance imaging (fMRI) or positron emission tomography (PET) scans.

In its current form, the Genetic Information Nondiscrimination Act would categorize the use of any of these genetic markers of personality or cognitive ability in an employee selection process as discriminatory. However, the assessment of the same personality traits or cognitive abilities through more traditional questionnaires or aptitude tests are perfectly acceptable, and proven to be effective predictors of job performance. The only difference between the use of questionnaires and genetic tests to measure personality factors is that questionnaires can be deceptive owing to their subjective nature. For example, an applicant for a sales job will likely recognize that extraversion would be a trait desired by the employer, and, therefore, respond more positively to questions about extraversion than they would under other circumstances (Morgenson et al. 2007). Why should neurogenomic tests, a potentially more reliable measure, be considered discriminatory whereas a less reliable measure of the same construct is perfectly acceptable?

13.3.3 Genetic Markers of Cognition

Beyond simple personality measures, genetic markers of more complex cognitive functions have been found as well. For example, Reinvang et al. (2010) discuss genetic factors that have been shown to influence cognitive decline due to aging. This research represents an ethical gray area somewhere between the use of genetic information to determine current cognitive abilities and using the same information to predict future health status. Should employers be permitted to include genetic-based predictions of future performance in their employee selection process? On one side of the argument, measures of current cognitive abilities are considered acceptable, and these measures are used because they are assumed to be predictive of future cognitive abilities, and, therefore, job performance. Thus, using genetic tests to derive the same predictions of future cognitive ability seems relatively innocuous. However, as with disease prediction, genetic prediction of age-related cognitive decline can never be certain, and will only provide an estimate of the employee's susceptibility to cognitive decline. Even someone who is genetically highly susceptible could potentially avoid falling victim if they make a conscious effort to preserve their mental faculties.

Legislative bodies are understandably hesitant to allow any genetic information to be included in the selection process; there is clearly a slippery slope linking the use of genetic measures of personality to the dystopian society described in the movie *Gattaca*, in which a person's future career path is determined at birth on the basis of their genetic makeup. If any genetic information is deemed allowable in the selection process, strict regulation will be necessary to ensure that the same genetic material is not also used to conduct prohibited tests. Despite this complication, the outright ban on the use of any genetic information seems heavy-handed and contrary to the great potential afforded by scientific discovery. Rather than completely removing the ability to use genetic information, a careful discussion of the benefits and potential risks of the use of individual genetic markers must be encouraged. In this way, we can promote the use of more objective measures to determine the most qualified candidate for a job, while prohibiting the use of measures that could potentially discriminate against a qualified applicant for illegitimate reasons.

Further, the passing of the Genetic Information Nondiscrimination Act was unprecedented in that it was passed before a single case of genetic-based discrimination was reported. Unlike previous forms of discrimination protection, no one was subjected to years of unnecessary prejudice before society recognized and supported their fight for equality. This is the result of those working in the genetic sciences maintaining a constant focus on the ethical consequences of their work, and being proactive to avoid the potential negative implications. This foresight has provided a valuable first step to ensure that American citizens do not face discrimination if they are qualified for a position, but this protection must not also restrict the ability of employers to determine which applicants are truly the most qualified. Doing so could undermine the very intention of the bill by allowing a less ideal applicant to be selected over one more qualified as a result of ineffective and easily manipulated selection tools.

13.4 Neuroethics in Clinical Diagnoses

13.4.1 Clinical Technology

Technological advances in bodily imaging have come a long way since the early developments of x-ray tubes and the gelatin photographic plates of the late 1800s. Since then, imaging science has significantly progressed in the ability to produce *in vivo* images of all types of biological tissues. However, in providing clinicians and scientists the ability to peer inside a living organism with clarity and detail, neuroimaging technologies are creating significant challenges for both clinicians and patients alike. Further, organizational and practical problems plaguing the modern health-care system can exacerbate neuroethical challenges for clinicians and patients. For example, the information age has increased the amount of both agreeable and disagreeable information for imaging technologies as well as direct marketing for diagnostic tests and treatments.

In a system already plagued by the fact that physicians have limited time with patients, it has become a real challenge for doctors to have adequate time to discuss the technologies accompanying these tests and possibly dispel any myths that may surround them. Further, complications also arise from the fact that there is evidence of a decline in not only examination skills but also communication skills among medical residents (Klitzman 2006; Stern et al. 2001). This is an especially important finding when considering the process by which physicians obtain informed consent. If there is a communication breakdown in the clinician–patient relationship, patients may misevaluate the risks or benefits of different neuroimaging diagnostic tests. In addition, physicians may misunderstand the motives that brought the patient to them in the first place. It becomes, then, an ethical imperative for physicians to correctly communicate with patients what claims to these devices are legitimate, how they should be used, and what inferences can be made of their use or even misuse.

13.4.2 How Informed Is Informed Consent?

In a clinical setting, informed consent is regarded as a continuous agreement to go forward with a particular treatment modality (Ford and Henderson 2006). That is, the patient or caretaker must not only voluntarily wish to proceed, but also have the capacity to understand the implications of agreeing to pursue a particular treatment. In terms of treatments such as functional neurosurgery, these are often elective, meaning that they are treatments for chronic disorders and not necessarily lifesaving procedures. Researchers Ford and Henderson (2006) described that many of these disorders manifest as impairments in cognitive functioning. Thus, ensuring that the patient fully understands the implications of treatment and thereby giving true informed consent can be somewhat ambiguous. That is, determining how well someone with a thinking impairment understands a suggested medical treatment can be considered questionable at best.

Thus, it is also imperative that physicians have a clear understanding as to the proper use, interpretation, benefits, and drawbacks of neuroimaging technologies. Although this seems like a somewhat obvious sentiment, there are no exact standards for specific neurotechnological interventions. Researcher Giordano (2010) explained that ongoing research is needed to enable clinicians to communicate the relative values, benefits, and risks of particular treatments and to enable patients to make well-informed decisions. As such, this research is instrumental in determining not only the practical but also the biomedical "good" of a particular technology. With that said, there is currently a question as to how research data should be incorporated into clinically applied practices. For example, a current trend in marketing neurotechnologies to clinicians has led to a tendency to ignore empirical evidence illustrating either the usefulness or uselessness of nuerotechnologies in making diagnoses. This marketing trend has relied mostly on anecdotal evidence and not empirically validated science, especially for pain management (Giordano 2010). This has also led to a rise in the number of undertrained or untrained individuals using these technologies for diagnoses.

Giordano (2010) also stated that it is not enough to simply know when a particular device is appropriate for a certain clinical case. It is equally important to understand the capacities and limitations of the technology, the pathology under investigation, and the physiological changes that coincide. He also states that this can only be accomplished though experience and time. As such, guidelines, policies, and standardized practices for training clinicians are a necessity. However, it is also necessary to discourage a one-size-fits-all approach to administering this technology. In the same way, how do we foster good contextual knowledge and practical wisdom? As neurotechnology certification programs that can be obtained in a weekend seminar or through an at-home course become more prevalent, how do we reflect the complexity of using and applying this technology? How do we help physicians acknowledge both the strengths and limitations of neurotechnology in making diagnoses?

13.4.3 Rise of Neurotechnologies: Linking Body and Mind

The oldest noninvasive form of neuroimaging is electroencephalography, which utilizes electrical signals to measure the firing of neurons in the brain. Since its inception in the 1920s, electroencephalograms have been extremely beneficial for diagnosing and monitoring epilepsy. By the 1960s, huge strides were made in neuroscience that allowed for measuring not only electrical activity within the brain but metabolic activity as well. Both PET and single-photon emission computed tomography (SPECT) are capable of measuring the metabolic activity of the brain and have been widely used in research studies of neurodegenerative disorders (Illes, Racine, and Kirschen 2006). The 1990s ushered in the decade of the brain, which focused on practical applications for neurotechnologies, especially in the diagnosis and treatment of pain (Giordano 2010). During this time, even more powerful techniques for measuring brain activity emerged, including magnetic resonance imaging (MRI) and fMRI. These have provided promising results for examining the brain on an even more detailed level. Further, both MRI and fMRI have contributed practical applications for speech and language as well as treatment for psychiatric disorders (Illes, Racine, and Kirschen 2006).

As such, the current trend in neuroimaging tends to focus on monitoring and interpreting very specific neurological processes (Keebler et al. 2010). With that said, our best efforts at noninvasively measuring mental activity can only measure the activity of about 100,000 neurons. Human brains, on average, have about 100 billion neurons and about 100 trillion individual synaptic connections.

Consequently, questions arise as to the quality of inferences made from measurements of brain activity. For example, assuming brain normality by using neurotechnologies uniformly across patients, presumes that most human brains function in roughly the same way. However, we know that there is large variation in brain activation in response to things like emotions and behaviors (Giordano 2010). This raises further questions about the relationship between structure and function, body and mind, normal and abnormal, and how to deal with the notion of brain normality.

13.4.4 Ethical Implications for Interpreting Brain Data

As neuroimaging technologies progress in their ability to catalog the human brain, there is a burgeoning concern for blurring the relationship between the biological and the psychological, the body and the mind. The mind/body debate is about as old as the study of the human condition itself. While there is mounting evidence that psychosocial factors can have physical manifestations in the brain (Astin et al. 2003), neurotechnologies may encourage clinicians to pursue a strictly biological cause for psychological disorders. This may greatly change the way clinicians and patients view the understanding of personality and how it is linked to the biological brain.

Although neuroscience has provided insight into both the structure and the function of the brain, there is still no clear understanding of how human consciousness and other mental processes actually occur (Giordano 2010). Therefore, making inferences as to the physical mechanisms of the mind is problematic. As such, drawing hard lines linking the involvement of brain structure and biology to psychological function may challenge a patient's notion of responsibility for symptoms and consequential actions. Klitzman (2006) described that if neurological structures become associated with predispositions for violence, violence may be seen as less volitional. As such, how should these predispositions be treated legally? Does giving a disease or behavior a definite cause allow a patient to assign blame for their actions? Does the disease now have a definite cure? While neuroimaging technologies may shed light on the biological underpinnings of things like alcoholism or aggression, they may also alter a patient's perception of what they can do to actively take control of their disease. In this respect, the patient is viewed as a passive piece of their own life, with the biological foundation of their disease in control.

Further, this brings about considerations for presenting and framing neuroimaging results. What should be said about incidental or clinically insignificant findings? A patient's particular neurological or psychological traits (like personality traits) may further complicate the interpretation of neuroimaging results. For example, should physicians disclose a clinically insignificant finding to a patient suffering from an anxiety disorder or paranoid schizophrenia? What if that person misinterprets these findings to mean that they are damaged? This may lead them to feel even more distraught or even depressed and exacerbate the reason they sought treatment in the first place. Additionally, the paranoid patient may misinterpret the motives of the physician, becoming more suspicious of their intentions, and damaging a patient–physician relationship that may have taken months or even years to develop. Who should be privy to these results once they are disclosed? Should a patient who shows a predisposition to Alzheimer's disease be required to inform their place of employment or insurance carrier?

While new developments in brain imaging technologies have provided clinicians the ability to better understand the human brain, using these technologies can be a double-edged sword for physicians and patients alike. Drawing inferences from neural images can be challenging and informing patients as to their meaning can be equally problematic. As such, several questions have been raised concerning the ethical nature of using these technologies. As we move forward, the hope is that the use of different neurotechnologies for clinical diagnoses will continue to be questioned in an effort to ensure their most ethical use. Further, we feel that this can only be done by continuing discourse concerning various neurotechnologies and their ability to be used as meaningful tools for clinicians and patients.

13.5 Neuroethics in Marketing

13.5.1 Rise of Neuromarketing

Advances in neuroscience combined with the understanding of the affective and cognitive associations linked to physiological measures have gained the attention of the advertising industry, giving rise to what has been coined neuromarketing. Lee, Broderick, and Chamberlain defined neuromarketing as "the application of neuroscientific methods to analyze and understand human behavior in relation to markets and marketing exchanges" (2007, 200). Although the use of such methods for marketing is not yet commonplace, it is becoming more prevalent. It is an understatement to say that advertising has become ubiquitous and unavoidable. We see them everywhere from product placement in entertainment and media, to user-tailored ads on social networking websites. Further, it is not uncommon for consumers to allow companies to collect individual data for the purpose of tracking their purchasing habits in exchange for rewards or discounts. Unfortunately, even though freely given, consumers may not understand the extent of the database in which their information is contained or the extent of data mining and analysis that is conducted on the basis of their personal information and purchasing habits. The information that companies compile on the basis of this data analysis is subsequently used to refine and target their marketing efforts to the individual (Wilson, Gaines, and Hill 2008).

Additionally, the social networking phenomenon, the power of portable information devices and ever-present marketing, has perhaps fueled consumers to relax their safeguarding of personal and private information. The combination of these factors makes one wonder whether consumers will also be willing to freely share information that may one day be a direct measure of their consciousness. Although neuroscientific advances are nothing short of astounding, it is still unclear whether a 1:1 ratio of brain measurement will ever be achieved (Keebler et al. 2010); however, this potential must be taken seriously when considering ethical neuromarketing practices.

13.5.2 Ethical Implications of Neuromarketing

The potential for scientific advances and their use for marketing, even if seemingly from the realm of science fiction, must be considered when discussing the ethics of neuromarketing. In their article "Neuroethics of neuromarketing," Murphy, Illes, and Reiner (2008) introduced the concept of "stealth neuromarketing." This futuristic neuroscientific capability would allow marketers the ability to manipulate consumers' brains without the recognition by the consumer that such manipulation has occurred. Although it can be argued that to some extent this already occurs in traditional marketing as advertisers utilize psychological and behavioral research to develop campaigns, the possibility of stealth neuromarketing treads on territory that has resounding implications. Consider the possibility that society's casual approach to personal information briefly noted above was extended to brain data. It does not take a great leap of imagination to envision a mobile electroencephalograph transmitting brain state data to a marketing system that could deliver targeted advertisements to an augmented reality device or adaptive displays at a shopping mall. Although a technology like this would require active participation obvious to the consumer, would the user be aware of the extent to which information about their moods, desires, biases, personalities, and insecurities were being manipulated to undermine their autonomous decision to make purchases? What if this unrealized technology could actively modify a consumer's cognitive state in order to achieve a desired marketing outcome? If used in a manner that could be perceived as beneficial to the consumer, would this capability be less alarming? Perhaps, an obese consumer struggling with weight loss was manipulated to purchase more expensive yet healthier choices at the market. Would it be justifiable to take advantage of these data because they were capitulated freely and it ultimately benefited the health of the consumer? How far removed is this from presently accepted practices in the use of psychopharmacology? Although extreme applications of stealth neuromarketing may never be realized, it does not require an extensive investigation to uncover potential ethical issues of using noninvasive technologies to gain access to the most invasive and intimate data.

Although a considerable amount of effort has been spent on the issue of neuroethics and "brain privacy" (Keebler et al. 2010), these ideas have yet to capture the sustained attention of the broader public. The ethical issues of neuromarketing is a deeply complicated issue and has recently been addressed in the academic and scientific realm at considerable length (see Canli 2006; Eaton and Illes 2007; Fugate 2007; Lee, Broderick, and Chamberlain 2007; Murphy, Illes, and Reiner 2008; Wilson, Gaines, and Hill 2008), yet there appears to be less of a philosophical debate from the general public or those who wish to utilize the advances of neuroscience to entice consumers and influence their decision making. It is, however, important to note that on occasion, public interest has peaked around the presentation of neuromarketing data. For example, Iacaboni et al.'s (2007) submission to the Op Ed section of the *New York Times* caused a minor stir with the results of an fMRI study that examined voters' neurological response to political candidates. While the merit of publishing simplified results with the potential for misinterpretation by the readers of a newspaper's opinion section can be debated, the net result was that the general populace was exposed to the potential of neuroscience to assess specific brain states. Perhaps fortuitously, there has yet to be a public outcry against neuromarketing akin to the response experienced by James Vicray's 1957 claim that he had developed a technique to subliminally influence unwitting consumers to "eat popcorn" and to drink "Coca-Cola." However, given the likelihood that the general public does not have a firm grasp on the nuances of neuroscience and the propensity to accept data from advanced technologies as accurate and indisputable, neuromarketing (and neuroscience as a whole) may be a mere Op Ed piece away from mass condemnation by the public accompanied by a long series of congressional hearings and subsequent legislative regulation.

13.5.3 Developing Standards

At the time of this edition, the Advertising Research Foundation (2010) embarked on an initiative they call Engagement 3: NeuroStandards Collaboration. This effort is in response to their recognition of the need for major validation studies to assess neuroscience and its application to media and advertising. The stated goal of Engagement 3 is to move toward a consensus for establishing standards of biometric research through competitive transparency through a peer review process conducted by neuroscience vendors who accepted their open invitation (thearf.org, 2010). Additionally, NeuroFocus, a neuromarketing company, assembled an advisory board comprising neuroscientists, marketing experts, and client executives and proposed a proprietary version of NeuroStandards (PR Newswire 2010). In the PR Newswire article, three core NeuroStandards were described:

- Standards for study design, protocols, and the establishment of statistical sampling processes and sample sizes.
- Standards for laboratory operations, including specialized design and construction techniques and materials, staffing and training, data collection and management, and laboratory processes and procedures.
- Safeguards for maintaining strict protections for consumers, their rights, and their data.

While both of these organizations should be applauded for recognizing the need for ensuring ethical standards for the use of neuroscience in marketing, it is not clear whether Engagement 3 or NeuroStandards will provide a publicly available set of neuroethical guidelines that will be necessary as neuromarketing becomes more widely accepted. As a way forward, neuromarketing professionals must maintain current capabilities and limitations of neuroscience and manage the expectations of their clients while adhering to freely available set ethical standards for the protection of consumers. Perhaps, a daunting task but one that neuromarketing professionals should be able to achieve if they are to maintain the balance of producing results for their clients while keeping the public trust.

13.6 Conclusions

The field of neuroethics is gradually gaining momentum as a realm for interdisciplinary scientific inquiry. The boundaries of using the technology explained in this chapter are, as of today, undefined. This is both unsettling and fascinating. In one sense, the emergence of neurotechnology demonstrates that mankind has reached a supreme apex. We are beginning to understand ourselves, and our brain/mind complex, in ways unimaginable even a few decades ago. In another sense, with the great power of emerging neurotechnologies comes great responsibility. This responsibility rests not only on the shoulders of scientists and governments but on individuals as well. We must be very careful as a species to ensure that these new technologies do not infringe on personal rights. This is not an easy task by any stretch of the imagination. To properly endure this coming century of technological explosiveness, we must be honest and clear about our past. The advancement of technology has almost always brought with it the most horrible permutations of human existence. A mental evolution must occur alongside the technological evolution, to ensure that technology is created when it is needed, and not simply because it can be.

Several examples have been cited throughout this discussion of scientists, practitioners, and politicians taking proactive action in the hope of minimizing the potential risks inherent in advanced neurotechnologies. These steps, such as the Genetic Information Nondiscrimination Act and the preliminary neuromarketing guidelines developed by NeuroFocus, are to be commended for their forward-thinking goals. However, as this chapter demonstrates, a great many ethical quandaries remain to fuel future debates. The only way we, as a scientific community, can hope to best improve society is to continue to foster this debate over the ethical implications of our work. This responsibility does not lie solely in the hands of the practitioners who apply the science, or the researchers who develop it, but in all people, including our politicians and individual citizens.

References

Acquisti, A. and R. Gross. 2006. Imagined communities: Awareness, information sharing, and privacy on the Facebook. In *Privacy Enhancing Technologies*, Vol. 4258, edited by G. Danezis and P. Golle, pp. 36–58. Berlin and Heidelberg: Springer.

Advertising Research Foundation. 2010. NeuroStandards: The next wave in advertising. http://www.thearf.org/assets/engagement-council/?fbid=RyHerCRbHTM

Ando, J., Y. Ono, and M. Wright. 2001. Genetic structure of spatial and verbal working memory. *Behavior Genetics* 31 (6): 615–24.

Astin, J. A., S. L. Shapiro, D. M. Eisenberg, and K. L. Forys. 2003. Mind-body medicine: State of the science, implications for practice. *Journal of the American Board of Family Medicine* 16: 131–47.

Boguski, M. S. and A. R. Jones. 2004. Neurogenomics: At the intersection of neurobiology and genome sciences. *Nature Neuroscience* 7 (5): 429–33.

Canli, T. 2006. When genes and brains unite: Ethical implications of genomic neuroimaging. In *Neuroethics: Defining the Issues in Theory, Practice, and Policy*, edited by J. Illes, 169–83. New York: Oxford University Press.

Chou, C., L. Condron, and J. Belland. 2005. A review of the research on Internet addiction. *Educational Psychology Review* 17 (4): 363–88.

Churchland, P. S. 2006. Moral decision-making and the brain. In *Neuroetchics: Defining the Issues in Theory, Practice and Policy*, edited by J. Illes, 3–16. New York, NY: Oxford University Press.

Driskell, N. 2010. The psychology of Farmville. *Psychomp*. Retrieved from http://www.psychcomp.com/psychology-farmville/

Eaton, M. L. and J. Illes. 2007. Commercializing cognitive neurotechnology—The ethical terrain. *Nature Biotechnology* 25 (4): 393–7.

Ford, P. J. and J. M. Henderson. 2006. Functional neurosurgical intervention: Neuroethics in the operating room. In *Neuroethics: Defining the Issues in Theory, Practice, and Policy*, edited by J. Illes, 214–28. New York, NY: Oxford University Press.

Friedman, D., R. Leeb, L. Dikovsky, M. Reiner, G. Pfurtscheller, and M. Slater. 2007. Controlling a virtual body by thought in a highly immersive virtual environment: A case study in using a brain-computer interface in a virtual-reality cave-like system. In Paper presented at GRAPP 2007 (*Proceedings of the Second International Conference on Computer Graphics Theory and Applications*), Barcelona, Spain, March 8–11, 2007, pp. 83–90. Portugal: INSTICC—Institute for Systems and Technologies of Information, Control and Communication.

Fugate, D. L. 2007. Neuromarketing: A layman's look at neuroscience and its potential application to marketing practice. *Journal of Consumer Marketing* 24 (7): 385–94.

Giordano, J. 2010. Neurotechnology. Evidence and ethics: On stewardship and the good in research and practice. *Practical Pain Management* 10 (2): 63–9. Retrieved from: http://www.potomacinstitute.org/attachments/604_PPM_Mar2010_Giordano_Neuro.pdf

Graimann, B., B. Allison, and A. Gräser. 2007. New applications for non-invasive brain-computer interfaces and the need for engaging training environments. Position paper presented at the *BrainPlay '07 Workshop of ACE 2007, International Conference on Advances in Computer Entertainment Technology*, Salzburg, Austria, June 13–25, 2007, pp. 25–8. http://hmi.ewi.utwente.nl/brainplay07_files/brainplay07_proceedings.pdf#page=33

Hancock, P. H. 2009. *Mind, Machine and Morality: Toward a Philosophy of Human-Technology Symbiosis.* Surrey, England: Ashgate Publishing.

Hudson, K., M. Holohan, and F. Collins. 2008. Keeping pace with the times—The genetic information nondiscrimination Act of 2008. *The New England Journal of Medicine* 358 (25): 2661–3.

Hunter, J. and F. Schmidt. 1998. The validity and utility of selection methods in personnel psychology: Practical and theoretical implications of 85 years of research findings. *Psychological Bulletin* 124 (2): 262–74.

Iacaboni, M., J. Freedman, J. Kaplan, K. H. Jamieson, T. Freedman, B. Knapp, and K. Fitzgerald. 2007. This is your brain on politics. *The New York Times.* Retrieved from http://www.nytimes.com/2007/11/11/opinion/11freedman.html?_r=1

Illes, J. and S. J. Bird. 2006. Neuroethics: A modern context for ethics in neuroscience. *Trends in Neurosciences* 29 (9): 511–7.

Illes, J., E. Racine, and M. P. Kirschen. 2006. A picture is worth 1000 words, but which 1000? In *Neuroethics: Defining the Issues in Theory, Practice, and Policy,* edited by J. Illes, 149–68. New York, NY: Oxford University Press.

Ilstedt, H. S. 2003. Research+ design: The making of Brainball. *Interactions* 10 (1): 26–34.

Keebler, J., S. Ososksy, G. Taylor, L. Sciarini, and F. Jentsch. 2010. Neuroethics: Protecting the private brain. In *Proceedings of the 3rd International Conference on Applied Human Factors and Ergonomics (AHFE '10).* Miami, FL, July 17–20, 2010.

Kim, K., E. Ryu, M.-Y. Chon, E.-J. Yeun, S.-Y. Choi, J.-S. Seo, and B.-W. Nam. 2006. Internet addiction in Korean adolescents and its relation to depression and suicidal ideation: A questionnaire survey. *International Journal of Nursing Studies* 43 (2): 185–92.

Klitzman, R. 2006. Clinicians, patients, and the brain. In *Neuroethics: Defining the Issues in Theory, Practice, and Policy,* edited by J. Illes, 230–41. New York, NY: Oxford University Press.

Lecuyer, A., F. Lotte, R. Reilly, R. Leeb, M. Hirose, and M. Slater. 2008. Brain-computer interfaces, virtual reality, and videogames. *Computer* 41 (10): 66–72.

Lee, N., A. J. Broderick, and L. Chamberlain. 2007. What is "neuromarketing"? A discussion and agenda for future research. *International Journal of Psychophysiology* 63: 199–204.

Luo, X., H. Kranzler, L. Zuo, S. Wang, and J. Gelernter. 2007. Personality traits of agreeableness and extraversion are associated with ADH4 variation. *Biological Psychiatry* 61 (5): 599–608.

Morgenson, F. P., M. A. Campion, R. L. Dipboye, J. R. Hollenbeck, K. Murphy, and N. Schmitt. 2007. Reconsidering the use of personality tests in personnel selection contexts. *Personnel Psychology* 60 (3): 683–729.

Murphy, E., J. Illes, and P. B. Reiner. 2008. Neuroethics of neuromarketing. *Journal of Consumer Behavior* 7: 293–302.

Ng, B. D. and P. Wiemer-Hastings. 2005. Addiction to the Internet and online gaming. *Cyberpsychology and Behavior* 8 (2): 110–3.

Nijholt, A., J. Erp, and D. K. J. van Heylen. 2008. BrainGain: BCI for HCI and games. In *Proceedings AISB Symposium* (Paper presented at the *AISB Symposium Brain Computer Interfaces and Human Computer Interaction: A Convergence of Ideas*), Aberdeen, UK, April 2, 2008, pp. 32–5. Brighton, UK: Society for Study of Artificial Intelligence and Simulation of Behaviour.

Nijholt, A. and D. Tan. 2007. Playing with your brain: Brain-computer interfaces and games. In *Proceedings ACE* (Paper presented at the *International Conference on Advances in Computer Entertainment Technology*), Salzburg, Austria, June 13–25, 2007, pp. 305–6. New York: ACM.

Nozick, R. 1974. *Anarchy, State, and Utopia.* New York: Basic Books.

PR Newswire. 2010. NeuroFocus announces NeuroStandards; Market research industry's sole set of principles for conducting scientifically-sound, full brain-based EEG studies. http://www.prnewswire.com/news-releases/neurofocus-announces-neurostandards-market-research-industrys-sole-set-of-principles-for-conducting-scientifically-sound-full-brain-based-eeg--studies-103993578.html

Reinvang, I., I. Deary, A. Fjell, V. Steen, T. Espeseth, and R. Parasuraman. 2010. Neurogenetic effects on cognition in aging brains: A window of opportunity for intervention? *Frontiers in Aging Neuroscience* 2:143. doi:10.3389/fnagi.2010.00143.

Rettew, D., I. Rebollo-Mesa, J. Hudziak, G. Willemsen, and D. Boomsma. 2008. Non-additive and additive genetic effects on extraversion in 3314 Dutch adolescent twins and their parents. *Behavior Genetics* 38 (3): 223–33.

Rueda, M., M. Rothbart, B. McCandliss, L. Saccomanno, and M. Posner. 2005. Training, maturation, and genetic influences on the development of executive attention. *Proceedings of the National Academy of Sciences of the United States of America* 102 (41): 14931–6.

Stern, D. T., M. S. Rajesh, L. D. Gruppen, A. L. Lang, C. M. Grum, and R. D. Judge. 2001. Using a multimedia tool to improve cardiac auscultation knowledge and skills. *Journal of General Internal Medicine* 16: 763–9.

Wilson, R. M., J. Gaines, and P. H. Hill. 2008. Neuromarketing and consumer free will. *Journal of Consumer Affairs* 42 (3): 389–410.

Wray, N., A. Birley, P. Sullivan, P. Visscher, and N. Martin. 2007. Genetic and phenotypic stability of measures of neuroticism over 22 years. *Twin Research and Human Genetics: The Official Journal of the International Society for Twin Studies* 10 (5): 695–702.

Index

A

ABM, *see* Advanced Brain Monitoring (ABM)
ACC, *see* Anterior cingulate cortex (ACC);
      Autonomous cruise control (ACC)
Accessory optic system, 130, 134; *see also* Eye
      movement tracking
    in eye stabilization, 128, 131
ACS, *see* Adaptive-compensative system (ACS)
ACT-R, 246–247
    driver model, 301–302
Action-monitoring functions, 143; *see also* Error
      monitoring
Action-perception model, 275
Activity diagrams, 318
Adaptive automation, 241–242
    ANN classification, 193
    in information processing, 243
    neural data and, 244
Adaptive data analysis techniques, 248
Adaptive-compensative system (ACS), 45, 46,
      50; *see also* Dorsolateral prefrontal
      cortex (DLPFC); Learning; Neural
      systems
    in action, 54–56
    BG, 52
    characteristics of, 61
    cognitive and motor processing, 55
    declarative memory theory, 52, 53
    DLPFC, 51–52
    goal achievement, 45
    hippocampus, 52–53
    interactions within system, 53–54
    neural substrates of, 51–53
    relational processing theory, 52–53
Adaptive training model, 190–191
ADHD, *see* Attention deficit hyperactivity
      disorder (ADHD)
Advanced Brain Monitoring (ABM), 193
Affective domain, 167
Affective states, 178
AI, *see* Artificial intelligence (AI)
AIP, *see* Anterior intraparietal (AIP)
aIPS, *see* Anterior intraparietal sulcus (aIPS)
ALS, *see* Amyotrophic lateral sclerosis (ALS)
Amygdala, 36, 56–57, 61, 324; *see also* Preventive
      system (PS)
    emotions, 58, 314
    in learning, 35, 37
    long-term potentiation in, 60
    negative stimuli response, 59
Amyotrophic lateral sclerosis (ALS), 204, 205
    BCI applications, 216
ANN, *see* Artificial neural network (ANN)
Anterior cingulate cortex (ACC), 15, 143; *see*
      also Dorsal anterior cingulate cortex
      (dACC)
    in conflict monitoring, 49
    dACC, 47, 48
    ERN, 157
    evaluative system, 46
    in executive control, 34
    in learning, 35
    parts of, 47
    role, 46–47, 143
    rostral, 148
    task-related interference and, 47
Anterior intraparietal (AIP), 77, 80
Anterior intraparietal sulcus (aIPS), 77, 86
    activation, 80
    bilateral engagement of, 83
    localizer, 84
Anterior ventral (AV), 36
AOI, *see* Areas of interest (AOI)
Apraxic patients, 88
Areas of interest (AOI), 258, 285
Artificial intelligence (AI), 11, 16
Artificial neural network (ANN), 193
Artificial selectional systems, 11
Attention, 14, 143; *see also* Brain; Inhibition of
      return
    anatomic-functional subsystems, 14–15
    attachment of, 287, 288
    BOLD feedback and, 221
    to cognitive scientists, 34
    as cognitive states, 168
    consciousness and sense of agency, 22
    control and, 21
    deficit, 142
    directions, 285
    executive, 15
    glance, 293, 296
    resources, 315
    response lapses, 149